Management
OF THE
Perimenopausal
AND
Postmenopausal Woman
A TOTAL WELLNESS PROGRAM

Barbara Kass-Annese
RNC, NP, MSN

*California Family Health Council
Nurse Practitioner Program
Harbor–UCLA Medical Center
Women's Health Department
Los Angeles, California*

Lippincott
Philadelphia • New York • Baltimore

Acquisitions Editor: Jennifer E. Brogan
Coordinating Editorial Assistant: Susan V. Barta
Production Editor: Virginia Barishek
Production Manager: Helen Ewan
Production Service: Berliner, Inc.
Printer/Binder: R.R. Donnelley & Sons Company/Crawfordsville
Cover Designer: Christine Cantera
Cover Printer: Lehigh Press

9 8 7 6 5 4 3 2 1

Library of Congress Cataloging-in-Publication Data

Kass-Annese, Barbara.
    Management of the perimenopausal and postmenopausal woman: a
total wellness program / Barbara Kass-Annese.
        p. cm.
    Includes bibliographical references and index.
    ISBN 0-7817-1654-3
    1. Menopause. 2. Climacteric. 3. Middle aged women—Health and
hygiene. 4. Middle aged women—Diseases. I. Title
    [DNLM: 1. Premenopause. 2. Menopause. 3. Postmenopause.
4. Women's Health. WP 580K19m 1998]
    RG186.K364 1999
    613'.04244—dc21
    DNLM/DLC
    for Library of Congress   98-26136
                                                            CIP

Care has been taken to confirm the accuracy of the information
presented and to describe generally accepted practices. However,
the authors, editors, and publisher are not responsible for errors or
omissions or for any consequences from application of the information in the book and make no warranty, express or implied, with
respect to the contents of the publication.

The authors, editors, and publisher have exerted every effort to
ensure that drug selection and dosage set forth in this text are in accor-
dance with current recommendations and practice at the time of publication. However, in view of ongoing research, changes in government regulations, and the constant flow of information relating to drug
therapy and drug reactions, the reader is urged to check the package
insert for each drug for any changes in indications and dosage and for
added warnings and precautions. This is particularly important when
the recommended agent is a new or infrequently employed drug.

Some drugs and medical devices presented in this publication
have U.S. Food and Drug Administration (FDA) clearance for limited use in restricted research settings. It is the responsibility of the
health care provider to ascertain the FDA status of each drug or
device planned for use in clinical practice.

CONSULTANTS

WILLIAM PARKER, MD
Chairman of Obstetrics and Gynecology
Santa Monica–UCLA Medical Center
Clinical Professor of Obstetrics and Gynecology
UCLA School of Medicine
Los Angeles, California

SHARON SCHNARE, RN, FNP, CNM
Private clinical practice
Seattle, Washington

REVIEWERS

HELEN A. CARCIO, NP
Infertility Case Manager
Community Health Plan/Massachusetts Region
Associate Clinical Professor
University of Massachusetts
Amherst, Massachusetts

GERI MORGAN, CNM, ND
Director of Provider Services
Certified Nurse-Midwife
Women's Healthcare Associates
Adjunct Faculty
College of Nursing
Arizona State University
Tempe, Arizona

ROSEMARY THEROUX, RNC, MS
Nurse Practitioner
Private Practice
Medway, Massachusetts
Clinical Instructor
Northeastern University
Boston, Massachusetts

ACKNOWLEDGMENTS

Several health care professionals generously gave of their time and expertise in the development of this book. I particularly express my gratitude to two friends and colleagues—William Parker, MD, and Sharon Schnare, FNP, CNM—for providing input, ongoing support, and review from the inception through the completion of the book and patient education materials. A warm thank you to Marie Lugani, President and Founder of the American Menopause Foundation, Inc.; Carlene Keller, RNCNP; Laurie Binder, RNCNP; and Maria Diaz, RNCNP, for critiquing the final draft and to Brenda Beeley, acupuncturist and practitioner of homeopathy, for reviewing the chapter about complementary health care practices. I would like to extend a very special thanks to Dr. Jerry Byrd, who edited the book; Lyle Sinkewich, who designed the front cover of the first version; and William Brown, who provided graphic design for the first version. And finally, I express my appreciation to Jennifer Brogan, Senior Editor, and Susan Barta, Editorial Assistant, both of the Nursing Division, Lippincott Williams & Wilkins, who provided support and guidance in the preparation of the book for this publication. They were a pleasure to work with during the collaborative effort.

PREFACE

Management of the Perimenopausal and Postmenopausal Woman was written to provide a comprehensive approach for the care of women over 30 and for women who are perimenopausal or post-menopausal. It is written with a strong emphasis on prevention, blending Western (conventional) medicine with complementary (alternative) health care practices that are in use by increasing numbers of women today.

This book was also written to add the missing pieces to existing protocols for women 30 to 40 years old. Typically, protocols for the care of women in this age group deal with contraceptive issues, routine gynecologic health care, and reproductive health care problems such as cervical, pelvic, and breast pathology, and sexually transmitted infections. Rarely do these protocols include information about a comprehensive approach to the prevention of osteoporosis, heart disease, and other chronic health problems and symptoms associated with the decline in hormones. This is truly unfortunate, because health care problems such as heart disease and osteoporosis do not magically appear because one becomes a senior citizen!

These diseases are, in part, a result of many years of inadequate nutrition, lack of exercise, and chronic stress. Consequently, women in their thirties and even younger need information essential to developing their own optimal health program. With this information they have the choice of making lifestyle changes that can contribute to the state of their present health as well as their health when they reach *menopause* (which is defined as the cessation of menses for 12 consecutive months).

Protocols for women who have entered their *climacteric* (the years from the onset of a decline in ovarian function until 15 or more years past menopause) usually focus on hormone replacement therapy (HRT) and calcium supplementation. As with protocols for women in their thirties, they generally do not include the key therapeutic interventions that contribute to the prevention of osteoporosis, heart disease, or other chronic health problems, and the symptoms associated with the climacteric. As you read this book, you will also learn how the same health care measures used for prevention can serve as the foundation for the treatment of many health care issues related to the climacteric and aging.

Over 43 million women today are nearing or have passed menopause, and 21 million more will be entering their climacteric over the next decade. Women can expect to live at least one third of their lives, if not more, beyond age 50. These years should be filled with great health and happiness. As a health care professional, you can contribute to making this a reality by educating women and by providing them with information that can enhance their lives.

INFORMATION YOU CAN USE

Reviewing articles, books, and research on health issues related to the climacteric is not an easy task. Information is contradictory, research is limited, and many questions are unanswered. In 1993 the National Institutes of Health initiated a 10-year study to compare hormone replacement therapy with a low-fat diet, calcium supplementation, and exercise to prevent cancer, heart disease, and osteoporosis. But don't try to tell a 45- or 50-year-old woman that she must wait several more years before answers are available. It definitely won't make her day!

However, even though more research is needed, the good news is that a considerable amount of valuable information exists for women right now. This information comes from research on aging, nutrition, exercise, heart disease, osteoporosis, and cancer. Also, you may feel comfortable sharing with your patients information that has been passed on for hundreds to thousands of years among health systems of various cultures.

CONVENTIONAL AND COMPLEMENTARY HEALTH CARE

Much has been written about the treatment of climacteric-associated and other health care problems using conventional (Western) and complementary (alternative) health care approaches. It is not the intent of this book to duplicate the work of other authors on these issues. Instead, this book is intended as a summary of key findings from the research, and an introduction to a comprehensive approach to women's health and to various aspects of complementary health care practices. It ends with the *Guidelines* section, which can serve as a foundation for protocols you may wish to develop for your practice or clinic.

The *Guidelines* summarize basic recommendations for the medical evaluation of women over 30 and outlines major nutritional, exercise, and stress reduction recommendations, including nutritional supplementation. It also presents basic recommendations for hormonal and drug therapies and for herbal and homeopathic treatments.

One of the major reasons for including information about herbal and homeopathic treatments and other complementary health care practices (besides the fact that they can work for some of your patients) is that they have woven their way into the fabric of American health care. Increasing numbers of people are taking a more active role in their own care by seeking the assistance of complementary health care practitioners. By doing so, they send a message to conventional health care providers that they are not particularly satisfied with a health system that relies primarily on surgery and pharmacology. Instead, people who use or are interested in complementary health care practices are asking for a different health system, one that focuses on less invasive approaches to treatment and the prevention of health care problems. This is evidenced by the fact that complementary health care now represents a multibillion dollar industry, with at least one in three Americans using complementary health care practices today.

ACCEPTANCE IS ON THE RISE

How has the medical field responded to this request for a change in focus? To mention only a few examples, disciplined inquiry into complementary health care practices is discussed in new peer-reviewed journals such as *Alternative Therapies in Health and Medicine* and *Complementary Therapies in Medicine: The Journal for Health Care Professionals*. Also, the National Institutes of Health now has an Office of Alternative Medicine, which funds research efforts in various aspects of complementary medicine. This office has released an extremely interesting and enlightening publication, *Alternative Medicine: Expanding Medical Horizons*, which discusses the history and current status of beyond-the-mainstream practices, explores new therapeutic claims, and makes recommendations for future research.

Seventeen other Public Health Service agencies, in addition to NIH's Office of Alternative Medicine, have granted and continue to award several million dollars for research activities in complementary therapies. For example, the National Institute of Drug Abuse has funded a study to determine the effectiveness of acupuncture for treatment of cocaine abuse, and the National Institute of Allergy and Infectious Diseases is funding testing of anti-HIV compounds found in plants. And, of course, a recent action of the Food and Drug Administration lifted the "investigational use" designation from acupuncture needles and reclassified them as "general use" medical devices.

Medical schools such as Harvard, Penn State, Yale, UC San Francisco, Temple, Tufts, Johns Hopkins, Boston University, Case Western, Columbia, and Emory now offer courses in complementary medicine. In fact, of the 135 medical schools in the United States, 50 have added acupuncture, homeopathy, nutrition, massage, and prayer to their curriculum. A few schools, including the University of Virginia, have mandated that every medical student learn about complementary treatments. The University of Arizona College of Medicine offers a variety of complementary health-based courses, from two-week programs to a two-year fellowship in complementary health care for physicians. Many programs in complementary health practices such as acupuncture, meditation, therapeutic touch, and herbal medicine are available to conventionally trained health care practitioners. Also, the numbers of physicians and nurses joining the American Holistic Physicians Association and the American Holistic Nurses Association are steadily increasing.

Insurance companies and health maintenance organizations (HMOS) are becoming more receptive to complementary medicine and the "Total Wellness Approach" to health care. American Western Life Insurance Company of Foster City, California offers a holistic hotline and the Mutual of Omaha Insurance Company pays for a nonsurgical, nonpharmaceutical approach to reversing coronary artery disease pioneered by Dean Ornish, MD. The Prudential in New Jersey reimburses for acupuncture and chiropractic therapies. A Blue Cross program in Washington State provides supplemental coverage for homeopathy, acupuncture, and naturopathy. Representatives from these companies indicate that there is enough evidence to suggest that insurance plans with a heavy emphasis on prevention and wellness, delivered within a holistic matrix, can bring down health care costs. It is no coincidence that Congress is being asked to pass the Access to Medical Treatment Act, which allows physicians to suggest non-

FDA approved remedies without fear of prosecution, resulting in an increase in access to complementary therapies for patients.

In another area of research, the National Cancer Institute has created a special department to scour the plant world for cancer and AIDS drugs. In addition, Pfizer, Inc., the pharmaceutical company, has an agreement with the Institute of Basic Theory at the China Academy of Traditional Chinese Medicine in Beijing to study Chinese herbs. The company already has a similar agreement with the New York Botanical Gardens regarding plants native to the United States.

THE TOTAL WELLNESS APPROACH: A CHALLENGE

Looking at health care from a different vantage point than the conservative, conventional Western medical approach in which you were probably trained is most likely a challenge for you, both as a health care professional and as a consumer. Yet it is an exciting challenge, as it calls on you to expand your knowledge base and to be open to new information that may be different from what you've encountered in your professional life thus far. Willingness to be open to a Total Wellness Approach will benefit you. Integrating aspects of this approach into your practice will help you to attain the goal you already strive for with your patients: helping them to achieve the quality of life that they deserve.

How does the dramatic shift towards a Total Wellness Approach impact the care of women who are approaching menopause, or those who are experiencing it, or those who have passed it? First, we know that hormone replacement therapy (HRT) will not prevent or treat heart disease, osteoporosis, and the many symptoms associated with the climacteric for all women. Although HRT certainly has benefits, some women who use it will still develop heart disease or osteoporosis. Other women do not experience complete relief from their symptoms, and some do not tolerate HRT well. Others are afraid of HRT, often because they are concerned about possible, unknown associated risks. Moreover, unless a woman has health insurance, the expense of HRT may be prohibitive. Others do not want to take hormones on a daily basis, and for those who have not had a hysterectomy, bleeding may be a bothersome event. Finally, some women have medical contraindications for using HRT.

Advertisements about HRT are found in a variety of women's magazines. HRT is discussed in several books about menopause, and it is advocated by the majority of health care professionals who provide gynecologic services. However, only about 25% to 35% of all women today who could use HRT chose to use this form of therapy. Many women, instead, are looking for ways to become healthier and to move through this transitional time without drugs or hormones. They do not view menopause as a disease (as discussed in some of the medical literature). Some women who use HRT choose to integrate other health care practices with this therapy to achieve the best available state of health.

As you read the information provided in this book, we hope that you will agree that a Total Wellness Approach—with exercise, nutrition, vitamin and mineral therapy, and stress management as its foundation—is the way to go.

A BIT MORE ABOUT THIS BOOK

Management of the Perimenopausal and Postmenopausal Woman is written for nurse practitioners, midwives, nurses, physicians, and physician assistants who are involved in women's health care or who would like to expand their focus to this field of health care. It can also be helpful for those working in other areas of health care who are interested in the subject.

This book provides:

- An overview of reproductive physiology of the premenopause and a discussion of the changes in this physiologic process with the onset of the perimenopause (Chapter 1).
- A discussion of the symptoms associated with the climacteric and an introduction to the various causes of these symptoms (Chapter 2).
- An overview of causes of cardiovascular disease, and a discussion of risk factors and the impact of a woman's lifestyle on the development of coronary artery disease (CAD). Symptoms of CAD and risk assessment and screening tests are also discussed (Chapter 3).
- An overview of bone development and causes and risk factors for the development of osteoporosis. The relationship of diet, exercise, and stress to osteoporosis is discussed, as are symptoms and screening recommendations (Chapter 4).
- A discussion of the psychosocial issues that can influence the

ways in which the climacteric is experienced. An overview of the indirect and direct effects of biologic factors on psychologically related symptoms is also presented (Chapter 5).

@ A discussion of the basics of a total wellness program for women over 30. Dietary guidelines are offered, along with information about vitamin, mineral, and other nutrient supplementation. Exercise recommendations and stress reduction techniques are also included (Chapter 6).

@ An overview of the use of estrogen, progesterone, testosterone, and dehydroepiandrosterone (DHEA). Plant-based hormonal therapies are also discussed, and information about nonhormonal therapies for hot flashes and osteoporosis is included (Chapter 7).

@ An introduction to several complementary health care practices and examples of research regarding these practices. Recommendations are also provided for integrating complementary therapies for prevention with treatment using conventional therapies (Chapter 8).

Barbara Kass-Annese, RNC, NP, MSN

CONTENTS

CHAPTER **4**

OSTEOPOROSIS AND OTHER HEALTH ISSUES   57

CHAPTER **5**

PSYCHOLOGIC, SOCIOLOGIC, SEXUAL, AND CONTRACEPTIVE ISSUES
RELATED TO THE CLIMACTERIC   85

CHAPTER 8

COMPLEMENTARY THERAPIES AND
HOLISTIC MEDICINE   195

CHAPTER 9

FINAL REMARKS   241

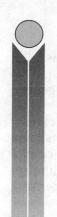

CHAPTER I

Reproductive Physiology from Premenopause Through the Climacteric

Perimenopause is a transitional phase in a woman's life. Like puberty, it represents the beginning of a gradual change in the reproductive system that ends in a major event. For puberty, this event is menarche; for perimenopause, it is menopause.

Ovarian function and fertility decline during the years of the perimenopause. This transition begins in the middle to late thirties or early forties and ends 10 or more years later with menopause. Women should be educated early about the physiologic effects of hormonal decline, rather than waiting until they are experiencing perimenopausal symptoms or until they are approaching the age of 50. To help prevent or ameliorate the effects of osteoporosis, heart disease, and other degenerative diseases associated with the climacteric, health care professionals must educate premenopausal women.

PERIMENOPAUSE AND CLIMACTERIC

Although the terms *perimenopause* and *climacteric* are often used interchangeably, climacteric describes the physiologic changes and symptoms associated with the change from a reproductive to a nonreproductive status.[1] Although the perimenopausal and climacteric phases both begin with a decline in ovarian activity, perimenopause ends at menopause, and the climacteric continues for 15 or more years beyond menopause. The climacteric usually ends after the age of 70, when there is generalized atrophy of all estrogen-dependent tissues.[2]

The onset of the climacteric or perimenopause probably is influenced by many of the same factors that affect menarche, such as genetics, race, ethnicity, body build, nutrition, exercise, and general health status.

Menopause occurs several years after the onset of the climacteric, usually between the ages of 49 and 55 (median, 51 years), and is experienced after menses have ceased for 1 year. The period of 1 to 2 years after menopause is known as *postmenopause,* although some authorities expand this term to include the remainder of a woman's life after menopause.

REPRODUCTIVE PHYSIOLOGY

THE MENSTRUAL CYCLE

The *menstrual cycle* is a result of a complex positive and negative feedback system comprising the hypothalamus, the pituitary, and the ovaries. The system is orchestrated by the hypothalamus through secretion of gonadotropin-releasing hormone, which stimulates the pituitary to increase or decrease its secretion of follicle-stimulating hormone (FSH) and luteinizing hormone (LH). Secretion depends on the three phases of the menstrual cycle: the follicular phase, ovulation, and the luteal phase.

FOLLICULAR PHASE AND OVULATION

The *follicular phase* of the menstrual cycle begins with the onset of menstruation. During this phase, an orderly sequence of events ensures that an adequate number of follicles is ready for ovulation.

In the beginning of the menstrual cycle, the pituitary increases its secretion of FSH, which stimulates a group of up to 1000 follicles to continue their development. As the follicles develop, they secrete increasing levels of estradiol. The elevated estradiol concentration reduces the pituitary's secretion of FSH. As the decline in FSH continues, the pituitary slowly increases secretion of LH.

About 12 to 18 hours after estradiol reaches its peak level, the concentration of LH sharply increases, causing usually one follicle to rupture and release its ovum; this is *ovulation.* These events usually occur over 10 to 14 days from the onset of menstruation; however, the follicular phase can vary according to the number of days required for follicular maturation.

THE LUTEAL PHASE

The *luteal phase* begins shortly after ovulation. It results from the transformation of the empty follicle into the corpus luteum. The corpus luteum secretes estradiol and progesterone, although progesterone is the dominant hormone of this phase.

The corpus luteum continues to secrete these hormones for about 9 to 11 days. If pregnancy does not occur, the corpus luteum begins to degenerate, causing the hormonal levels to decline. Without hormonal support, the endometrium begins to break down, and menstruation takes place. The luteal phase usually lasts 12 to 16 days.

During the premenopausal years, FSH is at its highest level a few days after the onset of menstruation, and LH is at its highest level shortly before ovulation. Estradiol is the dominant hormone until ovulation occurs, and progesterone is the dominant hormone from ovulation until shortly before the onset of menstruation.

FOLLICULAR LOSS

Approximately 1000 follicles are developing during each menstrual cycle. At the time ovulation approaches, these follicles cease their maturation process and undergo *atresia,* the egg-depletion process that occurs through retrogression and disappearance of follicles. This process does not begin with the onset of menarche; it begins in the fetus at about 15 weeks' gestation. Follicular maturation and atresia continue throughout the remaining months of fetal development.

At 4 months of fetal development, a peak number of at least 6 million germ cells exist in the ovary.[3] As a result of continuous follicular development and atresia, the number of germ cells at birth is 1 to 2 million. By puberty, this number is reduced to about 300,000, and by the mid-thirties, the number is about 25,000.[4] Follicular development and atresia during each menstrual cycle constitute a continuous process.

When the total number of follicles decreases to approximately 25,000, follicular loss begins to accelerate,[4] which correlates with increased secretion of FSH by the pituitary and a decreased level of the ovarian hormone inhibin. The concentration of estrogen may or may not decline at this time. Fewer follicles develop during each successive cycle as a woman ages. It is uncertain whether all follicles are depleted at menopause, although there is probably individual variation. Some researchers have found a few ovaries without follicles,[5] but others have reported ovaries containing follicles even 10 years after menopause.[6-8]

THE CLIMACTERIC

As a woman enters her late thirties or early forties, the frequency of ovulation usually declines, perhaps because the remaining follicles are less sensitive to stimulation by FSH. It was once believed that a decline in the production of estradiol before menopause was the major cause of elevated FSH levels. However, research has determined that the developing follicles secrete estradiol and inhibin, which influences (perhaps more than estradiol) FSH levels.[9]

The concentration of inhibin begins to decline in women in their mid-thirties, and the decline accelerates after age 40.[10-14] In women presenting with "incipient" ovarian failure, inhibin levels were found to be low, FSH levels were elevated, and estradiol levels were normal.[15,16]

Estradiol levels may or may not decline in women 40 years of age or older who are still experiencing regular menstrual cycles, even when inhibin levels have declined and FSH levels are elevated. In a large, longitudinal study, women who had not experienced a change in the frequency of their menstrual cycles were found to have levels of FSH above the normal range. Inhibin levels were so low in 28% of these women that they were undetectable, but only 9% had low levels of estradiol.[17] Among 233 women who had experienced a change in the flow of menses or frequency of menstrual cycles, more women had undetectable levels of inhibin than had low levels of estradiol (97 versus 48).[18]

As cycles become anovulatory, progesterone levels diminish,[19] and even when cycles are ovulatory, estrogen and progesterone levels are usually lower than they were during the premenopausal phase.[20-22] Women who experience elevated postmenopausal levels of FSH and irregular menstrual cycles can still experience endocrine changes compatible with normal ovulation.[18] An elevated level of FSH alone therefore may not indicate the end of a woman's fertility. The concentration of LH may increase before menopause in some women,[23] but despite the rise in FSH, the LH level usually remains in the normal range.[24] After about 12 months of amenorrhea, the LH level rises and then plateaus.[25] It may decline years later.[26,27]

With menopause, FSH levels are 10-fold to 20-fold higher than the usual menstrual levels, and LH concentrations are threefold to fivefold higher. Only when FSH levels are greater than 30 IU/L and LH levels are greater than 40 IU/L can it be assumed that fertility has ended.[28] The maximum increase in the FSH concentration is reached 1 to 3 years after menopause.

HORMONES

Estradiol is the major form of estrogen produced by the ovaries during the premenopausal and perimenopausal phases. When menopause occurs, estrogen levels decline steeply for the first 12 months and continue a slight decline as the years pass.[29,30] During the postmenopause phase, only about 10% of women's ovaries secrete significant quantities of estradiol.[31] Occasionally, estradiol concentrations are elevated, although the increase is not usually followed by menstrual bleeding.[32]

Estrone is an estrogen secreted during the premenopausal, perimenopausal, and postmenopausal phases. During the reproductive years, a small amount of estrone is produced by the ovaries. Additional estrone is derived from conversion of estradiol and androstenedione in peripheral tissues (principally blood and fat); in sites such as the muscles, liver, kidney, and brain; and possibly in other extraglandular sites.[33]

As a woman ages, the amount of available androstenedione decreases, which can cause a decline in estrogen to levels that are no longer sufficient to sustain estrogen-dependent tissues. Without estrogen, these tissues atrophy. Although the circulating levels of androstenedione decreases by about 50% after menopause, estrogen production can be sustained at an adequate level to maintain normal structure and function of estrogen-dependent tissues such as the vulva, vagina, urethra, and breasts well into a woman's seventies.[34]

One of the major sources of androgen precursors such as dehydroepiandrosterone sulfate, dehydroepiandrosterone (DHEA), androstenedione, and testosterone[35] is the adrenal gland. The ability of these glands to function properly before and after menopause may contribute to the amount of androstenedione and therefore to the amount of estrone produced.

DHEA is a hormone produced to some degree by the ovary, although its major source is the adrenal gland. The concentration of DHEA declines with age more than that of estrogen, progesterone, or testosterone. The reason for DHEA's significant decline is unknown, although it may also be related to the "health" of the adrenals. It has been proposed that DHEA has estrogen-like or androgen-like effects, depending on the hormonal milieu.[36] Some authorities believe that the decline in the concentration of this hormone will prove to be profoundly related to osteoporosis, cardiovascular disease, and other chronic, degenerative diseases and that it may underlie climacteric-related symptoms.

The level of testosterone produced by the ovary after menopause can remain the same or increase. However, for reasons not yet understood, the level may also decrease by as much as 50%.[37] As the frequency of ovulation decreases and periods of anovulation increase, progesterone levels begin to decline.

Another hormone that may affect menopause is melatonin. It is secreted by the pineal gland and has been found to inhibit the aging process in animals.[38] When nocturnal urinary excretion of melatonin was measured in women between the ages of 30 and 75 years, the concentration of melatonin was found to decline by 41% among women between the ages of 40 and 44 years.[38] Another decline of 35% took place in women between the ages of 50 and 54 years and in those between 55 and 59 years. Morning serum melatonin levels also declined with age. Because urinary melatonin levels correlated negatively with serum FSH levels in women during their menopausal years, this research suggests that melatonin may be linked to the initiation of menopause.

The levels of many hormones decline with age, and the once prevalent focus on estradiol levels in women with declining ovarian function is no longer appropriate. Research is beginning to unravel the complexity of the changes in and interactions of inhibin, estriol, estrone, progesterone, testosterone, DHEA, and melatonin. Although more research is needed to identify the roles these and other hormones play in the physiologic and psychologic well-being of women,

wise health care professionals should consider them in the health
intervention strategies for women as they age.

REFERENCES

1. Greendale G, Judd H. Menopause. In: Carr P, et al, eds. The medical care of
   women. Philadelphia: WB Saunders; 1995.
2. Glass R. Office gynecology. Baltimore: Williams & Wilkins; 1988.
3. Speroff L, et al. Clinical gynecologic endocrinology and infertility, 3rd ed. Baltimore: Williams & Wilkins; 1984.
4. Faddy MJ, et al. Accelerated disappearance of ovarian follicles in mid-life:
   implications for forecasting menopause. Hum Reprod 1992:7:1342.
5. Richardson SJ, Nelson JF. Follicular depletion during the menopausal transition. Ann N Y Acad Sci 1990;592:13–20.
6. Gosden RG. Follicular status at the menopause. Hum Reprod 1987;2:617–
   621.
7. Costoff A, Mahesh VB. Primordial follicles with normal oocytes in the ovaries
   of postmenopausal women. J Am Geriatr Soc 1975;23:193–196.
8. Thatcher SS, Naftolin F. The aging and aged ovary. Semin Reprod Endocrinol
   1991;9:189–199.
9. Byyny R, Speroff L. A clinical guide for the care of older women: primary and
   preventative care, 2nd ed. Baltimore: Williams & Wilkins; 1996.
10. Metcalf MG, Livesey J. Gonadotrophin excretion in fertile women: effect of age
    and the onset of the menopausal transition. J Endocrinol 1985;105:356.
11. Lenton EA, et al. Normal variation in the length of the follicular phase of the
    menstrual cycle: effect of chronological age. Br J Obstet Gynaecol 1984;91:681.
12. Lee J, et al. The effect of age on the cyclical patterns of plasma LH, FSH,
    oestradiol and progesterone in women with regular menstrual cycles. Hum
    Reprod 1988;3:851.
13. Musey VC, et al. Age-related changes in the female hormonal environment dur-
    ing reproductive life. Am J Obstet Gynecol 1987;157:312.
14. Hughes EG, et al. Inhibin and estradiol responses to ovarian hyperstimulation:
    effects of age and predictive value for in vitro fertilization outcome. J Clin
    Endocrinol Metab 1990;70:358.
15. Buckler HM, et al. Gonadotrophin, steroid, and inhibin levels in women with
    incipient ovarian failure during anovulatory and ovulatory "rebound" cycles. J
    Clin Endocrinol Metab 1991;72:116.
16. Cameron IT, et al. Occult ovarian failure: a syndrome of infertility, regular
    menses, and elevated follicle stimulating hormone concentrations. J Clin
    Endocrinol Metab 1986;67:1190.
17. Dennerstein L, et al. Med J Aust 1993;159:232–236.
18. Hee J, et al. Perimenopausal patterns of gonadotrophins, immunoreactive
    inhibin, oestradiol and progesterone. Maturitas 1993;18:9.
19. Longscope C. The endocrinology of the menopause In: Treatment of the post-
    menopausal woman: basic and clinical aspects. New York: Raven Press; 1994.

20. Sherman BM, et al. The menopausal transition: analysis of LH, FSH, estradiol, and progesterone concentrations during menstrual cycles of older women. J Clin Endocrinol Metab 1976;42:629–636.

21. Metcalf MG, et al. Pituitary-ovarian function in normal women during the menopausal transition. Clin Endocrinol 1981;14:245–255.

22. Metcalf MG. The approach of menopause: a New Zealand study. N Z Med J 1988;101:103–106.

23. Longscope C, et al. Steroid and gonadotropin levels in women during the perimenopausal years. Maturitas 1986;8:189–196.

24. Chakravarti S, et al. Hormonal profiles after the menopause. Br Med J 1976;2:784–787.

25. Kwekkeboom DJ, et al. Serum gonadotropins and a subunit decline in aging normal postmenopausal women. J Clin Endocrinol Metab 1990;70:944–950.

26. Metcalf MG, Livesay JH. Gonadotrophin excretion in fertile women: effect of age and the onset of the menopausal transition. J Endocrinol 1985;105:357.

27. Scott J, et al. Danforth's obstetrics and gynecology, 7th ed. Philadelphia: JB Lippincott; 1994:774.

28. Metcalf MG, Livesay JH. Gonadotrophin excretion in fertile women: effect of age and the onset of the menopausal transition. J Endocrinol 1985;105:357–362.

29. Meldrum DR, et al. Changes in circulating steroids with aging in postmenopausal women. Obstet Gynecol 1981;57:624–628.

30. Kwekkeboom DJ, et al. Serum gonadotropins and a subunit decline in aging normal postmenopausal women. J Clin Endocrinol Metab 1990;70:944–950.

31. Longcope C, et al. Steroid secretion by the postmenopausal ovary. Am J Obstet Gynecol 1980;138:564–568.

32. Metcalf MG. The approach of menopause: a New Zealand study. N Z Med J 1980;101:103–106.

33. Judd H. Menopause and postmenopause. In: Benson RC, ed. Current obstetric and gynecologic diagnosis and treatment, 4th ed. Norwalk, CT: Lange Medical Publications; 1982.

34. Meldrum DR, et al. Changes in circulating steroids with aging in postmenopausal women. Obstet Gynecol 1981;57:624.

35. Longscope C. Adrenal and gonadal androgen secretion in normal females. Clin Endocrinol Metab 1986;15:213–228.

36. Ebeling P, Koivisto VA. Physiological importance of dehydroepiandrosterone. Lancet 1994;343:1479–1481.

37. Glass R. Office gynecology. Baltimore: Williams & Wilkins; 1988.

38. Vakkuri O, et al. Decrease in melatonin precedes follicle-stimulating hormone increase during perimenopause. Eur J Endocrinol 1996;135:188–192.

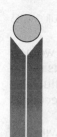

CHAPTER 2

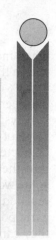

Symptoms of the Climacteric and Their Causes

VARIETY AND TIMING OF SYMPTOMS

Symptoms associated with the climacteric are experienced by about 80% of all women.[1] Although there is a wide variety of severity and duration of these symptoms, approximately 40% of all woman find them troublesome enough to seek medical assistance.[1]

The decline in ovarian function during the early years of the climacteric changes the characteristics of the menstrual cycle. This change may be subtle for some women, consisting of only a slight shortening of cycle lengths and a minimal decrease in the duration and amount of flow of menses. For others, cycle changes can be obvious. The cycle length may vary in length by several days, with a significant decrease in duration and flow of menses. Regardless of the degree of change in the cycle, the duration of the menstrual cycle decreases, and flow becomes significantly lighter as menopause nears. Women may experience different bleeding patterns, such as spotting after anovulatory cycles or occasional heavy menses. *Changes in the characteristics of the menstrual cycle* are usually the first indication that a woman has entered the climacteric.

HOT FLUSHES

Vasomotor instability, also called hot flushes or hot flashes, commonly is the second indication the climacteric has begun. Hot flushes are experienced by 10% to 20% of women during their forties,

9

when menstrual cycles are irregular, and by 40% to 58% of women within the 2-year period around menopause.[2] In one study, as many as 75% of women experienced some hot flushes.[2] Daily hot flushing has been reported by 15% to 20% of women.[3] In some cross-sectional surveys, 85% of the women reported hot flushes.[4]

Hot flushes are the most common symptom associated with the climacteric, and they begin to be experienced around the same time that the length and flow of the cycles begin to change. However, some women do not begin to experience hot flushes until they have reached menopause, and others experience them beginning in their early postmenopausal years. Regardless of when hot flushes begin, they can persist for 1 to several years. For a few women, hot flushes are persistent and disruptive problems that last 10, 20, or more years.[5] Most women find that their hot flushes subside over time and without intervention, because their bodies adjust to the decline in estrogen levels.

The physiology of hot flushes remains a mystery. They may be caused by a sudden, inappropriate excitation of heat-release mechanisms.[6] Whether this response results from the effects of decreasing estrogen levels on hypothalamic control of body temperature or from other causes has not been determined. However, hot flushes are associated with a decline in the estrogen level, and it seems that a gradual estrogen decline correlates with less severe hot flushes.

The result of the excitation of heat release mechanisms is a change in the diameter of the blood vessels near the skin surface. Vessels dilate and constrict irregularly and unpredictably. The blood flow to the skin, vital organs, and brain increases. Heat brought to the surface of the skin is often experienced first in the face and neck, then in the chest, and then sometimes throughout the rest of the body. The feeling can range from a warm sensation to a feeling of extreme heat. Perspiration may occur; if it does, it is followed by a cooling of the body as the perspiration evaporates. This physiologic response after perspiration can cause mild to extreme chills.

Hot flushes can be mild and occur for only a minute, or they can be moderate and cause significant discomfort. Severe hot flushes can disrupt every aspect of the woman's life. Hot flushes can last from a few minutes to 0.5 hour. Depending on the environment in which they are experienced (eg, during work, during a social engagement), they can be stressful or embarrassing. Pressure in the head, nervousness, and anxiety may be experienced shortly before the onset of a hot flush.

Hot flushes can occur once each week to several times each day. They may be experienced periodically over a few months and then not be experienced again for several months. They can occur during sleep (ie, night sweats) and awaken the woman one to several times during the night.

FATIGUE

Night sweats frequently lead to sleep deprivation. Even though hot flushes can occur at night without awakening the woman, her sleep pattern is still disrupted. She may feel fatigue and other symptoms associated with sleep deprivation but not know that the cause is nighttime hot flushes.

Hot flushes are not the only factor that can result in sleep deprivation. A study of nocturnal micturition and well-being in more than 3000 women between the ages of 40 and 65 determined that they experienced frequent nocturnal voiding and that their general state of health and feelings of contentment and of confidence in the future worsened with increasing numbers of nocturnal voiding episodes.[7] Women who did not void at night did not experience sleepiness during the day, but daytime sleepiness was more common among the women who voided three or more times during the night.

Symptoms of sleep deprivation include fatigue, inability to concentrate, irritability, and loss of memory. Depression can occur if sleep deprivation persists. These symptoms can also be unrelated to sleep deprivation, but it is difficult to determine to what degree they can be attributed directly to hormonal decline or to other factors, such as the woman's perception of menopause, aging, and the end of her reproductive years; relationship issues; life events during menopause; and her general physical health unrelated to the menopause. Only by taking a thorough physical, psychosocial, and sexual history is it possible to assist the woman in exploring potential reasons for these symptoms so that appropriate treatment can be initiated. Too often, hormone replacement therapy or antidepressants are offered as a quick fix, although another option may be more appropriate.

TISSUE ATROPHY

Atrophy of estrogen-dependent tissues (ie, vulva, vagina, uterus, cervix, ovaries, breasts, urethra, and bladder) is a direct result of the decline in estrogen concentration. The decline in estrogen is usually a slow and gradual process, and changes in estrogen-dependent tissues occur slowly over several years. The symptoms of these atrophic changes usually do not occur until a few years after menopause.

At some point during the postmenopausal years, the labia majora and minora become thinner, flatter, paler, and less elastic. The oil-secreting glands of the labia minora produce less of their moisturizing oil, resulting in a loss of moisture of the labia. All of these changes may result in *dryness of the vulvar area*. The vaginal canal becomes shorter and narrower. Without any form of treatment, vaginal tissues become thinner, paler, and less moist, and the rugal appearance of the vaginal vault may disappear completely. These changes can result in dyspareunia, which can also occur if the changes in the vaginal tissue progress to a state of inflammation known as *atrophic vaginitis*. If inflammation becomes severe, the tissues develop ulcers, which may bleed.

The declining estrogen concentration typically is associated with decreased elasticity of the vaginal tissues and alteration of the vaginal pH to a more alkaline or slightly more acidic state. The pH change results in a decrease in the glycogen content, which can decrease resistance to the growth of bacteria. Vaginal infections may have copious purulent discharges, and dyspareunia can result.[8]

Reduced estrogen levels result in a decrease in the size of the uterus, cervix, and ovaries. Atrophic changes in the bladder and urethra are similar to those of the vagina and vulva. The lining of the bladder and urethra become thinner and friable. Mucosal thinning of the urethra can promote inflammation that is characterized by symptoms of dysuria, urge incontinence, and frequency. This type of *urethritis* may be experienced after sexual activity.

Urinary incontinence also can result from relaxation of the pelvic floor; relaxation of the detrusor muscle, a muscular layer in the bladder; central nervous system conditions; Parkinson's disease; abdominal tumors; infection; obstruction; and atrophy of the urogenital tract as a result of hypoestrogenism.[8] Urinary incontinence is a common problem for postmenopausal women and is experienced even by some perimenopausal women. Because a woman may not be comfortable discussing the problem or may assume nothing can be done for her, careful evaluation and appropriate testing is essential.[9–12]

After menopause, the ligaments that support the uterus may lose tone. If significant loss results, partial or total prolapse of the uterus may occur. This change combined with the loss of strength of vaginal wall elastic tissue can result in bulging of the rectum (ie, rectocele) or bladder (ie, cystocele) into the vaginal canal. After menopause, the size, shape, and firmness of the breasts may change because of the reduction in fatty tissue. Nipples may become smaller.

OVARIAN, NEUROCHEMICAL, AND PSYCHOLOGIC CHANGES

Changes in the characteristics of the menstrual cycle, hot flushes, and changes in various tissues and organs are obvious signs of *decreasing ovarian hormone production*. However, several other symptoms associated with the climacteric may or may not result from declining ovarian activity. For example, they may be caused by months to years of poor nutrition, a lack of physical activity, and stressors, factors that cause the physiologic reactions commonly called stress. Symptoms such as fatigue, nervousness, headaches, insomnia, depression, irritability, joint and muscle pain, dizziness, and palpitations have been difficult to study because of the subjectivity of the complaints and because many other health problems such as hypoglycemia, hypothyroidism, hyperthyroidism, and premenstrual syndrome (PMS) share similar symptoms.

Neurochemical changes directly related to a decline in ovarian hormones can cause symptoms such as mental confusion, failing memory, and emotional changes. However, a decline in ovarian hormone levels may not be the primary cause of all symptoms; for some women, hormonal decrements may only worsen health problems that existed before the approach of menopause.

The worsening of PMS symptoms as menopause approaches provides a good example. More than 100 symptoms may be associated with PMS, ranging from irritability, fatigue, and breast tenderness to palpitations and dizziness. As with most health problems, the cause of PMS is multifaceted, and the theories developed to explain the causes vary. Women with PMS may experience different symptoms to various degrees during different cycles; some cycles may be symptom free. An estimated 75% of all women experience one or more symptoms associated with PMS at some point during premenopause. Because PMS symptoms can worsen with the approach of menopause and may correlate with the type of symptoms and degree of severity experienced with menopause, younger women should be provided with health information about the treatment of

PMS symptoms and about preventing them from worsening as they approach menopause.

Reported *psychologic symptoms* associated with the climacteric have included irritability, nervousness, tension, difficulty in concentrating, decreased energy, depression, headaches, insomnia, and decreased sexual desire. Are the causes of these symptoms physiologic, psychologic, or both? Chapter 5 has been devoted to the discussion of these important questions.

SYMPTOMS ASSOCIATED WITH THE CLIMACTERIC

Although the previous sections discussed some of the common symptoms of the climacteric, the following list provides a broader inventory of the symptoms associated with the perimenopause and early postmenopausal years:

- Fatigue
- Hot flushes
- Emotional changes (eg, irritability, nervousness, anxiety, depression)
- Restlessness
- Poor concentration
- Poor memory
- Headaches
- Joint and muscle pain
- Cold hands and feet
- Feelings of suffocation
- Pressure or tightness in head or body
- Dizziness
- Palpitations
- Insomnia
- Loss of appetite
- Tender or painful breasts
- Vaginal dryness
- Dyspareunia
- Increase or decrease in libido
- Constipation or diarrhea
- Dry skin
- Frequent bruising

- Formication (ie, prickly sensation, as if ants were crawling over the skin)
- Exacerbation of symptoms associated with other health problems (eg, diabetes, arthritis, migraine headaches)

The menopause site on the Internet[2] has added a few entries to the list of symptoms:

- Feelings of dread
- Changes in body odor
- Electric shock sensations
- Tingling in the extremities
- Gum problems
- Burning tongue

The following symptoms are associated primarily with the post-menopausal years:

- Vaginal and vulvar itching
- Abnormal vaginal discharge
- Vulvar dryness
- Urethritis
- Thinning of pubic and other body hair
- Wrinkling and loss of skin tone
- Redistribution of body fat
- Diminished muscle mass
- Decrease in energy
- Decline in libido

Hair thinning and diminished muscle mass, energy, and libido probably result from the lower estrogen and testosterone levels.

PUTTING THE SYMPTOMS INTO PERSPECTIVE

Can you imagine how your patients feel after they have read or heard about these symptoms? No wonder some women do not want to think or talk about menopause! You can help your patients put the symptoms associated with menopause into perspective.

They need to know that the symptoms previously discussed usually result only without intervention. Not all women experience symptoms to a degree that causes problems. Some women never experience even one hot flush; they just stop menstruating. Other women experience minimal hot flushes or other minor symptoms for a short period, stop menstruating, and never again experience any related symptom. A woman who has remained sexually active may not experience discomfort associated with sexual activity. Another woman may experience minimal vaginal dryness that causes vaginal pain during intercourse; for her, a vaginal lubricant may be the only intervention necessary. A variety of interventions are available to prevent or decrease the symptoms experienced and their degree of severity. These are discussed in Chapters 6 through 8 and summarized in the Guidelines section.

REFERENCES

1. Carr PL, et al. The medical care of women. Philadelphia: WB Saunders; 1995.
2. Locke M. Menopause in culture context. Exp Gerontol 1994;29:307.
3. Odenhave A, et al. Impact of climacteric on well-being. Am J Obstet Gynecol 1993;168:772.
4. Schwingl PJ, et al. Risk factors for menopausal hot flashes. Obstet Gynecol 1994;84:29.
5. Kronenberg F. Hot flashes: epidemiology and physiology. Ann N Y Acad Sci 1990;592.
6. Speroff L, et al. Clinical gynecologic endocrinology and infertility, 3d ed. Baltimore: Williams & Wilkins, Baltimore; 1984.
7. Asplund R, Aberg H. Nocturnal micturition, sleep and well-being in women ages 40–65 years. Maturitas 1996;1–2:73–81.
8. Byyny R, Speroff L. A clinical guide for care of older women: primary and preventative care. Baltimore: Williams & Wilkins; 1996.
9. Greendale G, Judd H. Menopause. In: Carr PL, et al, ed. The medical care of women. Philadelphia: WB Saunders; 1995.
10. Bergman A, Brenner P. Alterations in the urogenital system In: Mishell D III, ed. Menopause, physiology and pharmacology. Chicago: Year Book Publishers; 1987.
11. Parker W. A gynecologist's second opinion. New York: Plume Book; 1996.
12. Cardoza L, Kelleher C. Estrogen deficiency and urinary incontinence. In: The modern management of the menopause. New York: The Parthenon Group; 1994.

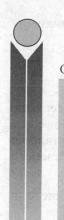
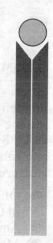

CHAPTER 3

Cardiovascular
Disease

*American hearts may be the warmest
in the world, but they are not the
healthiest.*[1]

When Dr. Paul Dudley White returned in 1914 to America from his medical studies in Europe, he brought with him an invention from Germany that he believed would help get his practice started: an electrocardiograph.[2] White had a junior teaching position at Harvard and was eager to share the machine with his colleagues. However, his superiors did not recognize the machine's potential applications and believed he should not waste his career on a minor anomaly.[3] White persisted, but he had to search to find patients with blocked arteries.[4] Thirty-five years later, White, by then a specialist, was chosen to treat President Eisenhower for his heart condition.[5] Ironically, Eisenhower's problem was no longer rare; by the 1950s, heart disease was America's leading cause of death.

One of four Americans has some form of cardiovascular disease (CVD), and one American dies of CVD every 34 seconds.[6] Every year, 1.5 million persons in the United States have heart attacks, and 6 million more are treated for angina or other forms of coronary heart disease.[7] Another 500,000 Americans suffer crippling strokes annually, and 60 million Americans have hypertension.[8] The figures attest to an epidemic. "In this nation's history, no other disease, no war, no epidemic has ever killed at anything like this suddenly rising, relentless pace of heart disease."[9]

WOMEN AND CARDIOVASCULAR DISEASE

Women assume that cancer is their worst foe. However, cancer is the leading cause of death only until about the age of 40, followed by CVD. By age 55, CVD overtakes cancer and becomes the number one cause of death of women. Statistics reported by the American Heart Association[10] offer some perspective:

- One of 9 women between the ages of 45 and 64 has some form of CVD
- Among women older than 65, 1 of 3 has some form of CVD
- More women than men die during the first year after a heart attack
- Women who have heart attacks are twice as likely as men to die within the first few weeks
- Heart attacks kill about 250,000 women annually

Circulation, the official publication of the American Heart Association, published study results that revealed that women who have experienced heart attacks have a significantly higher chance than men of dying before leaving the hospital.[1] A woman's risk of dying during or immediately after bypass surgery is double that of a man. A major reason for these findings is that women generally have not sought early diagnosis.

Historically, CVD has been considered a man's disease. Research has been conducted primarily with male subjects, and the fact that the medical profession neglected women sent the message that CVD was not something women should be concerned about. Because women have believed that CVD is not a major concern for them, the disease is more severe by the time they seek medical care, and treatment is less likely to be successful than for men. Because women tend to experience the symptoms of heart disease later (around age 65) than men, their overall health may be poorer, affecting the outcome of treatment. Another possible explanation for an increase in the death rate associated with cardiac surgery may be the operative difficulties encountered with the surgical instruments used, because they initially had been designed for the larger hearts and arteries of men.[6]

Some women who have gone to their health care providers complaining of symptoms associated with heart disease have not been taken seriously. In the past, women's chest pains were more likely to be diagnosed as psychiatric in origin, further delaying diagnosis and treatment of CVD. In one study, internists viewed videotapes of a male actor and a female actor portraying patients. Each "patient" complained of chest pain, each claimed to be a smoker, and each had a stressful job. Two thirds of the doctors recommended that the man undergo further evaluation, but only one third recommended evaluation for the woman. All of the doctors recommended that the man stop smoking, but none made such a recommendation for the woman. Two recommended that the woman see a psychiatrist.[7]

The difference between men and women regarding heart disease is not whether they are likely to develop it, but when they are most likely to experience the symptoms. Men have heart attacks about 10 years earlier than women, but women have been "catching up" and having more heart attacks at an earlier age. More American women than men have died of heart disease in the past 10 years. Some of the reasons cited for this shift are women's adoption of "male" living patterns, such as abuse of nicotine; adoption of a sedentary lifestyle; nutritional neglect; and increased mental stress. Gender plays a critical role because of the relationship between CVD and a decline in ovarian hormones.

Although the predominant mechanism is unknown, ovarian steroids have a variety of cardiovascular effects. Because of its antioxidant properties, estrogen has a direct effect on the vascular wall, probably protecting the lining from injury.[8-10] Estrogen also has beneficial effects on serum lipids and lipoproteins.[11,12]

CAUSES OF CORONARY ARTERY DISEASE

Although there are several types of CVD, this chapter focuses on coronary artery disease (CAD) because it is the most common form and the number one killer of Americans. It is also the CVD about which women most need to be concerned because of its correlation with the decline in ovarian function.

For many years, the search for the causes of CAD focused on excessive dietary intake of cholesterol, inadequate intake of dietary fiber, and nicotine abuse. The picture has become much more complex as the roles of lipoproteins, free radicals, and homocysteine have been identified. The deleterious effects resulting from intake of certain foods and substances and from deficiencies of various nutrients, inadequate exercise, and stress on the cardiovascular system are now better understood.

Although not all causes of CAD have been identified, enough is known to prevent or adequately treat most cases, many of which can be obviated through modifications in lifestyle. Dr. Castelli, director of the Framingham Heart Study, said, "Very few of us—in fact, almost none of us—have a family history of [heart disease] so strong we can't overcome it."[13] He stated that heart disease can be overcome if persons "know, monitor, and change controllable risk factors."

INJURY TO THE CORONARY ARTERIES

Injury to the lining of the arterial wall triggers a specific response that leads to development of atherosclerosis. When the lining of a coronary artery is injured, the body attempts to heal the area of injury through the deposition of cholesterol, collagen, calcium and other minerals, protein, platelets, fibrin, dead cells, and other materials (ie, plaque). However, the body's attempt to heal itself becomes destructive and even deadly if injury is chronic or repetitive. As plaque development continues, the injured arteries narrow, and flow of blood to the heart is reduced. Eventually (usually over decades), this process leads to complete blockage of one or more arteries. The imbalance that results between blood supply and the demands of cardiac muscle causes myocardial ischemia or damage. The atherosclerotic process also causes the arteries to lose their resilience, which results in hypertension.

There are many causes of injury to the arterial walls. Hypertension injures the lining through the forceful impact of blood against the arterial wall. Nicotine and other toxic substances in cigarettes directly injure coronary arteries, as can a significant spasm of a coronary artery. Injury also can be caused by oxidized low-density lipoproteins (LDLs) and cholesterol. Regardless of the cause, the physiologic response to injury is the same: plaque develops. If it continues to do so, blood flow to the heart is reduced or completely blocked. Blood flow can also be reduced by a thrombus or coronary artery spasm.

These mechanisms commonly interact. For example, if a coronary artery is significantly blocked already, a small thrombus can lodge in the artery, and blood flow is further reduced or completely blocked. If a spasm occurs in an already narrowed artery, reduction or complete blockage of flow can result.

RISK FACTORS FOR CORONARY ARTERY DISEASE

Lifestyle influences the risk for CAD. Specific factors include inadequate exercise, nutritional deficiencies and excesses, chronic stress, excess body fat, cholesterol, triglycerides, lipoproteins, free radicals, antioxidants, and homocysteine.

Age, sex, and genetic predisposition to CAD are nonmodifiable risk factors. Fortunately, they can be positively influenced by elimination or modification of other risk factors that stem from lifestyle, such as poor diet, sedentary habit, excess body fat, chronic stress, and toxic substances (eg, nicotine, alcohol, amphetamines, cocaine). These modifiable risk factors can lead to CAD by means of elevated levels of LDLs, triglycerides, and homocysteine; decreased levels of high-density lipoproteins (HDLs); hypertension; obesity; and diabetes mellitus.

CAD should not be considered a degenerative disease of old age. To a great extent, it is a behavioral disease of industrialized societies and one that can begin at an early age. The recommendations for lifestyle changes discussed in this section and in Chapter 6 are applicable to everyone at every age.

Autopsies performed on American soldiers during the Korean War revealed coronary artery disease in 77.3% of the hearts studied,[14] and autopsies of American soldiers killed during the Vietnam war revealed atherosclerosis in 45% of the soldiers; 5% had severe heart disease. Because of the decline in atherosclerosis from 77.3% to 45%, it was suggested that the prevalence of coronary atherosclerosis had declined over the years. However, autopsies of 111 victims of noncardiac trauma (average age of 26; 84% were white) conducted in 1992 found coronary atherosclerosis in 78%.[15] Twenty percent of the study group had a 50% narrowing of the arteries, and 9% had a 75% narrowing. The overall prevalence of coronary atherosclerosis in the young, predominantly white, male study group was comparable to that documented during the Korean War. Although these findings demonstrate that atherosclerosis often begins early in life, research has shown that this process can be significantly retarded and even reversed to a significant degree through a combination of proper nutrition, adequate exercise, and use of relaxation techniques.

DIET

Excessive intake or deficiencies of some nutrients can contribute to the development of CAD. Specific dietary recommendations and nutritional supplementation guidelines for CVD prevention and treatment are discussed in Chapter 6 and outlined in the Guidelines section.

A poor diet consists primarily of excessive intake of protein, fats, sugar, salt, refined carbohydrates, and processed foods. It also consists of an inadequate intake of essential fatty acids, vitamins, minerals, and other nutrients, particularly those that function as antioxidants.

Protein and Fat

Americans usually consume two to three times the recommended amount of protein,[16] usually in the form of animal products. Excess protein contributes to obesity, which is a major risk factor for CAD, because it is converted to fat that is stored in tissues.

A high content of saturated fat is converted into cholesterol. A high-saturated-fat diet also interferes with essential fatty acid functioning.[17] Essential fatty acids are precursors of prostaglandins, some of which inhibit platelet stickiness and affect the tone of involuntary muscles in blood vessels, thereby lowering blood pressure and relaxing coronary arteries.[17] The excess essential amino acids in animal protein cause hypersecretion of insulin, which contributes to elevated levels of cholesterol and triglycerides.[18]

Cholesterol

Cholesterol, the precursor of steroids and adrenal corticosteroids, promotes optimal cell membrane function. It is essential for the absorption and digestion of fats, oils, and fat-soluble vitamins from food. Secreted by glands in the skin, cholesterol helps protect skin from dehydration and the environment. It also may function as an antioxidant when the body's supply of antioxidants in the form of vitamins and minerals is insufficient.

The liver produces approximately 1000 mg of cholesterol each day for the body's needs.[17] When cholesterol is consumed in the diet, the liver compensates by decreasing its cholesterol output. However, consumption of excess cholesterol becomes a risk factor for CAD when the body can no longer maintain the equilibrium, and the excess cholesterol is deposited in arterial walls.

Cholesterol is transported through the circulatory and lymphatic systems in protein-encased globules, the lipoproteins. A few major lipoproteins and several subfractions of the major lipoproteins have been identified, and some have been linked to atherosclerosis. LDLs transport approximately two thirds of all cholesterol. In its natural state, LDL is quite harmless. Only when it becomes oxidized by free radicals in the arterial wall does it cause inflammation and injury, which eventually leads to plaque development and CAD. Maintenance of a low LDL level minimizes the possibility of oxidation of this lipoprotein and subsequent plaque accumulation.

The main function of HDL is to transport unused cholesterol back to the liver, where it is metabolized and then removed through stool in the form of cholesterol molecules and bile acids. HDL also assists in LDL transport out of cells and undergoes oxidization by free radicals, reducing its ability to transport LDL back to the liver.

Another key player that contributes to CAD is lipoprotein (a). It looks like LDL and carries apo(a), an adhesive repair protein. It can be oxidized by free radicals like LDL and incorporated into plaque, and it facilitates development of thrombi.

Free Radicals

Free radicals are unstable oxygen molecules whose movements are volatile and unpredictable. They have one or more unpaired electrons, which causes them to search out other molecules and bind with them to offset their extra charge and become chemically stable. Free radicals are biologic renegades that constantly attack organs and tissues. They can be activated by cigarette smoke, air pollution, pesticides, and excessive exercise.

Free radicals are necessary for many functions, including prostaglandin biosynthesis and phagocyte activity. However, when free radical reactions are uncontrolled, they cause a biochemical chain reaction of destruction, harming cells and damaging proteins, enzymes, and DNA. Most tissues of the body can be injured by free radicals, contributing to a multitude of health problems and speeding up the aging process. Oxidation of lipoproteins is one example of the work of free radicals. Free radicals are also implicated in the development of cancer because of their damaging effects on cell nuclei. Some injured cells grow uncontrollably and undergo malignant transformation.

Free radical–induced deterioration can be controlled substantially by a complement of antioxidants from foods and through supplementation. Antioxidants scavenge free radicals by donating electrons to them and thereby making them chemically stable. Antioxidants include vitamins B_6 and B_{12}, folic acid, vitamins C and E, beta-carotene, coenzyme Q10, selenium, and zinc.[19]

Triglycerides

Triglycerides are lipids produced by the liver and derived from dietary fat. More than 90% of the fat in the body and 98% of fat in foods are triglycerides. Saturated fats are one form of triglycerides. Elevated levels of triglycerides are associated with high LDL and low HDL levels.[20] Triglycerides tend to raise cholesterol levels more than dietary cholesterol.[21]

Triglycerides are transported by very-low-density lipoproteins, which are considered toxic to the arteries (although the mechanism is not understood). Triglycerides are an important risk factor for CAD. They appear to accelerate the atherosclerotic process and may contribute to the formation of thrombi. Elevated triglyceride levels may also indicate an underlying problem with fat metabolism. The Framingham Heart Study showed that elevated triglyceride levels are predictors for heart disease in women of all ages.[22]

Polyunsaturated fats are another form of triglycerides. They are found mainly in plants, and in their natural state, they are healthful. However, most Americans consume these fats through the intake of partially hydrogenated vegetable oils. When polyunsaturated fats are processed into oils, their molecular structure is changed to form *trans*-fatty acids. These compounds block the body's ability to use certain essential fatty acids such as linoleic acid, a fatty acid essential to the formation of prostaglandins. Deficiencies in these hormone-like compounds can result in hypertension, formation of thrombi, arterial degeneration, and other health problems. *Trans*-fatty acids have been associated with increased levels of total cholesterol and LDL and decreased levels of HDL.[23,24] They also have been implicated in elevated levels of lipoprotein (a).[25,26]

In the Nurse's Health Study, the risk of heart disease was doubled for women who consumed the greatest amount of *trans*-fatty acids.[27] Women who consumed the largest amounts of partially hydrogenated vegetable oils had 70% more heart attacks than women who consumed small amounts. Intake of foods that were major sources of *trans*-fatty acids (eg, margarine, cookies, biscuits, cake, white bread) was significantly associated with a higher risk for developing CAD. Although studies report various levels, it has been speculated that a diet in which 2% of caloric intake consists of *trans*-fatty acids increases the relative risk of heart disease by 7% to 35%. Using the more conservative estimate, consumption of *trans*-fatty acids may result in as many as 30,000 deaths from CAD each year[28] and an even greater number of cases of nonfatal heart disease.

Sugar

The effects of excessive sugar consumption on blood sugar levels include hypoglycemia, hyperglycemia, and diabetes. Sugar intake is not usually associated with CAD, except through its association with diabetes mellitus. However, excessive intake of sugar (including honey and maple syrup) is converted into triglycerides, which can contribute to a rise in triglyceride levels.[29] Triglycerides are stored in tissues as fat.

Because sugar lacks the vitamins and minerals needed for its own metabolism, the body's vitamin and mineral reserves are used for this process. This can result in a deficiency of vitamins and minerals essential for the metabolism of fats and cholesterol and for antioxidants needed to scavenge free radicals. If this occurs, cholesterol levels rise, the metabolic rate declines, fat is burned more slowly, and energy levels decline. The results of this chain of events are elevated cholesterol levels, a lack of ability to engage in physical activity, and obesity, which increase the risk of diabetes, CAD, and cancer.

Annual consumption of sugar in the United States is about 120 pounds per person. In the early 1900s, when sugar was treated as a condiment, annual consumption was 10 to 12 pounds per person. High intake of sugar can easily translate into excessive calories consumed and into a diet lacking nutritious foods. The result is a deficiency of vitamins and minerals such as magnesium, folic acid, vitamin B_6, copper, and manganese.

The sugar is often eaten in foods that are high in fat and cholesterol. Among 1500 men and women, an increase in sugar consumption was associated with an increase intake of sweetened fats, mainly in the form of pastries.[30] The investigators concluded that sugar could act as a vehicle for fat intake, thereby encouraging fat consumption by making it more palatable.

Salt

"Salt intake has been shown to be the most important determinant of blood pressure difference between populations and within populations as well as the main determinant of the rise in blood pressure with increasing age."[31] Intersalt, considered the largest and most comprehensive study on the connection between sodium intake and hypertension, showed that sodium intake of 2300 to 4000 mg per day did not demonstrate such an association.[32] However, reanalysis of the study findings concluded that the link between blood pressure and sodium intake was stronger than first thought, particularly in middle-aged and older populations.[33]

Some persons are sensitive to salt, and some are not. Those who are salt sensitive are more likely to develop hypertension as a result of their salt intake.[34] It is estimated that up to 60% of those with hypertension are salt sensitive,[35] a sensitivity that may be genetically determined. Pathophysiologic mechanisms suggest that the incidence of salt-sensitive blood pressure is higher among African Americans than other groups.[36] There are no reliable markers for predicting who falls into the salt-sensitive category. Only by restricting sodium intake for a few months and regularly monitoring blood pressure can it be determined who is in this category.

Salt is added to many foods during processing, and the salt shaker is used freely by many. Despite these obstacles, it is prudent to keep salt intake to a moderate amount—about 2400 mg per day. Moderate salt intake may also be important because of the associations among a high-sodium, low-potassium diet and CAD, hypertension, stroke, and cancer. As a result of food processing, it is easy to ingest twice as much sodium as potassium each day, which causes an imbalance in the ratio of these minerals. Because an adequate amount of potassium has been shown to reduce the number of deaths related to stroke in men and women, and can reduce hypertension, excess salt may reduce the protective properties of potassium.

Processed Foods

Three fourths of all calories consumed in a typical American diet come from processed fats, refined sugar, refined white flour, and meat. It is therefore not surprising that the processing of foods is regarded as the primary cause of the serious nutrient deficiencies in the American diet. Processing is everything done to foods, from peeling and canning fruit to cooking vegetables to toasting bread. These forms of processing lose nutrients. For example, 68% of vitamin C is destroyed when fruits are cooked in water, and 87% is lost when vegetables are cooked in water.[37] Likewise, 33% of B_1, 45% of B_2, and 61% of B_3 are lost in cooking roots and tubers such as carrots and potatoes.[37] Cooking meat depletes about 55% of B_6, and cooking vegetables loses about 30% of B_6.[38]

Forms of industrial processing are more deleterious to health than the day-to-day processing that occurs as a result of slicing, dicing, and steaming foods at home. Processing techniques that alter the molecular structure of substances such as fats and oils introduce known risk factors for CAD, such as *trans*-fatty acids and free radicals. In refining white flour, 70% to 80% of thiamin, riboflavin, niacin, and vitamin B_6 are lost, as are 80% to 90% of trace elements and most of the fiber.[39] This does not mean that an occasional serving of white flour pasta, bread, or white rice presents a problem. However, at least 30% of the average diet is composed of grains, and if these grains are primarily refined (even if they are enriched with a few nutrients), there can be a substantial impact on the daily intake of vitamins and minerals.

Dehydrated potato flakes that are reconstituted and kept on a steam table (eg, in a school cafeteria) have no vitamin C remaining, although potatoes are normally a good source of this vitamin.[2] Processed meats lose 15% to 60% of their B vitamins, depending on whether they are mildly cured or irradiated.[2] Vitamin E is lost during storage of foods cooked in vegetable oils, and 15% to 35% of vitamin A is lost in the processing of vegetables.[2] Persons who consume an average diet that incorporates many processed foods are probably consuming a diet that is seriously deficient in nutrients.

Various forms of industrial processing include additives. Some food additives are included to extend the shelf life of foods, but most can trigger free radical production. The nutritional value of foods is also compromised by the quality of the soils in which plants are grown and the feed given to animals.

Caffeine

Americans consume about 450 million cups of coffee each day. One half of the population between 30 and 59 years of age drinks coffee.[2]

An estimated 15 million are addicted, consuming 6 to 7 cups each day.[2] Other sources of caffeine include caffeinated sodas and teas, chocolate, and some weight loss products.

Caffeine consumption has been linked to effects that indirectly contribute to CAD, such as elevated blood pressure and peripheral vasodilation.[40] One study found that caffeine induced a higher increase in systolic and diastolic blood pressure in perimenopausal women than premenopausal women.[41] Caffeine has also been linked to headaches and nervousness and a decrease in the length and quality of sleep, causing stress reactions and diminishing a person's ability to deal with stress.

Diarrhea, constipation, and abdominal pain are additional side effects linked to excessive caffeine consumption. Gastrointestinal problems are indirectly linked to CAD, because they contribute to inadequate absorption and use of nutrients.

Essential Fatty Acid Deficiencies

Although most Americans consume an excess of saturated and trans-fatty acids, they may be consuming inadequate amounts of unsaturated fatty acids, which are vital to health. Low-fat and no-fat diets may compound the problem; persons may be becoming more deficient in the essential fatty acids than they are already are. The effects of essential fatty acid deficiencies include liver and kidney degeneration, loss of hair, compromised immune systems, and CVD.[17]

One important family of essential fatty acids is omega-3 fatty acids, which include alpha-linolenic, eicosapentaenoic, and docosahexaenoic acids. Another is the omega-6 fatty acids, which include linoleic, gamma-linolenic, and arachidonic acids.

The essential fatty acids lower LDL levels [42] and decrease the aggregation of platelets,[43] and they may help to lower homocysteine levels.[44] They have also been shown to decrease triglyceride levels.[45] In a meta-analysis of 65 controlled clinical studies, fish oil (an excellent source of omega-3 fatty acids) reduced plasma triglycerides by 25% in normal subjects and 25% to 34% in hypertriglyceridemic subjects.[46] After myocardial infarction, ingestion of omega-3 fatty acids appears to decrease the rate of cardiac death because of their antiarrhythmic properties.[47]

There are many sources of essential fatty acids, and experts seem to disagree on which ones are the best, the required ratio of the omega-3 to omega-6 fatty acids, and the amount and duration of supplementation. However, everyone seems to agree that the oils in fish (eg, salmon, sardines, trout, mackerel, orange roughy, tuna) are rich in omega-3 fatty acids. Flax (which appears to be the more favored source), soybean, pumpkin, canola, walnut, and wheat germ oils contain omega-3 and omega-6 fatty acids in various ratios. Sources that contain omega-6 fatty acids include rice bran, safflower, sunflower, olive, corn, sesame, borage, evening primrose, and black currant oils. Olive oil seems to be the favorite, with canola coming in second for cooking and dressings. Flax seed, borage, evening primrose, and black currant oils appear to be the favorites for supplementation.

Vitamin Deficiencies

Humans cannot synthesize most vitamins. Vitamins must be ingested as part of the diet, and they are essential for the metabolism of other nutrients and maintenance of a variety of physiologic functions. They often serve as coenzymes in metabolic reactions.

Some vitamin deficiencies are a result of genetic abnormalities or disease conditions that decrease the body's ability to absorb vitamins from food. However, inadequate dietary intake, combined with dietary excesses and poor lifestyle habits, are the most common causes of vitamin deficiencies.

VITAMINS B_6, B_{12}, FOLIC ACID, AND NIACIN   An intake of 400 micrograms of folate by pregnant women can greatly reduce the risk of neural tube defects. It has become common practice to "prescribe" folic acid supplementation and to recommend increasing consumption of foods high in folic acid for pregnant women. The assumption has been that folic acid deficiency is the cause of neural tube defects. However, these defects may be caused by elevated levels of homocysteine, a result of folic acid and other B vitamin deficiencies.[48]

Methionine is an amino acid found in milk, milk products, and red meat. Normally, it is converted to homocysteine, which is then converted into the harmless amino acid cystathionine. For this conversion to take place, sufficient levels of vitamins B_6 and B_{12} and folic acid are essential. Without an adequate amount of these vitamins, homocysteine levels rise and become a significant risk factor for CVD.[49] Moderately elevated levels of homocysteine are considered an established risk factor for CVD.[50] The link between CVD and elevated homocysteine levels has been recognized by some researchers for more than 30 years.

Elevated homocysteine levels are directly toxic to the endothelial cells that line vessel walls,[42] impairing their ability to dilate and contract. Affected endothelial cells cannot prevent thrombus formation at the wall of the vessel, and homocysteine can stimulate smooth muscle proliferation, important in the development of atherosclerosis. Killian Robinson, cardiologist at the Cleveland Clinic, believes that, "with regard to heart disease, high homocysteine [concentration] is about as dangerous as smoking. Each confers a twofold increase in risk." Homocysteine seems to endanger blood vessels in the heart, brain, and throughout the body.[51] Levels of homocysteine in men and women between the ages of 65 and 67 are significantly higher than those in men and women between the ages of 40 and 42 years.[52] This increase may be a major contributing factor to the rise in CAD in this population.

One reason that premenopausal women are at a low risk for CAD and menopausal women are at a high risk is that estrogen may help control the level of homocysteine. Peter Berger, cardiologist at the Mayo Clinic, stated, "We know now that homocysteine concentrations rise around the time of menopause."[53]

Postmenopausal women with high homocysteine concentrations experienced a 16.9% decrease in homocysteine concentrations during the first six cycles of hormone replacement therapy, with no additional changes observed during the subsequent 2 years of treatment.[54]

The folate-homocysteine link has been confirmed through other evidence. A study of about 1500 male physicians revealed that the risk of heart attack was three times greater for those whose folate intake was less than optimal for preventing CVD, although by current nutritional standards, they were not considered folate deficient.[55]

Reduced CVD mortality has been associated with long-term treatment of breast cancer patients with the antiestrogen tamoxifen, perhaps because it lowers homocysteine levels.[56] When plasma homocysteine levels were measured in women who had been using tamoxifen for 9 to 12 months, it was found that their homocysteine levels had decreased by about 30%; after 13 to 18 months of treatment, homocysteine levels had decreased by about 25%.[56] Inadequate levels of vitamins C, E, and beta-carotene and other antioxidants may also contribute to a rise in homocysteine levels.

The good news is that homocysteine levels can be reduced through an adequate intake of vitamins B_6 and B_{12} and folic acid.

Antioxidants also help to reduce damage to the arteries caused by homocysteine.

Niacin (B_3) can decrease the risk of CAD by helping to lower cholesterol levels.[57] Results of limited research have demonstrated that supplementation with niacin was beneficial in lowering the death rate and increasing the life span of subjects who had already had a heart attack.[58]

ANTIOXIDANTS   Antioxidants are nutrients that prevent damage by free radicals and are considered of primary importance in the prevention and treatment of CAD, in part because of their ability to inhibit the oxidation of LDL. Arterial damage from nutritional deficiencies and free radical damage may be just as important as the effects of dietary intake of fats and cholesterol.

> In recent studies involving the use of antioxidants to prevent CAD, researchers showed that we could reduce cardiac events for men and women by about 40%. Let's assume this number is too high. Let's be very conservative and cut it in half to 20%. In 1994, we are expecting over 1,500,000 heart attacks, over 500,000 cardiac deaths, about 400,000 bypass surgeries, and at least 350,000 angioplasties. With the addition of just vitamin E supplementation alone and using the conservative 20% reduction figure, we could lower the 1,500,000 heart attacks by 300,000, the 500,000 deaths by 100,000, the 400,000 bypass surgeries by 80,000, and the 350,000 angioplasties by 70,000! If we just calculate the dollar savings on bypass surgeries alone, we get $3.2 billion savings this year ($40,000 × 80,000 = $3,200,000)! Conservatively saving 100,000 deaths a year works out to 274 lives saved each day![59]

VITAMIN E   The question "Should you take vitamin E?" was answered with a definite "yes" in the March 1992 issue of the *Johns Hopkins Medical Letter,* entitled *Health After 50.* By 1992, the National Library of Medicine had included over 400 indexed articles about vitamin E.

Vitamin E has long been recognized as a potent antioxidant. Some of the mechanisms by which it helps to prevent CVD include the prevention of oxidation of lipoproteins and cholesterol and inhibition of platelet aggregation.[60] In moderately obese, nondiabetic, elderly subjects, vitamin E lowered fasting and 2-hour plasma insulin concentrations, plasma triglyceride levels, and the ratio of plasma LDL to HDL cholesterol.[61] In diabetic patients, vitamin E supplementation significantly lowered blood lipids.[62] In the Nurse's Health Study, the risk of CAD decreased by 46% among women who took 100 IU of vitamin E for more than 2 years but did not decrease among women who took the supplements for a shorter period.[63]

A World Health Organization study of 16 populations across Europe revealed that a low blood level of vitamin E may be a better predictor of CAD than elevated cholesterol or blood pressure.[64] If vitamin E levels are low and blood pressure or cholesterol levels are elevated, the risk for CAD appears to be greater.

BETA-CAROTENE   Beta-carotene, another nutrient that holds promise as an antioxidant, is a precursor of vitamin A, and although the mechanisms are unknown, it is believed to play a significant role in reducing CAD by inhibiting oxidation of LDL and increasing HDL levels.[65]

Low levels of beta-carotene may increase the risk of ischemic heart disease and stroke.[65] Diets high in beta-carotene have been associated with a reduction in deaths from CVD. An ongoing study of American male physicians showed that the group of physicians with a history of CAD who had been taking beta-carotene had 51% lower incidence of heart attack, stroke, bypass surgery, and cardiac death.[66]

VITAMIN C   Several mechanisms have been suggested for vitamin C's role in reducing CVD. Vitamin C plays a major role in collagen formation and is therefore necessary to maintain the integrity of arterial walls.[67] When a vitamin C deficiency exists, collagen synthesis is reduced, causing defects in the arterial walls that contribute to the development of atherosclerosis.[68,69] Vitamin C also participates in the metabolism of folic acid, some amino acids, and hormones, and it acts as an antioxidant. Vitamin C appears to regenerate the oxidized form of vitamin E and may therefore make it more available for antioxidant activity.[70]

Supplemental intake of more than 150 mg of vitamin C per day has been associated with less CAD progression,[71] and higher plasma levels of vitamin C have correlated with higher levels of HDL.[72] Vitamin C intake by a sample of more than 11,000 U.S. adults between the ages of 25 and 74 was associated with lower rates of mortality from CVD and all cancers.[73] Lower levels of LDL, higher levels of

HDL, and lower blood pressures were associated with vitamin C supplementation in men and women between the ages of 60 and 100.[74] In women between the ages of 45 and 75, plasma vitamin C concentrations positively correlated with HDL levels.[75]

BIOFLAVONOIDS   Although bioflavonoids are not vitamins, they enhance the action of vitamin C and are being studied as cofactors that increase the potency of antioxidants and assist in the maintenance of cell membranes. Deficiencies in bioflavonoids have been associated with CVD.

Bioflavonoids were originally named vitamin P, until it was determined that this class of compounds did not exhibit a true vitamin effect. Found only in plant foods, they were first identified as a substance that appeared to potentiate the action of vitamin C to prevent capillary permeability. It was later determined that vitamin P was a group of more than 500 compounds, flavones or flavonols called bioflavonoids.

Bioflavonoids work synergistically with vitamin C to protect and preserve the structure of capillaries, and they increase the uptake of vitamin C by the liver, kidneys, and adrenal glands to assist in preventing destruction of vitamin C. The 16-cohort Seven Countries Study found that antioxidant flavonoids contributed to a decrease in the rate of mortality from CVD.[76]

COENZYME Q10   Coenzyme Q10, also known as CoQ10, ubiquinol, or ubiquinone, may be one of the more potent antioxidants. Research suggests that the level of coenzyme Q10 in human plasma may represent a sensitive index of oxidative stress that is especially indicative of early oxidative damage.[77]

Coenzyme Q10 is fat soluble and able to penetrate the LDL molecule, protecting the molecule from oxidation.[78] Decreased levels of coenzyme Q10 were found in the myocardium and blood of patients with cardiopathies.[79]

Mineral Deficiencies

Minerals are nonorganic chemical substances found in the ground and other natural locations. They are absorbed by plants from the soil and are obtained by animals through the plants that they eat.

SELENIUM, CALCIUM, AND CHROMIUM   Several mineral deficiencies correlate with CAD. For example, selenium exerts an antioxidant effect, and low levels of selenium have been implicated as contributing to CAD.[80] Selenium may work synergistically with vitamin E.[81]

Calcium deficiency correlates with hypertension.[82,83] Calcium supplementation may decrease total cholesterol levels and inhibit platelet aggregation.[82]

Chromium has been shown to raise HDL and lower total cholesterol and triglyceride levels.[84] Its effectiveness increases when taken with niacin.[85]

MAGNESIUM   The U.S. Department of Agriculture Research Service has conducted extensive metabolic balance studies showing that the dietary ratio of calcium to magnesium is best maintained at 2:1.[86] Approximately 600 mg of magnesium intake is needed to achieve this ratio, but surveys of American diets during the past 10 years have found that the diets were inadequate, containing less than 300 mg of magnesium each day.[87,88]

Magnesium deficiency caused by a poor diet or errors in magnesium metabolism may prove to be a missing link between various cardiovascular risk factors and atherosclerosis.[89] Deficiency of this mineral is believed to contribute to CAD by increasing LDL levels and decreasing HDL levels.[90] Supplementation appears to be effective in helping to reverse this process. As a result of magnesium supplementation in patients with diabetes mellitus, elevated levels of LDL were decreased, and low levels of HDL were increased.[91]

The Atherosclerosis Risk in Communities Study of four U.S. communities included more than 15,000 African-American and Caucasian men and women between the ages of 45 and 65. Serum and dietary magnesium levels of the participants were found to be significantly lower in those with CVD, hypertension, and diabetes compared with levels in those free of disease.[92] Sudden cardiac deaths were 1.5 times more common in a group of subjects who were on a regular diet containing 300 to 500 mg of magnesium than in the high-magnesium diet group who consumed 900 to 1200 mg on a daily basis.[93]

Only a sampling of the numerous studies that demonstrate a direct correlation between nutrients and certain diseases have been discussed, but the association of diet and CVD is evident. As stated in the Surgeon General's Report on Nutrition and Health, there can no longer be any doubt that diet is crucial to health. "It is now time to move beyond dietary advice and to take action to put it into practice."[94]

EXERCISE

"Given the numerous health benefits of physical activity, the hazards of being inactive are clear. Physical inactivity is a serious, nationwide problem. Its scope poses a public health challenge for reducing the national burden of unnecessary illness and premature death!"[95] It probably came as no surprise to anyone when a 1989 article in the *Journal of the American Medical Association* reported that physical activity and physical fitness were directly correlated with a decreased risk of a number of common diseases: coronary heart disease, stroke, hypertension, obesity, diabetes, colon cancer, and depression.[96]

Most of the evidence for this information was derived from studies of men. However, Blair and colleagues[97] conducted an extensive, 8-year, prospective study involving 3120 women that showed that physical fitness was inversely associated with morbidity and with mortality from several chronic diseases in women and resulted in an overall decrease in mortality from all causes (ie, "all-cause mortality"). At the Cooper Institute for Aerobic Research, 32,000 men and women between the ages of 20 and 88 were followed for 8 years. A sedentary lifestyle was the strongest independent factor predicting an early death from heart attack or other causes.[98]

Other research has shown that physically active women have a lower incidence of CAD than their more sedentary peers.[99] Among women studied, the physically active group had a significantly higher maximal aerobic capacity, lower fasting plasma insulin and glucose concentrations, and favorable lipid profiles. Their total body and abdominal fat was lower than that of the sedentary group.

Lack of adequate exercise increases the risk of heart attack by 190%. At least 60% of American adults do not exercise at recommended levels, and at least 25% do not exercise at all. Inactivity increases with age and is more common among women than men and among those with a lower income and less education.[95] According to the Surgeon General's Report on Physical Activity and Health,[95] regular physical activity improves health in several ways:

@ Reduces the risk of dying prematurely
@ Reduces the risk of dying from heart disease

- ❧ Reduces the risk of developing diabetes
- ❧ Reduces the risk of developing high blood pressure
- ❧ Helps reduce blood pressure in persons who already have high blood pressure
- ❧ Reduces the risk of developing colon cancer
- ❧ Reduces feelings of depression and anxiety
- ❧ Helps control weight
- ❧ Helps build and maintain healthy bones, muscles, and joints
- ❧ Helps older adults become stronger and better able to move about without falling
- ❧ Promotes psychologic well-being

Research conducted by Evans and Rosenberg at the U.S. Department of Agriculture's Human Nutrition Research Center on Aging at Tufts University showed that loss of muscle is a primary factor in the development of cardiovascular and other chronic diseases and in the acceleration of the aging process.[100] It is the primary factor in the decline of other key biologic functions that deteriorate over time, but this decline can be prevented or reversed through exercise.[100] Exercise recommendations are discussed in Chapter 6.

Ten biomarkers associated with health status were identified by the Tufts group[100]:

- ❧ Lean body mass
- ❧ Strength
- ❧ Basal metabolic rate
- ❧ Body fat
- ❧ Aerobic capacity
- ❧ Blood pressure
- ❧ Glucose tolerance
- ❧ Cholesterol-HDL ratio
- ❧ Bone density
- ❧ Body temperature regulation

Exercise and Body Fat

Picture a marbleized piece of prime rib, and you have a picture of atrophying muscles with fat running through them. Lack of exercise causes this to occur long before fat appears as excess weight around the thighs and abdomen. As a result of lack of exercise, the typical American loses about 6.5 pounds of lean body mass each decade, beginning around age 20 and accelerating after age 45.[100] This change is a direct result of fat replacing dynamic, active, calorie-burning muscle.

The shift of muscle to fat is a catalyst for several other physiologic changes that contribute to CVD and other chronic diseases. One is the basal metabolic rate (BMR), or caloric expenditure at rest. Based on estimates of the average loss of lean body mass with age, a person's BMR drops about 2% per decade, starting at age 20.[100] As the BMR falls, caloric need is reduced, and from age 20 onward, if a person is not physically active, caloric intake should be reduced by about 100 calories per day each decade to maintain an appropriate body weight. However, people usually continue to consume as many calories as they did when they were younger. Coupled with reduced muscle mass and a decline in BMR, this continued calorie intake results in added body fat. Unless muscle mass is increased and lost BMR is restored, a person continues to accumulate excess body fat over time. Excess body fat can eventually translate into one of the major risk factors of CAD: obesity.

The area of the body in which body fat is stored is considered an independent risk factor for developing CVD and non–insulin-dependent diabetes. Persons who store much of their body fat above their hips have a greater risk of developing these diseases. A woman can be her ideal body weight for her height, but if the excess fat she is carrying is in the wrong place, she is still at a greater risk for developing CVD.

As early as 1956, Vague[101] proposed that obesity with a fat distribution characteristic of men (ie, "android" or upper body obesity) was more closely associated with diabetes, atherosclerosis, and gout than the more peripheral distribution characteristic of women (ie, "gynoid" or lower body obesity). It has been suggested that, because abdominal obesity has been linked to hypertension and CVD and is associated with other established CVD risk factors such as diabetes, this fat pattern should be included as a screening measure for all individuals.[102–106]

Exercise and Aerobic Capacity

Lack of exercise decreases muscle mass, strength, and aerobic capacity (ie, maximal oxygen intake [Vo_2max]).[100] The Vo_2max is considered a good index of overall cardiovascular fitness and does not have to decline with age if adequate physical activity is maintained during the younger years. It is an indicator of the amount of oxygen moving out of the lungs and into the red blood cells. It is also an indicator of the ability of the heart to pump oxygenated blood to the muscles and an indicator of how adequately blood is reaching the muscles. It indicates the ability of muscle cells to use oxygen needed for conversion of energy stored in carbohydrates and fat into the form of energy that supports physical activity. When the oxidative capacity is reduced through lack of exercise, extreme muscular fatigue is often experienced.

Vo_2max begins to decline at about 20 years of age in men. In women, this decline is often postponed until the early thirties.[100] However, by age 65, the aerobic capacity of women and men is typically 30% to 40% less than that of young adults unless the older person exercises regularly.

Other Effects of Exercise

Lack of exercise negatively affects lipid metabolism, which contributes to an alteration of glucose tolerance and increase in insulin resistance—factors that contribute to the development of diabetes.[100] Exercise can also reduce the physiologic and psychologic effects of stress as a result of repetitive motion (assuming that the exercise itself it not a cause of excessive stress).[107] Repeating an exercise for some time helps the person passively ignore thoughts from the day and can trigger the relaxation response identified by Benson about 20 years ago. During this response, the body relaxes after a period of rhythmic movement of at least 15 to 20 minutes.[107] Heart rate, blood pressure, and respiration rate decrease; blood flow to the extremities increases; and skeletal muscle tension and metabolism are reduced.

STRESS

"Stress is one of the driving forces of human life. But when prolonged, compounded, misunderstood, and poorly managed, stress becomes a threat to mental and physical health."[2] Although a correlation between stress and health (mind and body) has been discussed for centuries by philosophers and scientists, it is only in the past few years that stress has been considered a definite risk factor for ill health. Between 50% to 80% of all diseases are attributed to some form of stress.[108] These include peptic ulcer, ulcerative colitis, hay fever, arthritis, Raynaud's disease, hypertension, hyperthyroidism, amenorrhea, and migraine headaches.

There are complex biochemical interactions between how a person deals with various aspects of life and how well the body functions and is able to maintain a disease-free state. Realizations abut these complex interactions led to development of the field of psychoneuroimmunology (PNI), which considers how the psychologic self interacts with the nervous system and the immune system.[109] This 30-year-old medical research specialty began when researcher George F. Soloman studied chronic rheumatoid arthritis and determined that disease severity and progression were associated with certain personality types. Widespread acceptance occurred when research showed that immunosuppression could be behaviorally conditioned.[110] "Its clinical aspects range from an understanding of the biologic mechanisms [that underlie] the influence of psychosocial factors on the onset and course of immunologically resisted and meditated diseases to an understanding of immunologically induced psychiatric symptoms. PNI aims at clarifying the scientific basis for humanistic medicine and at developing new models of health and illness."[111]

"In its medical sense, stress is essentially the rate of wear and tear in the body. Anyone who feels that whatever he is doing—or whatever is being done to him—is strenuous and wearing knows vaguely what we mean by stress. But stress does not necessarily imply a morbid change: normal life, especially intense pleasure and the ecstasy of fulfillment, also cause some wear and tear in the machinery of the body. We define stress as the nonspecific response of the body to any demand."[112] Stress is not an event; it is the body's reaction to an event. It can be defined as specific biologic responses the body undergoes when being exposed to stress-producing factors. Called *stressors*, these factors include just about everything experienced in life. Some stressors cause strong emotional reactions experienced during the course of the day. They can range from an argument with a loved one or an unpleasant day at work to sitting in the middle of a traffic jam. Strong emotional reactions can also be caused by joy, fulfillment, and self-expression, as in taking a vacation, getting married, finally getting a desired job, or intensely working on a meaningful project. Stressors also include physical trauma, exposure to heat or cold, environmental toxins, noise, and poor nutrition. All pleasant and unpleasant stressors elicit essentially the same biologic stress response.

Stress can be determined by perception. What may affect one person in a negative way may not necessarily affect another person negatively. A person's adaptive response to stress is at least equally important as the stressor itself.

Dr. Hans Selye, perhaps the most well-known scientist in the area of stress, believed that stress is often beneficial (ie, eustress) and could bring out the best in people. However, if stress persists too long or if it is a result of unpleasant stressors, it develops into the type of stress (ie, distress) that can ultimately result in illness, disease, and death.[113] Research has demonstrated several effects of stress on the body:

- Suppression of the immune system
- Susceptibility to illness,[114] particularly to immune-related disorders and cancer[115,116]
- Increased platelet activity and aggregation and blood pressure[117]
- Increased epinephrine level, which moves fat into the bloodstream and increases blood levels of cholesterol[118]

General Adaptation Syndrome

The stress response was first described by the Harvard physiologist Walter B. Cannon at the turn of the 19th century.[119] He determined that a series of biochemical changes occurred to enable human beings to survive and to deal with threats, the roots of which stemmed from humans' need to fight or flee from predators.

It was further determined that these biochemical changes, or stress reactions, were meant to be short lived; reactions should fade after the stressor is gone. During investigations of stress-related illnesses, Selye recognized that, when stress is prolonged, persons undergo a general adaptation syndrome (GAS) consisting of three phases.[113]

In stage 1, the alarm reaction (ie, fight-or-flight response), the body prepares to fight or flee through complex biochemical interactions among the hypothalamus, pituitary gland, adrenal glands, and every system of the body. Physiologic changes ranging from constriction of blood vessels and involuntary muscles to release of norepinephrine, epinephrine, and mineralocorticoid and glucocorticoid hormones take place. Glucose metabolism, heart rate, and oxygen consumption increase; inflammation is suppressed; and immune responses are inhibited. The pituitary releases a variety of hormones, thereby influencing other endocrine glands and the release of endorphins. Stage 1 is usually of short duration and is the most dramatic response to a stressor because adrenocortical secretions rise sharply. The organ or system most capable of handling the stressor is selected, and the most appropriate channel of defenses is called into action.

In stage 2, the resistance stage, adrenocortical secretions decrease. The stressor is then dealt with by the system best suited to the task of coping with it.

In stage 3, the exhaustion stage, the organ system or process handling the stressor becomes worn out and breaks down, and natural defense systems are lowered. Adrenocortical secretions again rise, and the alarm reaction takes place again as the burden is shifted away from the worn-out system.

The frequency and duration of the GAS can lead to the body's inability to adapt to or overcome stress. "Adaptation diseases" can result. Selye stated that these were ordinary diseases that developed as a consequence of the unabated activity of the GAS.

Stress itself is not fully responsible for disease, but in the body's attempt to adapt to stress, physiologic conditions arise that predispose the body to disease. Heredity, environment, health habits, and past illnesses help to determine whether illness occurs because of prolonged stress. Prolonged stress can "wear out" the body's response system, depleting reserves, exhausting physiologic functions, and leading to cancer, CVD, and other health problems.

In the GAS, the kidney is an essential organ because of its crucial role in the maintenance of homeostasis.[113] Large amounts of corticosteroids in the system for an extended period increase blood pressure. Hypertension may then develop, causing injury to the coronary arteries, along with subsequent plaque buildup. Circulating levels of LDL are maintained as a result of stress, which further contributes to injury and plaque buildup. Platelet reactivity to psychologic stress may be a major mechanism in coronary events.[118] Over time, elevated blood pressure can cause serious kidney damage. The prolonged stress reaction can ultimately cause severe hypertension because of kidney damage, and hypertension aggravates the kidney damage.

Chronic stress can increase blood cholesterol levels independent of diet. Drivers at the Indianapolis 500 have higher cholesterol levels after the race than before, and cholesterol levels in tax accountants rise around April 15 compared with the rest of the year. Medical students' cholesterol levels rise during examinations.[120] Mental stress significantly increases heart rate and systolic blood pressure among patients with angina pectoris.[121]

The level of interferon-γ, which stimulates the growth and activity of natural killer cells, can decrease during times of stress considered a normal part of life. For example, interferon-γ levels decreased by as much as 90% during examinations taken by medical students. During examination time, levels of epinephrine and norepinephrine increased significantly during waking and sleeping hours. Students must repeatedly take examinations and do well on them before and during medical school. Over time, their immunologic function became regulated to a lower than normal level, despite their relative competence in this stressful situation.[121]

Another example of lowered immune system function was seen in the research project conducted at Ohio State University in which pencil eraser–sized wounds were made on the inner arms of 26 healthy women between the ages of 47 and 81. One half of these women were caring for a mother or husband with Alzheimer's disease. In the group of caretaking women, healing took an average of 9 days longer than for the other group; the difference in the healing process was most notable during the initial healing stages, when the risk of infection is greatest.[122]

Stress can affect human immunodeficiency virus (HIV) disease progression. Fatalistic beliefs regarding HIV status were negatively associated with health outcomes, such as shorter survival times and immune marker changes associated with HIV disease progression.[122] Another study that demonstrated the effects of stress on the immune system showed that gay men who were completely open about their sexual orientation with family and friends were healthier than those who were not. They experienced slower HIV disease progression, smaller declines in CD4 T-cell counts, longer periods before the diagnosis of acquired immunodeficiency syndrome, and longer periods of health.[123]

An example of the effects of stress on the cardiovascular system was demonstrated in a study that explored why African-American women experience a 60% greater risk of dying from heart disease than Caucasian women. This study, conducted at Duke University, exposed African-American women to racist comments.[124] Exposure resulted in feelings of anger, resentfulness, cynicism, and anxiety. The stress response was called into action, increasing the heart rate and elevating blood pressure. As one woman in the study stated, "If this is how strongly I reacted in the lab, I can only imagine how I react in real life."[124]

Newlywed couples were asked to discuss a topic known to be a source of conflict for them while blood measure, cortisol and norepinephrine levels, and white blood cell counts were monitored throughout the day. The effects of stress were more profound in women. Their blood pressure rose more than the men's, and they experienced a dramatic surge in cortisol and norepinephrine levels. By the next day, the women's white blood cell counts had declined. Most men remained physiologically unaffected.[125] The results of this test were duplicated with older couples married for an average of 42 years.[126] As the lead investigator acknowledged, "There may be no serious health consequences for our young female newlyweds. But for older women, hostile and chronic conflict might mean the difference between sickness and health."[127]

Depletion of dehydroepiandrosterone (DHEA) as a result of stress may play a significant role in the development of CVD, osteoporosis, and other chronic degenerative diseases, including cancer. A precursor of epinephrine and cortisol secreted by the adrenal cortex, it is a hormone whose functions are only beginning to be understood. DHEA circulates in the bloodstream in quantities thousands of times greater than estrogen and testosterone. Blood levels peak at age 25, decline rapidly with menopause, and fall to 5% of its maximum amount by the last year of life.[128] DHEA is the only hormone that declines linearly with age. Every time epinephrine and cortisol are secreted during times of stress, the reservoir of DHEA is depleted, potentially making DHEA a marker for the body's exposure to stress.

In a study of the effects of meditation on stress, 328 meditators were compared with 1462 nonmeditators of various ages. Results showed that, by independent factors such as diet, weight, exercise, and alcohol consumption, the meditators had higher levels of DHEA.[128] The men older than 45 who meditated had 23% more DHEA and the women had 47% more DHEA than the nonmeditators. The levels for meditators were estimated to be equivalent to those of persons 5 to 10 years younger.

Nutrients can be depleted by the demands of stress on the body, and free radicals can damage tissues if the diet does not adequately provide the nutrients essential for daily functioning and for dealing with the stress response. Deficiencies in nutrients can also result from stress-induced maldigestion and malabsorption.

Women and Stress

Chronic stress can inhibit ovulation. Psychologic stressors can significantly lower secretion of estrone, estradiol, and estriol.[129] The adrenals are the source of the hormone androstenedione, levels of which are low under conditions of chronic stress. Some research has demonstrated that, during the climacteric, women who have more stress in their lives also have more "climacteric complaints" than others. The climacteric and anxiety have in common the symptoms of insomnia, fatigue, shortness of breath, heart palpitations, hot flushes or chills, irritability, and difficulty in concentrating. Additional symptoms also are associated with stress:

- Anxious thoughts or fearful anticipation
- Poor concentration or difficulty with memory
- An inability to relax, feelings of tension, and restlessness
- Stiff or tense muscles, sweating, and tension headaches
- Frequency and urgency with urination
- Decline in libido
- Awareness of heart beat
- Gastrointestinal disturbances such as nausea, vomiting, diarrhea, and constipation

Depression is associated with stress, and "people who experience depression are more than twice as likely to have experienced stressful conditions in life."[130] This is an important relationship to consider in the care of women, because they are more likely than men to experience certain stressors such as sexual and physical abuse. Women increasingly must balance work, familial, and personal demands. Fatigue and emotional stress are caused by their multiple roles as mothers, spouses, caregivers for aging parents, and financial providers. Through repeated exposure to the stress response, women may experience exacerbations of symptoms associated with the climacteric, and they may develop hypertension, CVD, diabetes, and other health problems. Modern psychologic challenges can activate the archaic response to stress, with effects that eventually prove to be harmful.

Developing ways to relax deeply and changing perceptions of stressors are important aspects of a woman's health program. Stress responses can be controlled through the practice of several relaxation techniques.

PREVENTING AND TREATING CORONARY ARTERY DISEASE

OPENING YOUR HEART PROGRAM

No one knows whether nutrition, exercise, or stress is more important in preventing or treating CAD. By addressing all of these factors and more, Dr. Dean Ornish and his colleagues have developed a scientifically validated program that can reverse even severe CAD without using cholesterol-lowering drugs or surgery.

In describing the philosophical foundation for the Opening Your Heart program, Ornish said, "The further back in the causal chain of events we can address a problem, the more powerful the healing can be."[129] Symptoms should be addressed, but if the problem is treated only on the physical level, the patient's improvement will be less than it could be, and the illness is more likely to recur.

Ornish does not oppose lifesaving surgery or drugs. If these medical interventions are necessary, the Opening Your Heart program is used in combination with them. According to Ornish, "When a patient comes into the emergency room with severe chest pain, saying, 'Doc, please get this elephant off my chest,' I don't feed him broccoli and ask him to start meditating. I use whatever cardiac drugs, electrical shocks, and surgical procedures are necessary to treat the acute, life-threatening condition."[130]

Ornish and colleagues[131] studied two groups of patients with severe CAD. Patients in one group followed the Opening Your Heart program, and the other group followed their doctors' advice of making moderate dietary changes such as reducing intake of red meat, using margarine instead of butter, limiting eggs to no more than three each week, and stopping smoking. Follow-up angiograms of these patients were made 1 year later and sent to various independent experts for analysis. Eighty-two percent of the patients following the comprehensive heart program demonstrated measurable reversal of their coronary artery blockages. The women in the study, even those who made only moderate lifestyle changes, showed some reversal of arterial blockages. This finding suggests that women may experience reversal more readily than men. Most patients in the other group became measurably worse during the same interval.

The complete dietary and exercise recommendations of this program are not discussed here, because they have been integrated with other recommendations included in Chapter 6 and in the Guidelines section. However, a vital component of the Opening Your Heart program includes stress reduction techniques derived from yoga. The program also includes helping patients to address issues of isolation (from one's feelings, from others, and from a "higher force") that can lead to stress and illness. Various visualization techniques are also practiced by patients, as are techniques to enable them to communicate their feelings. Patients and their loved ones attend group support meetings.

Ornish believes it is not possible to determine the relative contribution of each component of the program, although some parts can be more important than others for some persons. The degree of reversal in coronary artery blockage was directly correlated to adherence to each component of the program. The success of this program may result from the low levels of cholesterol and fat, low levels of methionine (precursor of homocysteine), and ingestion of foods rich in antioxidants. Although the intent of this program is to reverse CAD in those already diagnosed with it, it is also reasonable to consider its value as a comprehensive approach to prevention of CAD by women of all ages. *Dr. Dean Ornish's Program for Reversing Heart Disease* is recommended reading for clinicians and their patients.

Atherosclerosis can begin in childhood, and the typical American lifestyle contributes to the development of CAD and other diseases. Approximately 40% of those who die of heart disease did not know they had a heart problem until they died of it—clearly not the best way to find out. So no matter how good we get at treating heart disease, the major focus should be on prevention.[131]

RECOGNIZING SYMPTOMS OF CORONARY ARTERY DISEASE

Symptoms of CAD include angina pectoris, palpitations, fainting,[132] edema, shortness of breath, great fatigue, and heart attack. Angina pectoris is the classic symptom of CAD, the incidence of which appears to be higher among women than in men. It is experienced by approximately 56% of women with CAD. Prinzmetal's angina, which primarily affects women, is more likely than angina pectoris to occur when a person is at rest.

Angina may be experienced as a feeling of pressure or heaviness in the chest, as a dull pain directly beneath the sternum, or as a band of pain across the chest. It may be experienced as back pain without any noticeable chest pain or pressure. Pain may or may not radiate down the arm. It can also radiate down the right arm instead of the more commonly experienced radiation of pain down the left arm.

Two thirds of syndrome X patients are women.[6] These otherwise healthy individuals, often with no risk factors for heart disease, sometimes experience agonizing anginal pain, but they do not have blockage in any major arteries. Angiographic and catheterization results can be normal.

The syndrome is caused by abnormalities of the small vessels. During physical or emotional stress, the distal blood vessels may not dilate sufficiently. The intense pain "may be caused by a hypersensitivity of the nerves leading to the heart, esophagus, and chest."[6]

RISK ASSESSMENT AND SCREENING TESTS

When assessing a woman's risk for CAD, the list of high-risk factors includes use of nicotine or alcohol, substance abuse, age, familial history, distribution of body fat and amount of excess body fat, medical history (eg, elevated levels of triglycerides, cholesterol, or LDL; decrease in the level of HDL), and previously diagnosed CVD, diabetes mellitus, or hypertension. Although these are extremely important factors to consider in assessing the level of risk for CAD, a more comprehensive approach should include obtaining information about the woman's lifestyle. What was her dietary intake and what was her level of regular physical activity from adolescence through adulthood? Does she feel that her life is stressful now, and were there periods of extreme stress in her life in the past? Is she at high risk for experiencing the negative consequences of stress? Because the atherosclerotic process can begin in childhood and be exacerbated by the typical American lifestyle of inactivity, poor nutrition, and chronic stress, the degree of risk can be better determined by obtaining as much information as possible about a woman's past and current lifestyle.

In the absence of any major risk factors, it is reasonable to obtain the following blood tests[133] for perimenopausal and postmenopausal patients:

@ Levels of total cholesterol, lipoprotein (a), HDL and LDL cholesterol ratio, total HDL, and triglycerides (after a 12 to 14-hour
  fast)
@ Fasting blood sugar level (after a 10-hour fast)
@ Thyroid-stimulating hormone concentration

If the results of these tests are normal and continue to remain normal, the tests should be repeated every 5 years. Additional tests, such
as an electrocardiogram, can be performed when the woman is
between the ages of 45 and 50.[130]

The echocardiogram is considered an excellent tool to evaluate
structural problems of the heart and probably is the first test to be
performed to evaluate symptoms such as fainting, palpitations, shortness of breath, and angina.[6] Chest radiography may be performed to
detect structural abnormalities, lung tumors, enlargement of the
heart, and congestion that may be caused by heart disease.

Routine health screening may soon include tests that measure
the serum levels of various nutrients such as homocysteine and vitamin E. Some health care professionals order them now, but until
they are affordable and reimbursable by health insurance companies,
these tests are unlikely to be fully integrated into preventive health
care practices.

If a woman 50 years of age or older is asymptomatic but has a
few risk factors and a family history of CAD, it is suggested that, in
addition to the tests previously mentioned, an exercise stress test
should be performed, possibly with echocardiographic imaging or
radionuclide tracer assessment.[6]

LIMITATIONS OF HEALTH CARE

Time and economics always limit health care. Few health care
providers have as much time as they would like to spend with their
patients. Within the current health care delivery system, complaints
by providers and patients alike focus on the lack of time available
and the resultant difficulty in making adequate assessments regarding any health issue or in providing patient education.

Because of time constraints during the course of an office or
clinic visit, the clinician may be able to conduct only a limited risk
assessment. If this is the case, educational materials and risk assess-

ment forms can be given to the woman to take home and review. By going through this process, she may identify factors that contribute to her risk that she had not considered before, and she would then be able to discuss them during her next office visit. She may then be motivated to make changes in her lifestyle that are essential in preventing CAD.

Health care professionals must assist women in evaluating their lifestyles and in identifying risk factors that contribute to CAD. Through this process, the health care professional can provide the necessary recommendations for the prevention and treatment of CAD and reinforce the fact that no hormone or medication can replace or compensate for prevention. A nutritional program consisting of minimal amounts of processed foods, animal sources of protein, refined carbohydrates, *trans*-fatty acids, and saturated facts is necessary for prevention and treatment of CAD, as is a program rich in antioxidants, vitamins, minerals, fiber, and essential fatty acids obtained through a variety of wholesome foods. Nutritional supplementation may be necessary, particularly for magnesium, calcium, the B vitamins, and vitamins C and E. An adequate nutritional program in combination with regular aerobic exercise and stress management yields the greatest promise of lowering a woman's risk for CAD.

REFERENCES

1. Simon HB. Conquering heart disease. New York: Little, Brown; 1994.
2. Beasley JD, Swift J. Kellogg report, the impact of nutrition, environment, and lifestyle on the health of Americans. Annandale-on-Hudson, NY: Institute of Policy and Practice of the Bard College Center; 1989.
3. Deinard L. Men of medicine: there's no end to what may be accomplished. Postgrad Med 1949;5:417–428.
4. Mayer J. A diet for living. New York: Pocket Books; 1977.
5. Kowalski R. Eight steps to a healthy heart. New York: Warner Books; 1992.
6. Ross E, Sachs J. Healing the female heart. New York: Pocket Books; 1996.
7. Health after 50. Johns Hopkins Med Lett 1990;Aug:4–5.
8. Adams MR, et al. Inhibition of coronary artery arthrosclerosis by 17-beta-estradiol in ovariectomized monkeys: lack of an effect of added progesterone. J Lipid Res 1985;30:1895–1906.
9. Keaney JF Jr, et al. 17β-Estradiol preserves endothelial vasodilator function and limits low-density lipoprotein oxidation in hypercholesterolemic swine. Circulation 1994;89:2251–2259.

10. Negre-Salvayre A, et al. Protective effect of 17β-estradiol against the cytotoxicity of minimally oxidized LDL to cultured bovine aortic endothelial cells. Atherosclerosis 1993;99:207–217.
11. Bush TL, Miller VT. Effects of pharmacologic agents used during menopause: impact on lipids and lipoproteins. In: Mishell DR Jr, ed. Menopause: physiology and pharmacology. Chicago: Year Book Medical; 1987:187–208.
12. Bush TL, et al. Cardiovascular mortality and noncontraceptive use of estrogen in women: results from the lipid research clinics program follow-up study. Circulation 1987;75:1102–1109.
13. Castelli W. Your healthy heart. Prevention 1996;April:102.
14. Enos, et al. Coronary disease among United States soldiers killed in action in Korea. JAMA 1953;152:1090–1093.
15. Joseph A, et al. Manifestations of coronary atherosclerosis in young trauma victims—an autopsy study. J Am Coll Cardiol 1993;22:459–467.
16. Gittleman A. Super nutrition for menopause. New York: Pocket Books; 1993.
17. Eramus U. Fats that heal, fats that kill. Burnaby BC, Canada: Alive Books; 1994.
18. Hubbard R. Chronic disease and the vegetarian diet. In: Hamilton K, ed. The experts speak: the role of nutrition in medicine. Sacramento, CA: IT Services Health Associates Medical Group; 1996.
19. Florence TM. The role of free radicals in disease. Aust N Z J Opthalmol 1995;23:3–7.
20. Hulley SB, et al. Epidemiology as a guide to clinical decisions: the association between triglycerides and coronary heart disease. N Engl J Med 1980;302, 1383.
21. Bass KM, et al. Plasma lipoprotein levels as predictors of cardiovascular deaths in women. Circulation 1993;153:2209.
22. Castelli WP, et al. Lipids and risk of coronary heart disease: the Framingham Study. Ann Epidemiol 1992;2:23–28.
23. Mensink RP, Ktan MB. Effect of dietary trans-fatty acids on high density and low density lipoprotein cholesterol levels in healthy subjects. N Engl J Med 1990;323:439–445.
24. Nestel PH, et al. Plasma cholesterol lowering potential of edible oil blends suitable for commercial use. Am J Clin Nutr 1992;55:46–50.
25. Nestel P, et al. Plasma lipoprotein lipid and Lp(a) changes with substitution of elaidic acid for oleic acid in the diet. J Lipid Res 1992;33:1029–1036.
26. Mensink RP, et al. Effect of dietary cis and trans fatty acids on serum lipoprotein (a) levels in humans. J Lipid Res 1992;33:1493–1501.
27. Willett WC, et al. Intake of trans fatty acids and risk of coronary heart disease among women. Lancet 1993;341:581–585.
28. Willett WC, Ascherio A. Trans fatty acids: are the effects only marginal? Am J Public Health 1994;84:722–724.
29. Bierman EL, Porti DJR. Carbohydrate intolerance and lipemia. Am Intern Med 1968;68:926.
30. Emmett PM, Heaton KW. Is extrinsic sugar a vehicle for dietary fat. Lancet 1995;345:1537–40.
31. MacGregor GA. Salt . . . more adverse effects. Am J Hypertens 1997;10(Suppl 5, Pt 2):37s–41s.
32. Intersalt Cooperative Research Group. Intersalt: an international study of electrolyte excretion and blood pressure. BMJ 1988;297:319–328.

33. Haddy FJ, Pamnani MB. Role of dietary salt in hypertension. J. Am Coll Nutr 1995;14:428–438.
34. University of California at Berkeley, School of Public Health. Don't let the salt news shake you up. Wellness Lett 1996;12:12.
35. Calloway W. Reexamining cholesterol and sodium restrictions. Nutr Today 1994;29:5.
36. Rutledge DR. Race and hypertension: what is clinically relevant? Drugs 1994;47:914–932.
37. Ang C, Livingston GE. Nutritive losses in the home storage and preparation of raw fruits and vegetables. In: White, Selvey, eds. 1974:51–64.
38. Borenstein B. Effect of processing on the nutritional values of foods. In: Goodhart, Shils, eds. 1980:497–505.
39. Schroeder H. Losses of vitamins and trace minerals resulting from processing and preservation of foods. Am J Clin Nutr 1971;24:562–573.
40. Lane JD, Manus DC. Persistent cardiovascular effects with repeated caffeine administration. Psychosom Med 1989;51:373–380.
41. Del Rio G, et al. Increased cardiovascular response to caffeine in perimenopausal women before and during estrogen therapy. Eur J Endocrinol 1996;135:598–603.
42. Kromhout D, et al. The inverse relation between fish consumption and 20-year mortality from coronary heart disease. N Engl J Med 1983;312:1169.
43. Renaud S, Nordy A. Small is beautiful: alpha-linoleic acid and eicosapentaenoic acid in man. Lancet 1983;8334:1169.
44. Olszewski AJ, McCully KS. Fish oil decreases serum homocysteine in hyperlipemic men. Cororn Artery Dis 1993;53–60.
45. Harris WN. Fatty acids and serum lipid/lipoprotein levels in humans: literature review. Presented at the ILSI workshop on individual fatty acids and cardiovascular disease; March 30–31, 1995.
46. Dolecek TA. Epidemiological evidence of relationships between dietary polyunsaturated fatty acids and mortality in the Multiple Risk Factor Intervention Trial. Proc Soc Exp Biol Med 1992;200:177–182.
47. Simopoulos AP. Omega-3 fatty acids in the prevention-management of cardiovascular disease. Can J Physiol Pharmacol 1997;75:234–239.
48. Mills J. Homocysteine metabolism in pregnancies complicated by neural-tube defects. Lancet 1995;345:149–151.
49. Stampfer M. Cardiovascular risk and homocysteine. In: Hamilton K, ed. The experts speak: the role of nutrition in medicine. Sacramento, CA: IT Services Health Associates Medical Group; 1996.
50. Brattstrom L. Vitamins as homocysteine-lowering agents. J. Nutr 1996;126(Suppl 4): 1276S–805.
51. Berger P. The B vitamin breakthrough. In: Mason M, ed. Health 1995;95:71.
52. Nygard O, et al. Total plasma homocysteine and cardiovascular risk profile: the Hordaland Homocysteine Study. JAMA 1995;274:1526–1533.
53. Berger P. The B vitamin breakthrough. In: Mason M, ed. Health 1995;Sept:73.
54. Van der Mooren MJ, et al. Hormone replacement therapy may reduce high serum homocysteine in postmenopausal women. Eur J Clin Invest 1994;24:733–736.
55. Stampfer MJ, et al. A prospective study of plasma homocysteine and risk of myocardial infarction in US physicians. JAMA 1992;268:877–881.
56. Anker G, et al. Plasma levels of the atherogenic amino acid homocysteine in post-menopausal women with breast cancer treated with tamoxifen. Int J Cancer 1995;60:365–368.

57. Seelig MS, Heggtveit HA. Magnesium interrelationships in ischemic heart disease: a review. Am J Clin Nutr 1974;27:59–79.
58. Canner PL, et al. Fifteen-year mortality in coronary drug project patients: long-term benefit with niacin. J Am Coll Cardiol 1986;8:1245–1255.
59. Goldstrich J, ed. The cardiologist's painless prescription for a healthy heart and a longer life. Dallas: 9-Heart-9 Publishing; 1994.
60. Jialal I, Grundy SM. Effect of dietary supplementation with alpha-tocopherol on the oxidative modification of low density lipoprotein. J Lipid Res 1992;33: 899–906.
61. Paolisso G, et al. Chronic intake of pharmacologic doses of vitamin E might be useful in therapy of elderly patients with coronary heart disease. Am J Clin Nutr 1995;61:848–852.
62. Jaen SK, et al. The effect of modest vitamin E supplementation on lipid peroxidation products and other cardiovascular risk factors in diabetic patients. Lipids 1996;(Suppl):587–90.
63. Stampfer M, et al. Vitamin E consumption and the risk of coronary heart disease in women. N Engl J Med 1993;328:1450–1456.
64. Grey KF, et al. Inverse correlation between plasma vitamin E and mortality from ischemic heart disease in cross-cultural epidemiology. Am J Clin Nutr 1991;63:326S–334S.
65. Sies HW, et al. Antioxidant functions of vitamins: Vitamins E and C, beta-carotene, and carotenoids. Ann N Y Acad Sci 1992;669:7–20.
66. Hennekens C, et al. Physicians health study. In: Goldstrich J, ed. The cardiologist's painless prescription for a healthy heart and a longer life. Dallas: 9-Heart-9 Publishing; 1994.
67. Ginter ER, et al. Vitamin C in the control of hypercholesterolemia in man. Int J Vitam Nutr Res 1982;23:S137–S152.
68. Rath M, Pauling L. Hypothesis: lipoprotein (a) is a surrogate for ascorbate. Proc Natl Acad Sci USA 1990;87:6204–7207.
69. Rath M, Pauling L. Solutions to the puzzle of human cardiovascular disease: its primary cause is ascorbate deficiency leading to the deposition of lipoprotein (a) and fibrinogen/fibrin in the vascular wall. J Orthomol Med 1991;6:125–134.
70. Gershoff SN. Vitamin C (ascorbic acid): new roles, new requirements? Nutr Rev 1993;51:313–326.
71. Hodis H. Atherosclerosis and antioxidant vitamins. In: Hamilton K, ed. The experts speak: the role of nutrition in medicine. Sacramento, CA: IT Services Health Associates Medical Group; 1996.
72. Hallfrisch J. High plasma vitamin C associated with high plasma-HDL-HDL2 cholesterol. Am J Clin Nutr 1994;60:100–105.
73. Enstrom JE, et al. Vitamin C intake and mortality among a sample of the United States population. Epidemiology 1992;3:194–202.
74. Jaques PF. Effects of vitamin C on high-density lipoprotein cholesterol and blood pressure. J Am Coll Nutr 1992;11:139–144.
75. Ness AR, et al. Vitamin C status and serum lipids. Eur J Clin Nutr 1992;50:724–729.
76. Hertog M, et al. Flavonoid intake and long-term risk of coronary heart disease and cancer in the Seven Country Study. Arch Intern Med 1995;155:381–386.
77. Kontush A, et al. Plasma ubiquinal-10 is decreased in patients with hyperlipidaemia. Atherosclerosis 1997;129:119–26.
78. Hanaki Y, et al. Ratio of low density lipoprotein cholesterol to ubiquinone as a coronary risk factor. N Engl J Med 1991;325:814–815.

79. Kucharska J, et al. Determination of coenzyme Q10 and alpha-tocopherol levels in patients with cardiopathies of unknown origin. Bratisl Lek Listy 1996;97:351–354.

80. Salonen JT, et al. Interactions of serum copper, selenium and low-density lipoprotein cholesterol on arthrogenesis. BMJ 1991;302:756–760.

81. Lehr D. Arrhythmias, selenium and magnesium. In: Hamilton K, ed. The experts speak: the role of nutrition in medicine. Sacramento, CA: IT Services Health Associates Medical Group; 1996.

82. Karanja N, et al. Plasma lipids and hypertension: response to calcium supplementation. Am J Clin Nutr 1987;45:60–65.

83. Calcium reduces blood pressure. Healthline 1984;Sept:20.

84. Press RI, et al. Effect of chromium picolinate on serum cholesterol and apolipoprotein fractions in human subjects. West J Med 1990;152:41–45.

85. Urberg M, et al. Hypercholesterolemic effects of nicotinic acid and chromium supplementation. J Fam Pract 1988;27:603–606.

86. Hathaway ML. Magnesium in human nutrition. Home economics research report #19. Washington, DC: USDA Agricultural Research Service; 1962.

87. Spillman DM. Calcium magnesium and calorie intake and activity levels of healthy adult women. J Am Coll Nutr 1987;6:454.

88. Morgan KJ, Stampley GL. Dietary intake levels and food sources of magnesium and calcium for selected segments of the US population. Magnesium 1988;7:225–233.

89. Altura BM, Altura BT. Magnesium and cardiovascular biology: an important link between cardiovascular risk factors and atherogenesis. Cell Mol Biol Res 1995;41:347–359.

90. Altura BT, et al. Magnesium dietary intake modulates blood lipid levels and atherogenesis. Proc Natl Acad Sci USA 1990;87:1840–1844.

91. Corica F, et al. Effects of oral magnesium supplementation on plasma lipid concentrations in patients with non–insulin-dependent diabetes mellitus. Mages Res 1994;7:43–46.

92. Ma J, et al. Associations of serum and dietary magnesium with cardiovascular disease, hypertension, diabetes, insulin, and carotid arterial wall thickness: Atherosclerosis Risk in Communities Study. J Clin Epidemiol 1995;48:927–940.

93. Singh RB. Effect of dietary magnesium supplementation in the prevention of coronary heart disease and sudden cardiac death. Magnes Trace Elem 1990;9:143–151.

94. U.S. Department of Health and Human Services, Public Health Service, Office of the Surgeon General. The Surgeon General's report on nutrition and health. Washington, DC: U.S. Government Printing Office; 1989.

95. U.S. Department of Health and Human Services. Physical activity and health: a report of the Surgeon General. Atlanta: U.S Department of Health and Human Services, Centers for Disease Control, and Prevention, National Center for Chronic Disease Prevention and Health Promotion; 1996:1.

96. Kaplan JP, et al. Physical activity, physical fitness, and health: time to act. JAMA 1989;262:2347.

97. Blair, et al. Physical fitness and all cause mortality: a prospective study of health in men and women. JAMA 1986;262:2395.

98. Vital signs, health, and medical news. Health 1996;October:4.

99. Hardman AE, Hudson A. Brisk walking and serum lipid and lipoprotein variables in previously sedentary women—efffect of 12 weeks of regular brisk walking followed by 12 weeks of detraining. Br J Sports Med 1994;28:261–266.

100. Evans W, Rosenberg I. The 10 determinants of aging. New York: Simon & Schuster; 1992.
101. Krotkiewski M, et al. Impact of obesity on metabolism in men and women: importance of regional adipose tissue distribution. J Clin Invest 1983;72:1150–1162.
102. Depres JP. Lipoprotein metabolism in visceral obesity. Int J Obes 1991;15:45.
103. Hartz AJ, et al. Relationship of obesity to diabetes: Influence of obesity level and body fat distribution. Prev Med 1983;12:351.
104. Kaplan N. The deadly quartet: upper body obesity, glucose intolerance, hypertriglyceridemia, and hypertension. Arch Intern Med 1989;149:1514.
105. Kannel WB, et al. Regional obesity and risk of cardiovascular disease: the Framingham Study. J Clin Epidemiol 1991;44:183.
106. Vague J. The degree of masculine differentiation of obesities: a factor determining predisposition to diabetes, atherosclerosis, gout, and uric calculous disease. Am J Clin Nutr 1956;4:20–34.
107. Benson H. The relaxation response. New York: Avon Books; 1976.
108. Pelletier K. Mind as healer; mind as slayer. New York: Dell Publishing; 1992.
109. Leiphart M. Psychoneuroimmunology: a basis for HIV treatment. Focus, a guide to AIDS research and counseling. 1997;12:1–7.
110. Ader R, Cohen N. Behaviorally conditioned immunosuppression. Psychosom Med 1975;37:333–340.
111. Soloman GF. Immune and nervous system interactions. Malibu, CA: Fund for Psychoneuroimmunology; 1995.
112. Seyle H. Stress and life. New York: McGraw-Hill; 1976:14.
113. Seyle H. Stress without distress. New York: Signet; 1974.
114. Soloman GF. Emotions stress the central nervous system and immunity. Ann N Y Acad Sci 1969;164:335–343.
115. Bahnson CB, Bahnson MB. Cancer as an alternative to psychosis: a theoretical model of somatic and psychologic regression. In: Kissen DM, LeShan, ed. Psychosomatic aspects of neoplastic disease. Philadelphia: JB Lippincott; 1964:184–202.
116. Levenson FB. The causes and prevention of cancer. New York: Stein & Day; 1985.
117. Bartrop RW, et al. Depressed lymphocyte function after bereavement. Lancet 1977;1:834–836.
118. Markovitz JH, Matthews KA. Platelets and coronary heart disease: potential psychophysiologic mechanisms. Psychosom Med 1991;13:642–668.
119. Goleman D, Guren J, eds. Mind-body medicine. Yonkers, NY: Consumer Reports Book; 1993.
120. Specchia G, et al. Mental stress as a provocative test in patients with clinical syndromes of coronary heart disease. Circulation 1991;83(4 Suppl):II108–114.
121. Kiecolt-Glaser J, Glaser R. Mind and immunity. In: Goleman D, Gurin J, eds. Mind-body medicine. Yonkers, NY: Consumer Reports Book; 1993.
122. Cole SW, et al. Stressful events, psychological responses and progression of HIV infection. In: Gloser R, Kiecolt-Glaser J. Handbook on stress and Immunity. New York: Academic Press; 1994.
123. Cole SW, et al. Accelerated course of HIV infection in gay men who conceal their homosexuality. Psychosom Med 1995;58:219–231
124. Vital signs: racism hurts the heart twice. Health 1996;October:26.

125. Glaser-Kiecolt, et al. Hostile arguing may compromise a woman's immune system. J Consult Psychol 1996;64:322–332.
126. Glaser-Kiecolt, et al. Marital conflicts in older adults: endocrinological and immunological correlates. Psychosom Med 1997;59:339–349.
127. McAuliffe K. More than just a spat. Self 1997;January:35.
128. Chopra DA. Ageless body, timeless mind. New York: Harmony Books; 1993.
129. Ballinger S. Stress as a factor in lowered estrogen levels in the early postmenopause. Ann N Y Acad Sci 1990;592:95–113.
130. Mazure C. Treat chronic stress as a serious medical problem. Am Health 1997;May:45.
131. Ornish D. Dr. Dean Ornish's program for reversing heart disease. New York: Ballantine Books; 1990:49.
132. Pashkovo F. The women's heart book. New York: Plume Book; 1994.
133. Castelli W. Your game plan for life. Prevention 1996;April:69–78.

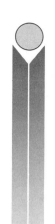
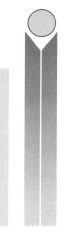

CHAPTER 4

Osteoporosis and Other Health Issues

The United States has the highest rate of osteoporotic fractures in the world.[1] Advertising sponsored by pharmaceutical companies and the American Dairy Council, articles in health in women's magazines, television, talk shows, and education provided by health care professionals have greatly influenced the number of women who have heard about osteoporosis. A 1991 Gallup survey found that 75% of the 750 women between the ages of 45 and 75 interviewed were familiar with osteoporosis. However, knowing about the disease had not made a substantial impact; 70% of those at highest risk had never spoken to their physicians about osteoporosis. Dr. Bernadine Healy, former director of the National Institutes of Health, states in *A New Prescription for Women's Health*, "Many of us, down deep, believe that osteoporosis is a disease of old women, that we are immune and by the time we reach the age at which it might strike us, surely 'they' will have found a cure."[2]

Do young women know about osteoporosis? In 1994, 100 young women students who were enrolled in a required undergraduate health course at a Midwestern state university participated in a survey. The results revealed that, although 90% had heard about osteoporosis, only 43% had received information about it from a health care provider or school.[3] Only 6.7% of the women reported getting "osteoprotective" exercise each week and adequate calcium each day. Respondents believed that it was unlikely that osteoporosis would develop in them and expressed little concern about osteoporosis, which they believed to be much less serious than other health problems such as heart disease and breast cancer.

"Healthy bones" have not been an issue for Americans, primarily because it was never a major issue within the medical community at large. The public was not informed that development of healthy bone can be compromised even in childhood as a consequence of inadequate nutrition and exercise, various diseases, and some medications. They were never made aware that, if development is hindered, the integrity of bone eventually becomes compromised, resulting in a chronic degenerative process that can lead to pain and disability caused by osteoporotic fractures.

The good news is that osteoporosis has become recognized as a devastating health problem, and many medical disciplines, including pediatrics, adolescent medicine, adult medicine, and gynecology, have recognized the importance of preventive measures. Increasing numbers of health care professionals are beginning to play an aggressive role in the education of patients. Health care professionals are also more conscious of the effects of certain treatments and medications (eg, cortisone therapy) on the integrity of bone. They are becoming more conservative in prescribing such treatments, and when they do, they also provide dietary and exercise recommendations.

BONE GROWTH

Rapid bone growth occurs during infancy. Adolescence is another phase of rapid growth, in which 37% of total bone mass is acquired.[4] The final phase of rapid growth occurs in the twenties, during which bone mass increases by 15%.[5]

Bone is made of two types of bone tissue: trabecular and cortical. Trabecular bone is the softer, loosely packed tissue found in the inner part of bones, and it is found primarily in the ends of the long bones of the body, the breastbone, the top of the pelvis, and the vertebrae of the spine. Cortical bone is the hard outer surface of bones and is responsible for 80% of total bone. Both tissue types are found in all bones, but the ratio of the two depends on the location of the bones. For example, each vertebra consists primarily of trabecular bone with a thin outer coating of cortical bone, but the femur is composed of about 80% cortical bone and 20% trabecular bone.

From the time of birth, bones are constantly being broken down and absorbed by the body and then built up again through the remodeling process. This process is made possible by osteoblasts (ie, cells within bone involved in laying down new tissue), osteoclasts (ie, cells that participate in breaking down old or damaged bone tissue), and an intracellular matrix. The intracellular matrix consists of an organic component (primarily collagen and other proteins) and an inorganic component. The inorganic component is composed mainly of calcium phosphate, calcium carbonate, magnesium fluoride, sulfate, and other trace minerals, which are responsible for rigidity of bones.

Through the remodeling process, new bone is added to the skeleton more rapidly than old bone is absorbed. Peak bone mass occurs by the age of 30. Peak bone mass is defined as the "highest level of bone mass achieved as a result of normal growth and within one's genetic potential."[5] A key to preventing osteoporosis later in life is the achievement of peak bone mass and the subsequent rate of bone loss throughout life.

OSTEOPENIA AND OSTEOPOROSIS

Osteopenia refers to reduced bone mass that has not yet resulted in fractures. It marks the first stage of bone deterioration and can develop in anyone at any age. The key to prevention or retardation of osteopenia is nutrition, exercise, and stress reduction.

For reasons not yet understood, spinal bone loss begins in the twenties. However, the overall change is quite small until menopause. Bone loss of the femur does not begin to increase until around the age of 30. The spine and femur are composed primarily of trabecular bone, and the resorption and formation of this bone occurs four to eight times as fast as cortical bone. The resorption of trabecular bone begins to exceed formation by about 0.7% after the age of 30, when the process of osteopenia may be initiated or worsen.

The rate of reabsorption becomes a major issue for women around the time of menopause, when the rate increases more rapidly in women than in men because of the decline in estrogen, progesterone, and probably dehydroepiandrosterone (DHEA).[6] Estrogen inhibits bone resorption and helps to control the rate of secretion of the parathyroid hormone (PTH), a vital regulator of calcium and phosphorus metabolism.[5] A decline in the estrogen level increases PTH secretion, which results in bone being broken down at a rapid rate. Excessive secretion of PTH can also occur when the parathyroid glands are enlarged or have developed a benign tumor. Progesterone also plays an important role in bone metabolism. Though data are limited, it appears that progesterone alters bone turnover or acts directly on the osteoblast to promote bone formation.[7] DHEA appears to be capable of inhibiting bone resorption and promoting bone formation.[7]

Up to 5% of trabecular bone loss and 1.5% of total bone loss occur during the approximately 10 to 15 years after menopause. The rate of loss diminishes considerably after this period, but it continues to some degree for the remainder of a woman's lifetime. The increased loss of trabecular bone results in a 50% reduction of this type of bone during the first 20 years after menopause; the total reduction in cortical bone is 30%.[8]

Although outer bone structure does not change as a result of bone loss, the internal structure becomes weaker and more fragile, eventually making the bone vulnerable to fracture and collapse. When osteopenia progresses to this point and symptoms such as pain and fractures occur, bone loss enters what is regarded by some as the disease state, also called the clinical syndrome of osteoporosis. Depending on nutritional and other lifestyle factors and the person's health status during childhood and adolescence, osteopenia can advance to the degree that osteoporosis can be well established before menopause.

Bone weakness, fragility, and vulnerability to fracture is devastating for millions of women. The risk of suffering an osteoporotic fracture during a woman's lifetime is higher than the combined risk of breast, endometrial, and ovarian cancer.[9]

Approximately one third of postmenopausal women have osteoporosis, and one third of all postmenopausal women experience a fracture of the hip. This type of fracture is serious; 12% to 20% die within 6 months of surgical, embolic, or cardiopulmonary complications associated with the fracture. At least 50% of women who experience a hip fracture are never again able to care for themselves and must spend the rest of their lives in nursing homes.

EVERYONE IS AT RISK

All women, men, and children of every age are at risk for osteopenia and osteoporosis if their nutrient intake and level of exercise is inadequate or interferes with the formation and strengthening of bone. Chronic stress can deplete the body of nutrients essential to bone mass, thereby contributing to the development of bone loss.

Certain women are at higher risk for developing osteoporosis during the climacteric:

- Caucasian (especially northern European) ancestry
- Oriental ancestry
- Small bones
- Experienced early menopause, naturally or surgically induced
- Have not had children
- Have a family history of osteoporosis
- Had or have an eating disorder, particularly to the point of developing amenorrhea

Other groups also are considered at high risk for osteoporosis:

- Female runners, ballet dancers, and other endurance athletes
- Male runners and other endurance athletes
- Young persons with eating disorders such as bulimia and anorexia nervosa
- Teenagers on "junk food" diets
- Heavy users of alcohol
- Cigarette smokers
- All men and women older than 65 years of age
- Anyone who has been on long-term bed rest or enforced immobility

ATHLETICS AND EATING DISORDERS

Amenorrhea, when experienced by premenopausal women, such as endurance athletes, some women on weight-reduction diets, and women with eating disorders, leads to loss of bone. Many of these women do not consume an adequate amount of nutrients essential to bone health. Add to amenorrhea and nutritional deficiencies the excessive stress commonly experienced by women who are athletes, who have eating disorders, or who frequently follow weight-reduction diets and the effects on bone integrity and other aspects of a woman's health can be disastrous.

OSTEOPOROSIS IN MEN

Men who are exposed to nutritional deficiencies, chronic stress, or lack of regular physical exercise can also lose bone. As with female athletes, male athletes can have bone loss if they consume a nutrient-deficient diet or experience excessive stress.

TEENAGERS AND THE ELDERLY

Teenagers are vulnerable to stress. They are easily influenced by peers and the media, and they are often poorly educated about nutrition and exercise. Eating disorders are at an all-time high among female teenagers and are rising in the male teenage population, as are intake of "junk foods" and use of drugs, alcoholic beverages, and nicotine. At a time when building healthy bone is particularly critical, the lifestyles of teens often accomplish the opposite.

As women and men age, exercise and nutrition are often severely inadequate because a reduction in the ability of the intestines to absorb nutrients, chronic and often debilitating diseases, lack of knowledge about exercise and nutrition, and lack of resources and support to provide this knowledge.

PREVENTION FOR EVERYONE

Although this is a guide about the care of women in their late premenopausal, perimenopausal, or menopausal years, I am mentioning other populations at risk for osteoporosis for two reasons. First, if you provide health care to any of these populations, you can play a major role in educating them about osteoporosis prevention and treatment with an emphasis on prevention. Second, evidence suggests that osteoporosis is easier to prevent than treat and that prevention can be accomplished only through the initiation of sound health behaviors (eg, adequate consumption of nutrients, regular physical activity) early in life and continuing them throughout life.[10]

In addition to educating women patients about how to prevent and treat osteoporosis for themselves, you can inform them about the development of osteopenia and osteoporosis in children, teenagers, and men and women of all ages. Because much of the information you present is applicable to others, they can share the information with their loved ones. This approach makes initiation and maintenance of an osteoporosis prevention and treatment program a family affair, following the model used successfully for prevention and treatment of coronary artery disease and other chronic degenerative diseases.

FACTORS CONTRIBUTING TO DEVELOPMENT OF OSTEOPOROSIS

The list of factors that are thought to contribute to the development of osteoporosis is continuously growing. As with coronary artery disease, most are intimately involved with the way in which women live their lives, such as the physical activities in which they engage, the foods and beverages they consume, and their ability to deal with stress in a way that positively affects their emotional and physical well-being.

The following sections discuss factors that contribute to development of osteopenia and osteoporosis and illustrate that treatment and prevention involve therapeutic intervention on several levels. Even if a woman did not develop maximum bone mass by her twenties or thirties or has lost a substantial amount of bone mass by her fifties, there is much that she can do to slow down and perhaps reverse the process.

The three major risk factors for the development of osteoporosis are lack of exercise, poor nutrition, and chronic stress. A fourth major risk factor is the decline in various hormones associated with the menopause, a topic that is discussed in Chapter 7.

LACK OF EXERCISE

German anatomist Julius Wolff stated in his 1892 book, *The Law of Bone Transformation,* that human beings could change their bone structure, for better or worse, by the amount of weight-bearing exercise performed. Wolff was correct. Athletes such as tennis and baseball players increase the size and bone mineral content of the dominant arm used in these sports. Bone mass is greater in the legs of long-distance runners. The beneficial effects of exercise on bone mass among postmenopausal women is becoming increasingly well documented.

Bone mineral content in the femur and lumbar spine has been greater in postmenopausal women who were physically fit than in women of the same age who were not fit.[11] Weight-bearing exercises were partly responsible for this. One study demonstrated that female long-distance runners between the ages of 50 and 72 had approximately 40% more bone mineral content than sedentary women of the same age.[12] Another study demonstrated that 20 minutes of moderate-intensity low-impact or high-impact exercises performed 3 days per week was effective in maintaining bone mineral density in early postmenopausal women.[13] The sedentary control group continued to experience a loss in bone mineral density.

Research conducted to evaluate the effects of high-intensity strength training exercises demonstrated that these exercises, when performed 2 days per week by postmenopausal women, led to increases in femoral neck bone and lumbar spine mineral density and total-body bone mineral content.[14] The sedentary control group of the study had decreased total-body mineral content and bone mineral density.

Women between 50 and 70 years of age took part in a study of a supervised physical activity program consisting of aerobic dancing, flexibility exercises, and weight-bearing exercises (eg, walking, stepping up and down from benches) for 60 minutes three times each week for a year.[15] Spinal bone mineral density stabilized in the exercisers and decreased significantly in the controls. Self-perceived health increased in the exercise group, as did a sense of well-being. Those who had experienced back pain found that its intensity decreased with exercise. Another study demonstrated an increase in lumbar spine density among postmenopausal women performing non–weight-bearing exercises (ie, exercising with bicycle ergometers) for 8 months.[16]

Swimming may have a beneficial effect on bone mass, and research has shown that postmenopausal women who performed water exercises experienced an increase in bone mineral density.[17] This is important, because some women with osteoporosis may have limited mobility or may experience pain, making it difficult for them to perform weight-bearing exercises. Water exercises and swimming may be comfortable alternatives for them. Others who have not exercised at all or regularly may find swimming helps them to regain strength so that they eventually are able to add weight-bearing exercises to their exercise program. Women who have physical limitations for weight-bearing exercises unrelated to osteoporosis may have an exercise option available to them that can help decrease their loss of bone mineral density.

One particularly interesting study compared bone mineral content in four groups of postmenopausal women.[14] Group 1 performed brisk walks 4 days each week for 45 minutes; they also drank a dietary calcium supplement that brought their daily calcium intake to 1200 mg. Group 2 walked with the first group but was given a placebo drink so that their calcium intake was only 600 mg. Group 3 did not exercise but consumed the same high-calcium drink as the group 1. Group 4 remained sedentary and drank the placebo. The results demonstrated that the calcium supplement had virtually no effect at all! The active women, even those with lower calcium intake, increased their bone mineral content. The sedentary group of women all experienced a decrease in bone mineral content. These results were confirmed in another study conducted over a 3-year period.[18]

This finding about exercise is consistent with the results of research on some populations in Africa, Central America, and various areas in Asia. These people develop and maintain strong bones on levels of calcium considerably lower than the amount currently recommended in the United States.

POOR NUTRITION

A diet that causes osteopenia and osteoporosis is one that includes excessive intake of protein (particularly from animal sources), phosphorus, caffeine, alcohol, sodium, and sugar. It is also a diet that is deficient in vitamins and minerals.

IMPORTANCE OF CALCIUM

It is hard to escape the conclusion that calcium has been oversold as a weapon against osteoporosis.[19] Adequate calcium is essential for healthy bones, and calcium supplementation is probably necessary for most women in the United States. The average calcium intake of women is about 450 mg per day, which is about 350 mg below the recommended dietary allowance. If calcium intake is insufficient for other vital functions, secretion of PTH increases, which draws calcium from the bones' reserves so that it can be used elsewhere. However, issues important to consider include whether calcium is the only major nutrient about which women should be concerned when it comes to osteoporosis prevention, the amount and kind of calcium supplementation that should be taken, the ways in which it should be taken, and the amount of other essential nutrients that should be consumed with calcium.

It was recommended at the 1984 National Institutes of Health Consensus Conference that the daily calcium intake should be 1000 mg for perimenopausal women and 1500 mg for postmenopausal women.[20] This recommendation has been highly publicized, and as a result, women's focus has been primarily on calcium supplementation. Women often take 1500 mg without considering the amount that they are already ingesting with food. These women may assume that supplementing with this dosage of calcium alone provides adequate protection against osteoporosis, although this is probably not true for most women.

Mixed results and mixed conclusions are the themes of the research conducted to assess the efficacy of calcium supplementation alone. Some of the confusion regarding the benefits of calcium supplementation may result from combining trials conducted with younger women (less than 5 years past postmenopause) with trials conducted with older postmenopausal women into a single group.[21] One study demonstrated that calcium supplementation retards bone loss in older women but not in younger postmenopausal women.[22]

Another factor contributing to the confusion is that the skeletal sites evaluated have varied among the studies. In general, the hard cortical bone (eg, shaft of forearm or thigh) appears to be more responsive to calcium supplementation, and the softer trabecular bone (eg, spine) appears to be not as responsive or not at all responsive.[23] Other factors that contribute to mixed results and confusion include the bioavailability of the calcium supplementation used (which can affect the amount of bone loss), how many of the subjects in any given study were calcium deficient at baseline, whether their general diets consisted of adequate fiber and the nutrients essential to the absorption and use of calcium, and the subjects' circulating levels of calcitonin, the active form of vitamin D.

For example, in a group of women given 2000 mg of calcium carbonate, cortical bone loss was minimal. This group did not experience a reduction in trabecular bone loss compared with the placebo group.[24] In another study, women who took calcium supplements lost more bone mass than the placebo group.[25]

When calcium deficiency was assessed in postmenopausal women with osteoporosis, it was found that only 25% of the patients had a skeletal calcium deficiency.[26] Supplementation with calcium and vitamin D corrected the skeletal calcium deficiency, but did not improve bone mass in the 75% of the women who had normal skeletal calcium levels. In a group of postmenopausal women whose mean calcium intake was about 1900 mg each day (including supplementation), bone was not lost at the hip and ankle sites.

Supplementation of 1000 mg of calcium citrate malate taken by older postmenopausal women slowed spinal bone loss by 65%. However, spinal bone loss was completely attenuated in the group of women taking the trace minerals manganese, zinc, and copper in addition to 1000 mg of calcium citrate malate.[27] Vertebral crush fractures in postmenopausal women with osteoporosis were reduced by one half as a result of calcium supplementation.[28] Loss of bone mineral density of the lumbar spine was less among women who consumed more than 777 mg of calcium per day and greater among women who consumed less than 405 mg per day.[29]

The studies cited here and many others have looked at the effects of calcium supplementation and bone mass. However, whether calcium supplementation and high dietary intakes of calcium reduce the rate of fractures is still debatable. For example, a study monitored almost 10,000 women 65 years of age or older for approximately 6.5 years and found no important associations between dietary calcium intake and the risk of fractures of the hip, ankle, proximal humerus, wrist, and vertebra.[30] In another study, approximately 78,000 women between the ages of 34 and 59 were followed in a 12-year prospective study, during which dietary intake was assessed to determine if higher intakes of milk and other calcium-rich foods during adult years could reduce the risk of osteoporotic fractures.[31] The results revealed no evidence that fracture incidence of the hip or forearm were reduced as a result of higher intakes of milk or calcium from food sources.

Although there are conflicting research results, the general consensus is that supplementation does slow the rate of decline of postmenopausal bone loss by 30% to 50%.[32] When 17 studies that included measurements of calcium intake and how exercise effects bone density were reviewed, certain patterns emerged. When calcium intake was higher than 1000 mg per day, exercise made bones measurably stronger, and only when a person was moderately active did calcium increase bone density.[32]

The results of these and other studies show that bone health is a multifactorial affair, with calcium being only one of the factors. If other critical factors are missing, intake of the recommended amount of calcium cannot guarantee adequate absorption and use of it, nor can it guarantee optimal bone growth or protection against bone loss.

A critical issue for calcium and all nutrients is the maintenance of balance, the difference between the amount of a nutrient entering the body and the amount leaving. A woman who is in positive calcium balance is excreting less than she is taking in, and her total-body calcium content is increasing. The body's total calcium content declines when more calcium is excreted than consumed, which creates a negative calcium balance. The goal of osteoporosis prevention therefore should be one of preventing excessive calcium excretion and maintaining a positive calcium balance.

Vitamin D

Vitamin D is essential for calcium absorption and deposition into bone tissue, and it has been associated with a significant reduction in hip fractures.[33] Vitamin D plays an essential role in maintaining a healthy mineralized skeleton. Its major biologic function is one of keeping serum calcium and phosphorus concentrations within the normal range to promote mineralization of the skeleton and maintain essential cellular functions.[34] As a result of the aging process, vitamin D synthesis is often compromised, causing functional alterations in the intestines and kidneys that can lead to calcium malabsorption.

Vitamin D is obtained through the intake of foods such as fish liver oils, fatty salt-water fish, egg yolks, milk fortified with vitamin D, oatmeal, sweet potatoes, and liver and through exposure to sunlight. The skin manufactures a form of vitamin D from a cholesterol derivative under the influence of solar ultraviolet radiation. This form of vitamin D is relatively inactive until it undergoes metabolic processes in the liver and then the kidneys which result in an active form that increases calcium and phosphate absorption in the small intestine and decreases calcium excretion in the urine.

Persons who are most susceptible to vitamin D deficiency are those who are not exposed to adequate sunlight on a regular basis (about 20 to 30 minutes per day). This is particularly true for persons with limited mobility and for those living in areas of the country in which sunlight is limited for most of the year.

Magnesium

Magnesium deficiency may contribute greatly to a decrease in bone density, in part because of its effect on the parathyroid glands.[35] Magnesium deficiency impairs secretion of the PTH, an action that can reduce calcium absorption and retention.[36] A magnesium intake of 600 mg should be sufficient to maintain an adequate magnesium reserve in bone (50% of all magnesium is found in bone) and substantially reduce trabecular bone loss.[36]

A study of postmenopausal women with osteoporosis demonstrated that 90% of them had significant magnesium deficiencies and abnormally large and abnormally shaped calcium crystals.[37] The women with adequate magnesium status had normal crystals. These findings suggest that magnesium deficiency is common in women with osteoporosis and is associated with abnormal calcification of bone.[5] When the women in this study supplemented their intake with 250 to 750 mg of magnesium per day for 2 years, 75% of them experienced an increase in bone density of 1% to 8%.

Other Nutrients

In addition to calcium, magnesium, and vitamin D, several other nutrients are essential for bone health. Vitamin K plays a crucial role in the formation, remodeling, and repair of bone, in part because it helps to build the protein matrix on which calcium crystallizes.[5] Subtle deficiencies, perhaps not detectable through the testing of prothrombin, may be more common than originally thought. In one study, vitamin K levels in patients with osteoporosis and hip fractures were about 74% less than the levels in the healthy control group.[38] Another group of patients with vertebral crush fractures had a 56% reduction in serum vitamin K.[38] In yet another study, vitamin K supplementation reduced excessive calcium excretion by 33%.[39]

Boron is a trace element that may prove beneficial in preventing bone loss and may have a powerful influence on the metabolism of calcium, magnesium, estrogen, testosterone, and DHEA. Boron supplementation can markedly increase the concentrations of 17ß-estradiol and testosterone and decrease urinary calcium excretion in postmenopausal women.[40]

Other nutrients important to bone health include manganese, folic acid, vitamin B_6, zinc, strontium, copper, silicon, and vitamin C. Recommendations for the amounts to be taken are included in the

Guidelines section, and sources discussing the effects of these nutrients on bone health and related research regarding osteoporosis are
included in the References.

EXCESS URINARY EXCRETION OF CALCIUM

Many dietary factors contribute to increased urinary excretion of
calcium. These include excessive intake of phosphorus, caffeine,
sodium, and protein (particularly animal sources), and sugar.

Phosphorus

The ratio of phosphorus to calcium is a critical factor in bone health.
Excessive intake of phosphorus causes calcium to be drawn from
bone, and consumption of a high-phosphorus diet in combination
with adequate or low intake of calcium can lead to secondary hyperparathyroidism, with subsequent progressive loss of bone.[41]

Phosphorus is found in abundance in many high-protein and
processed foods and in beverages such as colas. Cola drinks are
processed with phosphoric acid and may be a leading cause of osteoporosis.

Data from the National Health and Nutrition Examination Survey revealed that the ratio of calcium to phosphorus for most Americans is below the ideal 1:1 ratio, primarily as a result of high intake
of high-phosphorus foods and beverages and low intake of calcium-
rich foods.[42]

Sodium

Excessive salt intake increases urinary calcium excretion[43] and may
reduce bone demineralization and contribute to hip fractures.[44] In a
2-year longitudinal study of postmenopausal women, sodium-
induced urinary calcium loss correlated with reduced bone mass of
the hip and ankle.[45]

Protein

Excessive protein appears to increase urinary excretion of calcium,
particularly if the protein source is animal meat. Dietary intake was
measured among the almost 86,000 women who participated in the

Nurses' Health Study. Protein intake was associated with an increased risk of forearm fracture among the women who consumed more than 95 g of protein per day compared with those who consumed less than 68 g per day. A similar increase in risk was observed for animal protein. No association was found for consumption of vegetable protein. A significantly increased risk of forearm fracture was found among women who consumed five or more servings of red meat per week.[46]

It has been suggested that 70% of the variance in osteoporosis among people of different countries can be explained by the difference in animal protein consumed.[47] Consumption of animal protein is higher in the United States, Norway, Sweden, and New Zealand than in Singapore, Africa, or New Guinea. People in the latter group of countries consume much less animal protein and have considerably lower osteoporosis rates.

Some research has shown "better bones" in vegetarians, but other research has not confirmed this finding. When the bone mineral density of women who had been vegetarians for at least 20 years was compared with that of women who had consumed a typical American diet, the loss of bone mineral density by age 80 was 18% for the vegetarian group and 35% for the typical American diet group.[48]

Caffeine

Daily consumption of caffeine in amounts equal to or greater than that obtained from two to three cups of brewed coffee has been shown to accelerate bone loss from the spine and total body in women whose calcium intakes were below the recommended dietary allowance of 800 mg.[49] Lifetime coffee consumption equivalent to two cups each day has been associated with a decrease in bone density of the hip and spine in women 50 years of age or older who did not drink milk on a daily basis.[50] It has also been demonstrated that an intake of more than two cups of coffee each day or four cups of tea modestly increased the risk of hip fracture.[51]

Even though caffeine increases urinary excretion of calcium and several studies have correlated caffeine consumption with bone loss, it is still controversial whether caffeine contributes to osteoporosis, in part because some of the coffee drinkers also smoked or were past smokers. However, it is probably better to err on the safe side and recommend limiting caffeine intake.

Sugar

A high-sugar diet can cause a significant increase in urinary excretion of calcium[52] and can significantly increase the fasting level of serum cortisol produced by the adrenal glands.[53] As with corticosteroids, an increase in cortisol can contribute to the development of osteoporosis.

CHRONIC STRESS

The chapter about coronary artery disease (CAD) introduced some basics regarding stress and its effects on CAD. These effects are applicable to osteoporosis as well. The physiologic reaction to stress can contribute to the depletion of many nutrients essential to maintaining the integrity of bone. Stress can also contribute to addictions to drugs, alcohol, caffeine, and nicotine, all of which have been linked with nutritional deficiencies that contribute to osteoporosis.

Women with a past or current history of depression were found to have a decrease in bone density of 6.5% at the spine and 10% to 15% at the hip, which translates into a 40% rise in the risk of hip fractures in a 10-year period.[54] Though the reason for this has not been clearly established, the principal investigator of the study suspects that cortisol, one of the hormones that increases as a result of chronic stress, may be one of the factors. An increase in urinary cortisol levels was found in the study group. Elevated cortisol concentrations can interfere with the activity of osteoblasts.

OTHER FACTORS CONTRIBUTING TO OSTEOPOROSIS

NICOTINE AND ALCOHOL

Smoking decreases estrogen levels in blood and tissues and affects the parathyroid glands, which regulate calcium levels. Smoking also interferes with vitamin absorption.

Excessive, regular intake of alcohol can contribute to an increase in urinary excretion of calcium and a deficiency of magnesium and other nutrients essential to bone health. Prolonged, moderate drinking decreases the function of osteoblasts, and chronic alcoholism results in low serum levels of vitamin D metabolites.[55]

MEDICATIONS

Bone loss is one of the most devastating side effects of corticosteroids. It has been proposed that the medications inhibit osteoblastic activity, impair calcium absorption, and cause secondary hyperparathyroidism.[56] Thyroxin, certain anticonvulsant agents, diuretics, and high doses of heparin over a long period can contribute to the development of osteoporosis.

Chronic renal disease alters bone resorption, which contributes to the development of osteoporosis.[57] Any disease that affects the functioning of the intestines (eg, Crohn's disease, ulcerative colitis) and therefore contributes to poor absorption of calcium and other nutrients is also considered a risk factor for osteoporosis. Corticosteroids are often used in the treatment of such diseases, which further impairs absorption of nutrients.

Diseases that decrease the ability to undertake regular and adequate exercise contribute to osteoporosis, and endocrine disorders such as hyperparathyroidism negatively affect calcium absorption and absorption of other essential nutrients.

SYMPTOMS OF OSTEOPOROSIS

Many women do not experience any symptoms associated with osteoporosis until a fracture occurs. An example is acute back pain as a result of a vertebral fracture. However, other women can experience pain at any site of excessive bone loss and chronic aching along the spine and in the muscles of the back. A loss of height and curvature of the back are two symptoms of osteoporosis that result from fracture and collapse of vertebrae.

RISK ASSESSMENT AND DIAGNOSIS

Although the risk factors of age, body build, race, family history, and medical history (eg, past or current use of corticosteroids, other medications, other illnesses) are important to consider in assessing the level of risk for osteoporosis, a comprehensive risk assessment for osteoporosis should obtain information from the woman about her

lifestyle from a historical point of view. The following questions
should be asked when assessing the risk for osteoporosis:

@ What was her dietary intake in adolescence, in her early twen-
  ties, and now?
@ Has she ever abused substances such as nicotine, alcohol, and
  other drugs, or has she found it difficult to deal with stress?
@ How does she deal with stress?
@ Has she ever followed a weight-reduction plan and, if so, what
  was it?
@ Has she ever had or does she currently have an eating disorder?

The level of risk is assessed by going back in time. Osteopenia is
a progressive loss of bone density that can begin many years before
menopause, and assessment of the many factors that might have
contributed to loss of bone density is essential.

Understanding the level of risk can help to determine at what
point bone density screening should be performed. Some authorities
recommend that bone density screening be performed when a
woman has experienced menopause. Others suggest that this be
done when she begins to experience the obvious symptoms associated with a decline in ovarian function, such as hot flushes. Some
health care professionals recommend that women from age 25 to the
time of menopause be screened only when one or more of the following major risk factors exist[58]:

@ Familial history of osteoporosis (ie, grandmother, mother, sister)
@ History of or current hyperthyroidism or hyperparathyroidism
@ Amenorrhea for at least 6 consecutive months
@ Surgical menopause without subsequent hormone replacement
  therapy
@ History of restricted mobility for 3 to 6 months, particularly if
  this occurred during adolescence
@ Long-term use of thyroxin or corticosteroids or any medications
  that are associated with possible loss of bone density
@ Fracture during adult life that was caused by a modest trauma

Considering all the factors that affect bone formation and resorption, this appears to be a reasonable approach to screening of premenopausal and perimenopausal women. However, an osteoporosis-
contributing lifestyle of poor diet, substance abuse, or lack of regular
exercise should be added to the list. The information obtained
through the screening process enables the woman to determine
whether she needs to make significant lifestyle changes, perhaps

beyond those that she already has made, to reduce the possibility of further loss in bone density. If the results show that a significant loss has already taken place, you can recommend a more aggressive course of action.

If the results of the screening reveal a minimal loss of bone density and the woman is not yet menopausal, assessment does not need to be repeated until she is postmenopausal. However, it should be repeated before that time if something occurs in the woman's life that increases her risk for loss of bone density (eg, she must undergo a course of corticosteroid therapy, prolonged period of restricted physical activity).

If a woman has not been screened before menopause, the screening should be performed when she reaches that stage. The second test should be scheduled according to the results of the first test. Also determined at that time is any hormone or drug therapy intervention and other interventions that might be undertaken. This is true for the postmenopausal woman, regardless of the length of time that has passed since she experienced menopause.

Although these recommendations may seem extreme, consider the following scenario. You recommend that your 30-year-old patient undergo screening because of her regular soda consumption, a calcium- and other nutrient-deficient diet throughout her teenage years to the present, and her use of corticosteroid therapy for asthma for a few years during her early twenties. The test reveals that she has loss of bone density in her hips consistent with that of a 46-year-old woman. She then has concrete information that could be the turning point for her in making the lifestyle changes that can offer protection from further loss in bone density.

Another scenario is the 45-year-old woman who appears to be in good health and has no symptoms associated with the climacteric. She learned about osteoporosis prevention strategies at age 42 and has integrated them, to some degree, into her life. However, her previous lifestyle definitely contributed to osteoporosis. The test reveals a 25% loss in bone density. With this information, she may be inclined to reevaluate the health program that she is following to determine whether she is doing everything she can to slow down the bone loss. Five years later, when she experiences menopause, she has another test. It shows that her bone density loss has increased to 35%. Because she has the baseline information and has followed an excellent osteoporosis prevention program, she may consider adding hormone replacement therapy or one of the bone-building drugs such as alendronate to her health program (see Chapter 7). She has essential information to make an informed choice about her bones.

PATIENT'S UNDERSTANDING OF SCREENING RESULTS

One important issue is how women may react to the results of bone density screening. If results are normal at menopause, a woman may assume that she is not at risk for developing osteoporosis and may not aggressively follow a bone-strengthening program. If the results show a significant loss in bone density, a woman may feel that, despite the use of therapeutic measures to slow or halt continued loss, she is doomed to bone fracture.

Neither view is correct, but to put this issue into perspective and to educate women appropriately, it is essential that they understand that bone density screening identifies women at increased risk for developing a fracture in the future. It does not identify with certainty women who will develop a fracture in the future. This is an important fact for women to understand, because a women with normal bone density at age 50 can develop osteoporosis later in life.

BONE DENSITY SCREENING TESTS

Bone density screening is a *diagnostic test,* but recommendations for screening expand the definition to a *preventive health test*—one that provides women information that may change the way they think about and behave toward osteoporosis. Several tests are available to assess bone density:

- Radiographic absorptiometry uses a specialized x-ray assay of the hand to calculate bone density.
- Quantitative computed tomography measures the bone density of the spine. This test is expensive and exposes a woman to a higher dose of radiation than other screening tests.
- Single-energy x-ray absorptiometry measures the bones of the wrist or heel.
- Dual-energy x-ray absorptiometry, which uses a very small dose of radiation to measure the spine, hip, total body, and wrist, is considered the gold standard for measuring bone density.

At least two sites should be measured: one in which cortical bone is dominant, the other in which trabecular bone is dominant.

LIMITATIONS OF SCREENING

If only a minimal evaluation can be conducted because of time constraints, a woman still can be provided educational materials about bone health and an osteoporosis risk assessment instrument that she can take home to complete. By doing this, you are encouraging her and giving her an opportunity to view her past and current lifestyle in terms of bone health. Through this process, she is able to assess her level of risk for developing osteoporosis, and this information can motivate her to make the necessary lifestyle changes. It may also encourage her to further discuss with you the risks that she has identified and talk about treatment options.

Financial issues frequently play a major role in selecting tests to be recommended. The average cost for bone density screening is $100 to $200. Only about half of the private health insurance companies cover a percentage of the cost of screening, and the same is true for Medicare. The deciding factor regarding who has the test and at what age may be determined by the woman's ability to pay for it.

OTHER HEALTH ISSUES

Cardiovascular disease (CVD) and osteoporosis are not the only health problems about which women in their climacteric should be concerned. Others are obesity, diabetes, and breast cancer.

OBESITY

Obesity is an epidemic in this country that affects several million more women than men and affects more poor and minority women than other groups. It is perhaps one of the most profound factors contributing to increased mortality. Obesity contributes to heart disease, diabetes mellitus, gallbladder disease, and hypertension.[59–61] Reproductive abnormalities, gout, and osteoporosis are a consequence of obesity, as is the increased risk for endometrial and breast cancer.[61] Obesity can lead to impaired psychosocial function resulting from social isolation, loss of job mobility, economic and social discrimination, and increased employee absenteeism,[61] stressors that can have profound psychologic and physiologic effects.

DIABETES

Between 80% and 90% of patients with non–insulin-dependent diabetes mellitus are obese.[62] As with obesity, diabetes is more common among women than men. It has been estimated that, of the 5 million persons who are unaware that they have diabetes, 70% are women.[63] Diabetes is the seventh leading cause of death, and its incidence is on the rise. The number of persons with this disease is estimated to double every 15 years.

By preventing and assisting in the treatment of diabetes through lifestyle changes, women can prevent blindness, kidney disease, amputations, and CVD. Fortunately, all of the lifestyle recommendations for CVD and osteoporosis prevention and treatment are the same as those for obesity and diabetes.

CANCER

Approximately one third of the 500,000 cancer deaths that occur annually in the United States result from dietary factors.[64] Two of the most modifiable determinants of cancer risk are diet and physical activity. "Cancer risk can be reduced by an overall dietary pattern that includes a high proportion of plant food (fruits, vegetables, grains, and beans), limited amounts of meat, dairy, and other high-fat foods, and a balance of caloric intake and physical activity."[65]

Increased intake of vegetables and fruits has been associated with a lower risk of lung and colon cancer.[65] The risk of cervical cancer appears to be related to deficiencies in several nutrients as well, including carotenoids and vitamin C,[66] vitamin E,[67] and folic acid.[68] High-fat diets are associated with an increased risk of cancers of the lungs,[69] colon and rectum,[70] prostate,[71] and endometrium,[72] and consumption of meat, especially red meat, has been linked to several types of cancers.

The number of women diagnosed with breast cancer greatly increases after the age of 40, and it is this disease, rather than CVD or osteoporosis, that concerns most women. Some women may embark on lifestyle changes only when they know that these changes can help to reduce their risk of breast cancer.

Societies in which the Western lifestyle—low levels of physical activity and an energy-dense diet rich in total and saturated fat and refined carbohydrates—is prevalent have a high incidence of breast cancer.[73] Diet has long been considered a significant cause of breast cancer,[74] and breast cancer has been directly correlated with the intake of milk, table fats, beef, calories, protein, and fat.[75] Among patients newly diagnosed with cancer (including breast cancer) in one study, levels of vitamins E and C and beta-carotene were significantly lower than in the control group.[76]

A study comparing more than 2000 women with breast cancer and a similar number of women without breast cancer showed a significant inverse association between breast cancer risk and levels of beta-carotene, vitamin E, and calcium. The conclusion of the investigators was that a diet rich in several micronutrients, including the ones previously mentioned, may protect against breast cancer.[77] Preliminary findings suggest that vitamin D may also have a protective effect against breast cancer,[78] and long-term calcium restriction may promote the development of breast cancer.[78] Among women older than 50 years of age, selenium supplementation has been found to have a preventative effect against breast cancer.[79]

Exercise may also prove to reduce the risk of breast cancer. Greater leisure-time activity has been associated with a reduced risk of breast cancer.[80] One to 3 hours of exercise each week has been shown to reduce the risk of breast cancer among premenopausal women by about 30%,[81] and 4 hours or more of weekly exercise could lower the risk by 50%. Although not well defined, there are several proposed mechanisms for the prevention of estrogen-dependent cancer by physical activity[82]:

- Maintenance of low body fat and moderation of extraglandular estrogen
- Reduction in the number of ovulatory cycles and subsequent decrease of lifetime exposure to endogenous estrogen
- Enhancement of natural immune function
- Association of other healthy lifestyle habits

A discussion about breast cancer risk would not be complete without mentioning some of the latest research regarding the association of breast cancer and bone mass. When approximately 1300 women between the ages of 47 and 80 underwent evaluations of their bone mass, the incidence of breast cancer was shown to increase among women who were in the highest quartile of bone mass group compared with those in the lowest quartile.[83] A relationship between the risk of breast cancer and an increase in bone mineral density was again shown among a study of more than 6500 women 65 years or older. The mechanisms for this relationship are not understood, although a cumulative exposure to estrogen may play a role.[84] The effects these results have on the health recommendations for women have not been determined.

Research has clearly shown, as with CVD, that the greatest impact on the prevention and treatment of osteoporosis is achieved through exercise, stress management, and nutrition, and that, contrary to popular belief, calcium supplementation alone is not the answer. Excessive intake of animal protein, sodium, phosphorus, and salt, which increase urinary secretion of calcium, must be avoided to maintain a positive calcium balance. Calcium is only one of many nutrients needed for bone health. A woman's diet must include optimal amounts of other nutrients, including vitamin D, magnesium, and several other vitamins and minerals if osteoporosis is to be prevented. If it is determined that a woman's daily food intake does not provide her with recommended amounts of these nutrients, nutritional supplementation should be taken in dosages to compensate for the nutrients deficients. Adequate nutrition, exercise, and stress management are the foundation for the prevention and treatment of many health problems.

REFERENCES

1. Tolstoi LG, Levin RM. Osteoporosis: the treatment controversy. Nutr Today 1992;August:6–12.
2. Healy B. A new prescription for women's health. New York: Penguin; 1996.
3. Kasper MJ, et al. Knowledge beliefs and behaviors among college women concerning the prevention of osteoporosis. Arch Fam Med 1994;3:696–702.
4. Key JD, Kely LL Jr. Calcium needs of adolescents. Curr Opin Pediatr 1984;6:379–382.
5. Jasminka Z, Matkovic V. Osteoporosis: its pediatric causes and prevention opportunities: primary care update. Obstet Gynecol 1997;4:15–20.
6. Gaby A. Every woman's essential guide to preventing and reversing osteoporosis. Rocklin, CA: Prima Publishing; 1993.
7. Division of Endocrinology and Metabolism. Progesterone as a bone-trophic hormone. Endocr Rev 1990;11:386–398.
8. Lindsay R. Prevention and treatment of osteoporosis. Lancet 1993;341:801.
9. Ettinger B. Prevention of osteoporosis: treatment of estradiol deficiency. Obstet Gynecol 1988;72:125.
10. Anderson JJ, et al. roles of diet and physical activity in the prevention of osteoporosis. Scand J Rheumatol 1996;(Suppl 103):65–74.
11. Pocock NA, et al. Physical fitness is a major determinant of femoral neck and lumbar spine bone mineral density. J Clin Invest 1986;78:618–621.

12. Lane NE, et al. Long-distance running, bone density, and osteoarthritis. JAMA 1986;255:1147–1151.

13. Grove KA, Londeree BR. Bone density in postmenopausal women: High impact vs low impact exercise. Med Sci Sports Exerc 1992;11:1190–1194.

14. Nelson ME, et al. Effects of high-intensity strength training on multiple risk factors for osteoporotic fractures: a randomized controlled trial. JAMA 1994;272:1909–1914.

15. Bravo G, et al. Impact of a 12-month exercise program on the physical and psychological health of osteopenic women. J Am Geriatr Soc 1996;44:756–762.

16. Bloomfield SA, et al. Non-weightbearing exercise may increase lumbar spine bone mineral density in healthy postmenopausal women. Am J Phys Med Rehabil 1993;72:204–209.

17. Tsukahara N, et al. Cross-sectional and longitudinal studies on the effect of water exercise in controlling bone loss in Japanese postmenopausal women. J Nutr Sci Vitaminol (Tokyo) 1994;40:37–47.

18. Smith EL, et al. Physical activity and calcium modalities for bone mineral increase in aged women. Med Sci Sports Exerc 1981;13:60–64.

19. Calcium: oversold. Harvard Med School Health Lett 1987;April:1–2.

20. National Institutes of Health Consensus Conference statement on osteoporosis. JAMA 1984;252:799.

21. Heaney RP. Thinking straight about calcium. N Engl J Med 1993;328:503–505.

22. Dawson-Hughes B, et al. A controlled trial of the effect of calcium supplementation on bone density in postmenopausal women. N Engl J Med 1990;232:878–883.

23. Pak C. Nutrition and metabolic bone disease with special emphasis on the role of calcium. Med Grand Rounds (SW Medical School, University of Texas Health Sciences Center) 1986;6:1–22.

24. Riis B, et al. Does calcium supplementation prevent postmenopausal bone loss? N Engl J Med 1987;316:173–178.

25. Ettinger B, et al. Postmenopausal bone loss is prevented by treatment with low-dosage estrogen with calcium. Ann Intern Med 1987;106:40–45.

26. Burnell JM, et al. The role of skeletal calcium deficiency in postmenopausal osteoporosis. Calcif Tissue Int 1986;38:187–192.

27. Strause L, et al. Spinal bone loss in postmenopausal women supplemented with calcium and trace minerals. J Nutr 1994;124:1060–1064.

28. Reggs BL, et al. Effect of the fluoride/calcium regimen on vertebral fracture occurrence in postmenopausal osteoporosis. N Engl J Med 1982;306:446–450.

29. Dawson-Hughes BP, et al. Dietary calcium intake and bone loss from the spine in healthy postmenopausal women. Am J Clin Nutr 1987;46:685–687.

30. Cumming RG, et al. Calcium intake and fracture risk: results from the study of osteoporotic fractures. Am J Epidemiol 1997;145:926–934.

31. Reid JR. Therapy of osteoporosis: calcium, vitamin D, and exercise. Am J Med Sci 1996;312:278–286.

32. Soy may cool down a hot flash. Health 1997;Jan/Feb:18.

33. Finkelman RD, Butler WT. Vitamin D and skeletal tissues. J Oral Pathol 1985;14:191–215.

34. Holick MF. Vitamin D and bone health. J Nutr 1996;126(Suppl 4):1159S–64S.

35. Abraham G. The importance of magnesium in the management of primary postmenopausal osteoporosis. J Nutr Med 1991;2:165.

36. Rude RK, Olerich M. Magnesium deficiency: possible role in osteoporosis associated with gluten-sensitive enteropathy. Osteoporos Int 1996;6:453–461.
37. Cohen L, Kitzes R. Infrared spectroscopy and magnesium content of bone mineral in osteoporotic women. Isr J Med Sci 1981;17:1123–1125.
38. Hart JP, et al. Electrochemical detection of depressed circulating levels of vitamin K1 in osteoporosis. J Clin Endocrinol Metab 1985;60:1269–1269.
39. Knapen MHJ, et al. The effect of vitamin K supplementation on circulating osteocalcin (bone GLA protein) and urinary calcium excretion. Ann Intern Med 1989;111:1001–1005.
40. Nielsen FH. Boron—an overlooked element of potential nutritional important. Nutr Today 1988;Jan/Feb:4–7.
41. Calvo MS. The effects of high phosphorus intake on calcium homeostasis. Adv Nutr Res 1994;9:183–207.
42. Human Nutrition Services, U.S. Department of Agriculture. Food intakes: individuals in 48 states: nationwide food consumption survey 1977–78. Report I-1. Washington, DC: U.S. Department of Agriculture; 1983.
43. Antonios TF, MacGregor GA. Deleterious effects of salt intake other than effects on blood pressure. Clin Exp Pharmacol Physiol 1995;22:180–183.
44. MacGregor G, Cappuccio FP. The kidney and essential hypertension: a link to osteoporosis? J Hypertens 1993;11:781–785.
45. Devine A, et al. A longitudinal study of the effects of sodium and calcium intakes on regional bone density in postmenopausal women. Am J Clin Nutr 1995;62:740–745.
46. Feskanich D, et al. Protein consumption and bone fractures in women. Am J Epidemiol 1996;143:472–479.
47. Abelow B, et al. Cross-cultural association between dietary animal protein and hip fracture: a hypothesis. Calcif Tissue Int 1992;50:14–18.
48. Marsh AG, et al. Vegetarian lifestyle and bone mineral density. Am J Clin Nutr 1988;48:S837–S841.
49. Harris S, et al. Caffeine and bone loss in healthy postmenopausal women. Am J Clin Nutr 1994;60:573–578.
50. Barrett-Connor E, et al. Coffee-associated osteoporosis offset by daily milk consumption: the Rancho Bernardo Study. JAMA 1994;271:280–283.
51. Kiel DP, et al. Caffeine and the risk of hip fracture: the Framingham Study. Am J Epidemiol 1990;132:675–684.
52. Lemann J Jr, et al. Possible role of carbohydrate-induced calciuria in calcium oxalate kidney-stone formation. N Engl J Med 1988;280:232–237.
53. Yudkin J. What you eat affects your bones. In: Gaby A, ed. Every woman's essential guide to preventing and reversing osteoporosis. Rocklin, CA: Prima Publishing; 1993.
54. Michelson D, et al. Bone mineral density in women with depression. N Engl J Med 1996;335:1176–1181.
55. Laitinen K, Valimaki M. Bone and the "comforts of life." Ann Med 1993;25:413–425.
56. Lukert BP, Raisz LG. Glucocorticoid-induced osteoporosis. Rheum Dis Clin North Am 1994;20:629–650.
57. Morio K, Koide K. Secondary hyperparathyroidism and tertiary hyperparathyroidism chronic renal failure uremia. Jpn J Clin Med 1995;53:958–964.
58. Bilezikian J. Size up your bones now. Prevention 1996.
59. Sjostrom LV. Mortality of severely obese subjects. Am J Clin Nutr 1992;55:516S.

60. Berg F. Risks of obesity. In: Hettinger ND, ed. Health risks of obesity, 2nd ed. 1993:9–33.
61. Bray GA. Health hazards of obesity. Endocrinol Metab Clin North Am 1996;25:907–919.
62. Felber J-P, et al. From obesity to diabetes. New York: Wiley; 1993:213–231.
63. Snyderman N. Dr. Nancy Snyderman's guide to good health. New York: William Morrow; 1996.
64. Frazo E. The American diet: health and economic consequences. Agriculture information bill 711. Washington, DC: U.S. Department of Agriculture; 1995.
65. World Cancer Research Fund. Food, Nutrition and the Prevention of Cancer: A Global Perspective. Washington, DC: American Institute for Cancer Research; 1997:1–16.
66. Btieha AM, et al. Serum micronutrients and the subsequent risk of cervical cancer in a population-base nested case-controlled study. Cancer Epidemiol Biomark Prev 1993;Jul/Aug:3359.
67. Huda SN, et al. Plasma level of antioxidant nutrients (retinol and alphatapapheral) in patients with different grades of cervical carcinoma. Bangladesh Med Res Coun Bull 1993:Dec:79–85
68. Vanenwyk J, et al. Folate, vitamin C and cervical intraepithelial neoplasia. Cancer Epidemiol Biomark Prev 1992;1(2):119–120.
69. Ziegler RG, et al. Nutrition and lung cancer. Cancer Causes Control 1996;7:127–146.
70. Potter JD. Nutrition and colorectal cancer. Cancer Causes Control 1996;7:127–146.
71. Kolonel LN. Nutrition and prostate cancer. Cancer Causes Control 1996;7:83–94.
72. Hill HA, Austin H. Nutrition and endometrial cancer. Cancer Causes Control 1996;7:56–68.
73. Kaaks R. Nutrition, hormones, and breast cancer: is insulin the missing link? Cancer Causes Control 1996;7:605–625.
74. MacMahon B, et al. Etiology of human breast cancer: a review. J Natl Cancer Inst 1973;50:21.
75. Gaskill SP, et al. Breast cancer mortality and diet in the United States. Cancer Res 1979;39:3628–3637.
76. Town M, et al. Serum beta-carotene, vitamin E, vitamin C and malondialdehyde levels in several types of cancer. J Clin Pharmacol Ther 1995;20:259–263.
77. Ferraroni M, et al. Intake of selected micronutrients and the risk of breast cancer. Int J Cancer 1996;65:140–144.
78. Barager-Lux MJ, Heaney RP. The role of calcium intake in preventing bone fragility, hypertension, and certain cancers. J Nutr 1994;124(Suppl 8):1406S–1411S.
79. Haradell L, et al. Levels of selenium in plasma and glutathione peroxidase in erythrocytes and the risk of breast cancer: a case-controlled study. Biol Trace Elem Res 1993;36:99.
80. McTiernan A. Exercise and breast cancer time to get moving? N Engl J Med 1997;336:1311–1312.
81. Kramer MM, Wells CL. Does physical activity reduce the risk of estrogen-dependent cancer in women? Med Sci Sports Exerc. 1996;28:322–334.
82. Bernstein L. Physical activity and the risk of breast cancer. N Engl J Med 1997;336:1269–1275.

83. Zhang Y, et al. Bone mass and the risk of cancer among postmenopausal women. N Engl J Med 1997;336:611–617.

84. Cauley JA, et al., the Study of Osteoporotic Fractures Research Group. Bone mineral density and the risk of breast cancer in older women: the study of osteoporotic fractures. JAMA 1996;276:1404–1408.

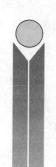

Psychologic, Sociologic, Sexual, and Contraceptive Issues Related to the Climacteric

The association between psychologic symptoms and menopause has been one of the most contentious issues in menopause research. Opinions have varied widely and often reflect the discipline of the investigator. Gynecologists have swung from declaring all such symptoms as the "ills" arising from an estrogen-deficient state to maintaining that only vasomotor symptoms and vaginal atrophy were "true symptoms of the menopause." Social scientists have maintained the view that psychologic symptoms occurring in midlife are not related causally to underlying biologic changes but rather reflect expectations and attitudes of the particular sociocultural group. Some common meeting ground for disciplines seems to have been found with a recognition of the interactive effects of endocrine changes with sociocultural and psychologic factors in any individual.[1]

Several psychologic symptoms have been associated with the climacteric, including anxiety, irritability, nervousness, changes in mood, depression, loss of concentration, headaches, decreased energy, insomnia, and decreased sexual desire. The causes of these and other psychologic symptoms typically are multifaceted. What might be the cause of symptoms experienced by one woman may not be the cause for another. A physical problem can cause psychologic distress, and psychologic distress can cause or significantly contribute to physical problems. As frustrating as this may be for the clinician, an appropriate therapeutic intervention may need to be one that integrates a variety of approaches. The clinician should consider a woman's menopausal status and the broader context of a woman's life.

CAUSES OF PSYCHOLOGIC SYMPTOMS

Research to determine specific causes of psychologic symptoms associated with the climacteric is limited and sometimes appears to be flawed by methodologic problems. For example, some studies mention chronologic age and deduce a potentially inaccurate relationship with endocrine status.[1] It is difficult to measure psychologic symptoms, and the psychologic testing methods used vary among the research studies conducted. Another difficulty is that research in this area must deal with the climacteric, a phase that spans many years and that is affected by myriad factors, including varying rates of decline in steroids, nutritional status, level of physical activity, and degree of stress.

Other confounding factors include general societal influences and a woman's own "personal society," such as her community, culture, and religion. These societal influences sometimes conflict with each other, and cause disharmony for the woman. Research has shown that sociologic, psychologic, and biologic factors should be considered when assessing and treating psychologically related symptoms.

SOCIAL FACTORS

"If there is one single factor that influences a woman's experience of menopause, it is the attitude of the society in which she lives."[2]

SOCIETAL INFLUENCES

The major milestones in the history of menopause provide a fascinating background to understand attitudes and prognosticating future trends in the perception and management of this event through which all women will inevitably pass. *Menopause* is a word of multiple meanings. Once the subject of taboo; now almost in danger of overexposure. Once neglected, now recognized by multiple groups as the entry to a "market." The result is a new level of confusion and even exploitation in the minds of the health profession and the public alike. A historical survey of issues relating to the menopause is therefore an ideal vehicle for providing information and perspective into this fascinating and extremely important component of a woman's health care."[3]

There is no doubt that lack of discussion about menopause and the difficulty of attaining factual information about it contribute to women's negative perceptions about menopause. Research in 1982 revealed that about 56% of the women studied expected to be depressed and that 67% expected to be nervous and irritable. Thirty-five percent of the women did not know what their mothers' experiences of menopause were like.[4] In the United States, society's view of the menopause and aging has its roots in centuries-long beliefs about women and their limitations as productive members of society.

Historically, women have not been permitted to have intellectual, artistic, or other interests of their own outside of their home. Their primary purpose was to bear children and take care of them and their husbands. The literature is rich with stories of women who were poets, writers, scientists, political leaders, and founders of all-female colleges when universities were closed to them. However, these women were in the minority. Their successes were not considered the norm, and men in these fields were given greater recognition than their female counterparts. As Florence Nightingale wrote in 1852, "Why have women passion, intellect, moral activity—these three—and a place in society where not one of the three can be experienced?"[2]

In the early 19th century, physicians and psychoanalysts believed that too much intellectual activity was unhealthy for women. Women who were not content with being a mother and caretaker of the home were often diagnosed as mentally ill. Because a woman's major purpose in life was to bear children, when menopause arrived, a woman who still desired a sexual life needed to be "cured" of this unnatural and unhealthy desire. Medical treatments included applying leeches to the vulva and packing ice into the vagina. No wonder menopause was a dreaded time for women and certainly not to be talked about!

The 20th century brought with it similar negative attitudes within the medical profession. From the 1940s through the 1980s, some of the medical literature and presentations by physicians at medical conferences described menopause as "partial death"[5] and "a chronic and incapacitating deficiency disease that leaves women with flabby breasts, wrinkled skin, fragile bones, and loss of ability to have or enjoy sex."[6]

It may not be the case today, but in 1979, the medical faculty at the University of Louvain still used a medical text that stated, "Women in the climacteric have a strong tendency to aggressiveness and pettiness. They are jealous and possessive and they acquire a 'mother-in-law mentality.'"[7] In the late 1970s, a ruling by an American judge disqualified a woman witness on the grounds that she was in the climacteric.[7]

It is not unreasonable to consider that a substantial number of the women who are perimenopausal and postmenopausal today grew up with negative messages from society about becoming an older woman—messages that are still being perpetuated. Their grandmothers and mothers did not talk about what it felt like to become older, and they often lived sedentary, inactive lives because that was expected of them. Menopause was not discussed, and an older woman was not considered to have sexual needs at all.

The effects of a strong negative history about menopause is still with us to some degree, as is our society's negative attitude toward aging. Our society remains youth oriented and one in which older persons are not revered as the wise ones to "look up to." Aging may be feared by many women as a period fraught with illness and disability and loss of their youthful appearance. These fears may have an impact on climacteric-related symptoms and their severity.

Some anthropologic studies have shown that, in cultures in which the elderly are revered and supported, physical and mental health greatly surpasses that of the elderly of the Western world and that women have fewer symptoms associated with menopause. One example of this can be seen among the Rajput women in India.[8] In Rajasthan, the women live veiled and secluded before menopause. The women of Himachal Prasdesh, although not living in seclusion, are not allowed to be in the company of men other than their husbands. Before marriage, they can be in the company of only their fathers. Both of these groups of women live a restricted life because of their culture's taboos regarding menstruation and childbirth. However, with menopause, the women of Rajput cease to live a restricted life. They can leave the women's quarters and talk with men. Women living in Himachal Prasdesh can visit and joke with men in public. Menopause elevates them to a status considerably higher than that held when they were menstruating. In a sense, they are rewarded for becoming menopausal.

In addition to the Rajput citizens' attitudes toward menopause, their view about aging is extremely different from that in Western countries. Unemployment and inactivity are not an issue among older Rajputs, because they are fully involved in their farming economy and are models of wisdom or experience.

A cross-cultural study of Mayan women offered another example of minimal or no menopause-related symptoms. Demographic information, history, physical examination, hormone concentrations, and radial bone density measurements were obtained. None of the women in this study admitted to hot flushes, and they did not recall significant menopausal symptoms. These women experienced menopause approximately between the ages of 40 and 49. The study determined that all of the women experienced the same endocrinologic changes as women in the United States. For example, they experienced a decline in estrogen. They also experienced age-related bone demineralization but did not experience symptoms common among women in the United States and had a low incidence of osteoporotic fractures.[9]

Each woman is influenced by the unique cultural, religious, and psychosocial dynamics of her life. Some women may have been brought up to believe that their fertility is what makes them women. If this is the case, menopause can be viewed as the end of their "womanliness." This can even be the case for the woman who has had the children that she desired. Just knowing that she cannot bear any more children can be traumatic.

Women whose identity is synonymous with motherhood may also find it difficult to cope with menopause. Having spent most of their adult life caring for their children, some women may experience feelings of sadness and loneliness when the children leave home. Even though research has not demonstrated a significant relationship between the "empty nest syndrome" and climacteric-related symptoms, it is important to acknowledge a relationship can exist for some women.

For the woman who is infertile or who never had children but wanted them, menopause represents the final point. There is no turning back. A sense of loss may be experienced unless these issues were resolved earlier in life and the woman feels that her life is complete and fulfilling even though she was unable to have children.

If a woman's worth is synonymous with attaining certain professional goals but she has not yet achieved them as she approaches menopause, she may experience negative feelings that affect her experience of menopause. The woman who abandoned her educational, creative, or professional pursuits to care for her family may feel that she is too old to pursue them again. She may also not be in a financial situation to do so. The feelings she experiences as a result of this situation can negatively affect her experience of menopause.

This is also true for the woman who may need to enter the work force, but being a homemaker for many years has made her feel that she is not "marketable." Unfortunately, these feelings may prove accurate, not because the woman has no potential, but because society does not reach out to these women to provide affordable employment training programs and employment opportunities.

These are only a few examples of the ways in which women respond to societal influences and their personal expectations and perceptions. A woman may not even be consciously aware of how she is feeling; nevertheless, these feelings can translate into the powerful physiologic effects of stress, which can influence the type and severity of menopausal symptoms experienced by the woman.

MIDLIFE AND OTHER FACTORS

Several major events that characterize the middle period of the life span also influence a woman's experience during the climacteric: illness and death of parents, having to care for ailing parents, retirement, and loss of a partner through death or separation. These events alone can be stressful, alter the woman's social role, and sometimes involve much psychologic and sociologic readjustment, regardless of the effect menopause has on a woman. They can cause some women to undergo profound changes in their lives, their expectations about the future, and their perceptions about themselves.[10]

Epidemiologic studies have demonstrated that gender, social class, income level, employment status, and educational attainment are generally associated with many psychologic, physiologic, and psychiatric conditions.[10] To what extent do these and other psychosocial factors cause or exacerbate symptoms of the climacteric?

Several cross-sectional epidemiologic studies have provided some reasonable answers. These studies, conducted in the United States and in other countries, have investigated groups of women of various ages and menopausal statuses and compared them with some measure of well-being, usually symptoms. "Interpretations were then made as to how well-being changed in relation to age and menopausal status."[11]

Several studies demonstrated that women of low sociodemographic status, low family income, low educational level, and limited employment opportunities experienced more symptoms and greater severity of symptoms than women with higher social status, greater income, better education, and more rewarding employment.[7,12–25] Women of a low socioeconomic status generally reported more psychologic symptoms than women of a higher status, and women of low sociodemographic status who were employed suffered the most compared with employed women with a higher income. These findings suggest that only when employment is career oriented and rewarding does it have beneficial effects on a woman's emotional status, unlike the situation for the woman whose primary purpose in working is to provide income for the family.

Many of the studies also revealed that negative attitudes toward menopause, poor social support, stressful life events, a recent death in the family, and poor marital relations were associated with climacteric-related symptoms.[7,16,25–32] The event of children leaving the home has not been found to correlate with symptom severity, and "emptying the nest" does not result in a woman being more prone to depression. Children leaving the home can often have a positive effect on a woman's life.[33]

When researchers reviewed 94 articles from 30 years of research that examined the relation of natural menopause with depression, they concluded that "there is insufficient evidence at present to maintain that menopause causes depression."[34] A review of studies of health and ill-health experiences during the menopausal transition found no increase in the incidence of major depression with menopause.[35] Factors associated with negative moods included surgical menopause, prior depression, health status, menstrual problems, social and family stress, and negative attitudes toward menopause.

Another study determined that a woman's health status, not menopause, had the most influence on depressed mood.[36] A change in menopausal status was unrelated to depressive symptoms experienced by study subjects between the ages of 42 and 50.[37] In this study, depressive symptoms were higher among women who reported stressful events, especially of a chronic nature; those who scored highly on the trait of anxiety; and those who were pessimistic and subsequently experienced a stressful, ongoing problem. The investigators concluded that midlife stress, optimism, and anxiety are important predictors of depressive symptoms during midlife.

Midlife may be problematic for women with certain female gender role traits.[38] Depressive symptoms were more common in women who tested higher for the trait of self-consciousness. These women were the most vulnerable to subsequent ongoing stress. Women who tended to suppress angry feelings and who used hormone replacement therapy (HRT) when they were postmenopausal had more symptoms than other women. For women who reported having hot flushes and night sweats once each week or more, it was determined that depressed mood, anxiety, and low self-esteem—not the frequency of the symptoms—discriminated between those who viewed the symptoms as problematic and those who did not.[39]

The psychologic symptoms associated with menopause appear to be related more to a variety of psychosocial factors such as family and socioeconomic experiences in midlife and personality traits than to endocrine changes.

A conceptual framework for the findings of many of the studies conducted is the vulnerability model.[10] This model implies that women who are vulnerable at the time of the climacteric because of adverse sociodemographic and psychosocial factors are more likely to experience nonspecific physical and psychologic symptoms. The model implies that the symptoms and their severity are determined by the way in which a woman has coped with problems in the past, her earlier life experiences, and her biologic and psychologic makeup. As illustrated in Figure 5-1, there is no typical climacteric profile for the symptoms that women experience. Some women may experience more psychologically related symptoms, and others experience more physically related symptoms.

Stressors such as inadequate income; unhappiness in one's job or relationships; not being involved in a supportive, loving relationship; and having a poor social support system can detrimentally affect psychologic and physiologic well-being. If a woman has been experiencing any of these or other stressors for years, by the time she reaches her forties or fifties, she may feel "emotionally drained," and

FIGURE 5-1
Vulnerability model

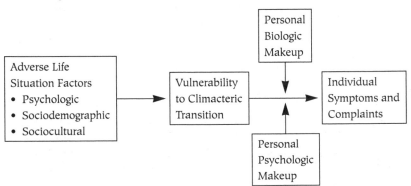

her physical and psychologic health may be compromised. It is not surprising that whatever the woman experiences can be exacerbated by the physiologic changes associated with the climacteric and compounded by a negative attitude toward aging or menopause.

BIOLOGIC FACTORS

Biologic factors can directly or indirectly cause psychologic symptoms, but how and to what degree remain unanswered questions. Some women in the United States experience no symptoms or minimal symptoms associated with the climacteric, as is the case for women of various cultures throughout the world.

INDIRECT EFFECTS OF BIOLOGIC FACTORS

Biologic factors can indirectly cause psychologic symptoms through a "domino effect." For example, sleep deprivation resulting from night sweats or nocturnal micturition can lead to fatigue and irritability. These symptoms can lead to lack of concentration and can negatively affect the woman's life in several ways. Over time, as the effects of sleep deprivation escalate, a woman may find that her ability to function is compromised and her relationships are affected. Depression may be the result of the cascade of events that began with sleep deprivation, which came from physiologic changes associated with a decline in ovarian hormones.

Another example of the ways in which biologic factors can indirectly contribute to psychologic symptoms is dyspareunia. A woman may experience anxiety from the physical pain and from the impact of dyspareunia on her sexuality and her relationship. Experiencing these symptoms can also remind her that she has entered a phase in her life that she may not welcome. This can lead to anxiety, irritability, and depression.

DIRECT EFFECTS OF BIOLOGIC FACTORS

Significant changes in mood and a variety of nonreproductive behaviors from cognitive function, motor activity, seizure susceptibility, pain sensitivity, and pathologic processes such as Parkinson's and Alzheimer's diseases are associated with alterations in circulating levels of estradiol and progesterone.[40] Estrogen and progesterone receptors are located in various areas of the brain.[41-46] When estradiol levels are high, an excitatory action is exerted on the central nervous system.[47] Some women notice an increase in energy, an enhanced sense of well-being, a euphoric state, or high activity states.[48] Estradiol can have antidepressant effects[49] and cause an increase in sensory perception.[50] Elevated progesterone levels exert an inhibitory or depressant effect on the central nervous system.[47,51–54] During the luteal phase, some women experience a tranquilizing or mood-stabilizing effect, and others experience depressant effects.[55,56]

Estrogens and progesterone also influence amines such as norepinephrine, epinephrine, serotonin, dopamine, and phenylethylamine, all of which affect moods.[57–62] However, it is not known to what degree alterations in the levels of these hormones ultimately cause mood changes or the extent to which these changes happen.

Some women experience a profound change in their psychologic status after childbirth (ie, "postpartum blues") that appears to be directly related to endocrine changes. Some women report feelings of euphoria, anxiety, and an increase in energy associated with the rise in estradiol before ovulation. Some women experience anxiety, irritability, and depression premenstrually, and negative mood changes can be experienced by women taking progestogens, oral contraceptives, progestin-only contraceptives, or HRT. It has been suggested that women who experience significant psychologic symptoms related to a reproductive event (eg, postpartum depression, premenstrual syndrome, oral contraceptive use) are more vulnerable to having recurrences during the climacteric.[63,64]

The relationship between ovarian hormones and neurotransmitters began to be discussed more vigorously in the literature when premenstrual syndrome became an acknowledged, physiologically based problem. During this debate, other causes of psychologic symptoms were discussed, such as magnesium and B vitamin deficiencies.[63] It has been suggested, for example, that magnesium deficiency may be involved directly in deficiency of central nervous system dopamine, the neurotransmitter that contributes to feelings of relaxation and mental alertness.[65] Vitamin B_6 deficiency has also been linked with dopamine deficiency.[66] As discussed in Chapter 3, deficiencies in these and other vitamins and minerals are commonplace in the typical American diet.

Chronic stress may be a major contributor to the psychologic symptoms that some women experience during the climacteric, because stressful life events have been found to be significant predictors of premenstrual syndrome and menstrual problems.[67,68]

There is evidence of a close relationship with changes in estrogen levels and the hormones and enzymes most commonly implicated in biologic stress responses.[68] Animal studies have shown that estrone, estradiol, and estriol secretions were reduced in response to biologic stressors.[69] Reduced levels of estrogens can affect the levels of mood-related neurotransmitters.

Chronic stress can cause inadequate functioning of the adrenal glands. Because these glands secrete the androgens that are precursors of estrogens, progesterone, and testosterone, some symptoms may result from an inadequate level of androgens being produced during the climacteric.

Many of the symptoms caused by chronic stress can be experienced by anyone of either gender or any age and are similar to those associated with the climacteric: anxiety, irritability, depression, hot flushes, dizziness, headaches, heart palpitations, decreased libido, insomnia, and lethargy (see Chapter 3). Chronic stress is often a result of the way in which a person perceives and copes with life stressors, absence of regularly practiced methods of stress reduction, lack of regular exercise, and nutritional deficiencies. A woman may enter the climacteric with her adrenal glands compromised by stress and may already be experiencing one or more of the stress-related symptoms. This situation, combined with a decline in ovarian hormones and the inability of the adrenals to secrete adequate amounts of androgens, may cause or exacerbate psychologic symptoms.

Another possible scenario is one in which a woman experiences stressful events related to midlife situations. This can contribute to nutritional deficiencies, some of which affect secretion of neurotransmitters that affect mood and the adrenal glands' ability to secrete androgens. Because a woman may already be vulnerable to the psychologic effects of a decline in ovarian hormones, she begins to experience psychologic symptoms. Woman are physiologically, emotionally, and spiritually different, and climacteric-related symptoms should continue to be viewed in the context of interactions of social, psychologic, and biochemical factors.

POSITIVE ATTITUDES

For some women, menopause is a positive experience. Some women are elated about not having to be concerned with pregnancy. They look forward to the end of menstruation, relish the thought of no longer contributing to Johnson and Johnson, and like the fact that they have a couple of hundred dollars more each year to spend on things that are more enjoyable than tampons or sanitary napkins.

Many women have been waiting eagerly for their children to leave home and, with much love in their hearts, do not want them to return! The time that a couple gains to devote to themselves and to each other enables them to develop and nurture their own and other relationships in a way that was not possible before. A woman may return to school or embark on the pursuit of interests she has had for years or only recently considered. She may take better care of herself physically and emotionally, and she views this time as an opportunity to change careers or become involved in various activities. Some women leave a relationship that they have wanted to end for years but took no action because of the children. Some divorced and widowed women truly enjoy living alone. They feel free in ways that they never experienced before.

SEXUALITY

Human sensuality and sexuality encompass more than the anatomy and physiology of sexual intercourse, the levels of hormones, the frequency of orgasm, more than the interaction of genital systems; [they are] an integral part of the human being at any age. As one form of connection to other persons and as a symbol of reaffirmation of self, the freedom and opportunity for sexual expression are basic to mental and physical well-being.[70]

I'm 62 and sex has never been better. The kids are gone. I don't have to worry about getting pregnant and we're retired, so we can make love any time of day, even all day, anywhere we want. Every day is a celebration; we've made it this far and we're still alive. I wouldn't trade in this time of my life for anything.[71]

It is not unusual to find that many women share similar positive feelings and experiences. Research conducted by Masters and Johnson, Kinsey, and others supports these ideas. By observing and documenting the physiologic changes of the sexual response cycle in women 40 through 78 years old, Masters and Johnson demonstrated that the aging woman is physiologically fully capable of sexual activity, intercourse, and orgasm, particularly if she experiences regular and effective sexual stimulation. They found no physiologic reason why the frequency of sexual expression found satisfactory in the younger years should not be carried into the postmenopausal years.[72]

> There is every reason to believe that maintained regularity of sexual expression coupled with adequate physical well-being and healthy mental orientation to the aging process combine to provide a sexually stimulative climate within a relationship. This climate can improve sexual tension and provide a capacity for sexual performance that frequently extends beyond the 80-year level.[72]

The Duke University Center for the Study of Aging and Human Development found that 40% to 65% of the subjects between the ages of 60 and 71 engaged in intercourse with some frequency and that 10% to 20% of those 78 years old or older still experienced some form of sexual activity.[73] A significant portion of the elderly subjects showed rising patterns of sexual activity and interest, and women 78 years of age or older showed a greater interest in sex than did men of that age group.

A cross-sectional study conducted in 48 states and launched in 1988 undertook the enormous task of examining a broad spectrum of issues related to sexuality in the context of daily life among Americans.[74] Some of the results of this research is found in Tables 5-1 and 5-2. These results enable us to compare various aspects of the sexual lives of women and men of all ages and to put into perspective certain aspects of sexuality and aging, particularly when compared with the sexual lives of women and men between the ages of 18 and 38.

As illustrated in Table 5-1, when *active* was defined to mean a few times weekly or daily, 18 to 26 year olds did not have a more active sex life than their parents or their grandparents. The combined frequency of all sexual activity declined among women between the ages of 27 and 64, although it increased after the age of 65, indicating that the women had an active sex life as they entered and passed middle age. Although decline in those between the ages of 51 and 64 was about twice that for those between the ages of 27 and 38, interviews with women supported the investigators' assumption that this was related to increased rates of widowhood, women's reluctance to enter into a sexual relationship soon after divorce, and not knowing how to find a new sex partner after experiencing a loss.

TABLE 5-1
Frequency of All Sexual Activity

	Participation (%) by age group*									
	18 to 26		27 to 38		39 to 50		51 to 64		65+	
	M	F	M	F	M	F	M	F	M	F
Frequency	(254)	(268)	(353)	(380)	(282)	(295)	(227)	(230)	(212)	(221)
a. Daily	15	13	16	8	15	10	12	4	14	1
b. A few times weekly	38	33	44	41	39	29	51	28	39	40
c. Weekly	19	22	23	27	29	29	18	33	16	33
d. Monthly	15	15	8	12	9	11	11	8	20	4
e. Rarely	13	17	9	12	8	21	8	27	11	22
Active = lines a+b	53	46	60	49	54	39	63	32	53	41
At least weekly = lines a through c	72	68	83	76	83	68	81	65	69	74

*Absolute numbers of women and men in each category are given within parentheses.
From Reinisch J. The Kinsey Institute new report on sex. New York: St. Martin's Press; 1990

TABLE 5-2
I Have Orgasm During Lovemaking

	Orgasm frequency (%) by age group*									
	18 to 26		27 to 38		39 to 50		51 to 64		65+	
	M	F	M	F	M	F	M	F	M	F
Frequency	(254)	(265)	(352)	(373)	(283)	(293)	(226)	(231)	(213)	(221)
a. Daily	68	18	68	16	60	14	77	21	55	8
b. Often	25	39	26	51	34	52	18	44	38	42
c. Sometimes	3	22	3	18	4	22	1	22	4	37
d. Rarely	1	8	1	9	1	7	2	10	1	4
e. Never	3	13	2	6	1	5	2	3	2	9
Frequently = lines a+b	93	57	94	67	94	66	95	65	93	50
At least sometimes = lines a through c	96	79	97	85	98	88	96	87	97	87

*Absolute numbers of women and men in each category are given within parentheses.
From Reinisch J. The Kinsey Institute new report on sex. New York: St. Martin's Press; 1990

Interviews with men and women older than 65 years of age revealed that their sexual lives were "more deeply gratifying; being unhurried, they shared to a greater degree with their partner[s] and had more time to spend on a seductive buildup. They also reported that they experienced more warmth and intimacy after the sex act."[74]

As shown in Table 5-2, the rates for the *frequently* category remained fairly constant across all age groups. Although the frequency of sexual activity declined somewhat with age (see Table 5-1), the data in Table 5-2 show that women's and men's ability to reach orgasm diminished very little from the levels of their earlier years.

A study to determine the relation of sexual functioning to age, menopausal status, and hormone levels was conducted among 201 women between the ages of 48 and 58.[75] The results revealed that most aspects of sexual functioning were not affected by age, menopausal functioning, or hormone levels.

These studies and others have demonstrated that enjoyment of sexual activity can and often does continue throughout a person's lifetime. However, a sexual life is not enjoyable in the face of dyspareunia and pain. These symptoms are experienced by an estimated 50% of postmenopausal women and to a much lesser extent by perimenopausal women.

PHYSIOLOGIC CHANGES AFFECTING FEMALE SEXUALITY

Dyspareunia and changes in vaginal lubrication, orgasms, response to touch, and libido result in a decline in estrogen, testosterone, and perhaps progesterone, which affects a woman's intimate life.

DYSPAREUNIA

Dyspareunia as a result of vaginal changes caused by a decline in estrogen and perhaps progesterone has also been related to frequency of sexual activity. Regardless of hormone levels, maintenance of overall health of the vagina and genitalia is to some degree related to sexual activity.[76,77] Vaginal vasculature and circulation are maintained through regular intercourse or other forms of sexual activity such as masturbation. Women who continue to have regular intercourse during the climacteric have a significantly lower vaginal pH than age-matched women who do not have intercourse.[77] A lower pH helps to protect against the development of vulvovaginitis.

VAGINAL LUBRICATION

The decrease in the amount and duration of vaginal lubrication may cause a woman to experience irritation, burning, and discomfort or significant pain during intercourse. These symptoms can also occur from thinning of the lining of the vaginal mucosa as estrogen begins to decrease. This results in an inadequate "cushion" against the friction caused by the penis during intercourse. These initial changes in vaginal mucosa are usually not detectable during a vaginal examination.

In one study, postmenopausal women not on HRT and who continued to engage in intercourse three or more times per month or who masturbated had less vaginal atrophy than women who engaged in intercourse less than 10 times per year or did not masturbate.[76] According to Masters and Johnson, at some point after the age of 40 the vasocongestive response experienced during sexual activity can begin to decrease because of a decline in estrogen.[76a] This results in less vaginal lubrication. During a woman's premenopausal years, she may have experienced vaginal lubrication within several seconds after beginning to feel sexually aroused. However, at some point during the perimenopause, even when the intensity of sexual arousal is the same as that experienced during younger years, the onset of lubrication may be delayed for a couple of minutes after feelings of sexual arousal begin. The amount of vaginal lubrication may be less and last for a shorter period than during the premenopause. About 40% to 60% of women experience an increase in the amount of time and stimulation required to experience vaginal lubrication.[78]

Vaginal lubrication is affected by the decrease in estrogen levels and by anxiety.[79] Research has demonstrated that vaginal blood flow and therefore the amount of vaginal lubrication decrease as a result of anxiety.

ORGASM

The characteristics of a woman's orgasm can change during the climacteric. For some, orgasm becomes more intense, but for others, it can take longer to experience orgasm, or orgasm may not be experienced as frequently as during the premenopausal years. Vaginal contractions can decrease in number and intensity. If this occurs, it does not mean that a woman's enjoyment of sex has decreased. Some women still experience intense pleasure during orgasm, although others experience less pleasure and are disappointed that the quality of the orgasm has diminished.

A decline in hormones may affect a woman's response to physical affection and caressing. For example, during their premenopausal years, women may have enjoyed softer caresses of particular areas of the body. With the climacteric, firmer caresses in those areas become more pleasurable.

A decline in sexual desire for some women may be caused by a decrease in testosterone.[80,81] Decreased sexual desire, although it can occur early in the climacteric, is more common several years after menopause.

POSTMENOPAUSAL CHANGES

After a woman has been postmenopausal for a few years and without some form of treatment, she usually experiences significant changes in the genitalia. There is loss of superficial cells of the vaginal epithelium, which results in a thinner, drier, and less elastic vaginal mucosa. The vaginal pH becomes less acidic. The increase in pH and decrease in epithelial thickness create a favorable environment for growth of microorganisms, contributing to the development of vulvovaginitis.

Loss of elasticity can result in narrowing of the introitus and decreased width and length of the vaginal canal. The mons and labia become thinner so that the clitoris and urethra are not as well protected and are more vulnerable to irritation from sexual activity. The clitoris may also become smaller and sometimes more sensitive to touch. All of these changes can cause dyspareunia, and women experiencing them may complain of symptoms such as burning pain and tightness in the vagina and clitoral pain with stimulation.

The effects of declining estrogen levels have been associated with specific changes in the sexual response cycle. These include a decrease in the lengthening and ballooning of the vaginal canal, delayed and reduced vaginal expansion, less constriction of the introitus, and no enlargement and poor elevation of the uterus. During orgasm, there are usually fewer contractions, and painful uterine spasms occasionally are experienced.

As with the perimenopausal woman, discomfort or pain associated with sexual activity and a change in the physical response can cause feelings of sexual inadequacy and fear that the ability to be a sexually responsive woman and enjoy a sexual relationship is no longer possible. Because she is not able to respond to her partner in ways that she had before, her partner may experience feelings of inadequacy as a lover. Unless both partners obtain information about these physiologic changes and are able to discuss how to cope with them in positive, loving ways, the impact on the relationship can be quite traumatic.

With thinning of the urethral mucosa, some women are more prone to developing urethritis from sexual activity. They may feel the need to urinate right after sexual activity and can experience urinary symptoms such as dysuria.

Loss of pelvic support that may have initially resulted from childbirth can increase with declining estrogen levels. This can lead to development of a urethrocele or rectocele, uterine prolapse, stress incontinence, and the loss of some sensation in the vagina during intercourse. These physiologic changes can cause a woman to feel less desirable and make intercourse difficult or uncomfortable.

With aging comes the loss of elasticity of the skin and a decrease in size and flattening of the breasts caused by fibrous tissue replacing fatty tissue. A decrease in elasticity of supporting muscles and ligaments results in "drooping" of the breasts, depending on the size of the breasts and the health of the woman. The physical changes associated with aging can result in the development of a poor self-image, particularly as it relates to sexuality. These reactions are typical in a society in which youth, desirability, and sex are synonymous.

CHANGES AS A RESULT OF HYSTERECTOMY

The abrupt decline in production of estrogen and androgens as a result of a complete hysterectomy can produce a variety of symptoms that can affect a woman's sexuality. A decrease in libido and the ability to have orgasm have been reported in some women who have had a hysterectomy without ovary removal.[82,83] This response has also been reported by some women who have had their ovaries removed. In addition to hormonal changes associated with a hysterectomy, depending on how the surgery was performed, sexual problems can arise from shortening and narrowing of the vaginal vault and from vaginal scarring.[84–87]

Some women experience a decrease in pleasurable sexual feelings because they are no longer able to experience the uterine contractions that occur during orgasm. This may also be true for those women who enjoyed pleasurable feelings when pressure was applied to the cervix during intercourse. Another reason for a decline in sexual feelings experienced by some women who have had a hysterectomy is psychologic fear, because they believe that the surgery affected their level of sexual satisfaction and caused a loss of attractiveness. The frequency of desire, intercourse, and orgasm and the woman's attitude toward her partner before the surgery are some of the best predictors of how a woman will respond sexually after a hysterectomy.[88]

Many women who experienced pain with intercourse or orgasm because of endometriosis, fibroids, and other uterine pathology find that, because they are pain free as a result of having a hysterectomy, they are able to enjoy their sexual life. Because the fear of pregnancy is eliminated, some women find that their enjoyment of sexual intercourse is increased.

EDUCATING WOMEN ABOUT SEXUALITY

Hormonal and complementary therapies are available to treat many of the symptoms discussed in this chapter. If the woman is given facts about these physiologic changes before they take place, some symptoms can be prevented. For example, if a 40-year-old woman receives education about the physiology of sexual functioning associated with the climacteric, she is prepared for possible changes such as a delay in and decreased amount of vaginal lubrication. She is then able to understand this is a normal change and will not fear it as a signal of the "beginning of the end" of her being a sexually responsive woman.

The woman should be encouraged to discuss these changes with her partner. The couple is then able to experiment with their lovemaking techniques so that the woman's pleasure is enhanced. Her sexual life, instead of becoming less fulfilling as a result of the physiologic changes, can become more fulfilling and satisfying.

It is also important that a woman involved in a heterosexual relationship be educated about the normal physiologic changes of the man's sexual responsiveness as he ages. Masters and Johnson's research revealed that, as a man enters his mid-forties or early fifties, it usually takes longer for him to achieve an erection.[72] The amount and force of ejaculation decreases, while the refractory or resting stage between ejaculations increases. Longer and more intense stimulation is needed to achieve erection and ejaculation. As a man enters his late fifties or sixties, he may find that, after ejaculation, he is unable to achieve another erection for 12 to 24 hours. If adequate education about normal physiologic changes does not occur and communication among couples is inadequate, it is easy to see how their sexual life, instead of becoming more enriched with age, can become disastrous.

With women, as with men, it is difficult to separate the effects of changes in sexual functioning associated with aging and the effects caused by lifestyle, health, and psychosocial factors. The change in the man's sexual response cycle occurs at a time in his life when he may be experiencing physical and emotional difficulties associated with the midlife. This can lead to sexual problems. The physiologic changes, with or without midlife stressors, may adversely affect a man's feelings about his own sexuality and tap into his negativity about aging. He may fear becoming impotent, and because he may not know the facts about the normal physiologic changes of the man's sexual response cycle associated with aging, he may withdraw from his partner sexually and in other aspects of their relationship. This is particularly true for the man who equates his ability to enjoy a sexual relationship and be a good lover with his ability to have and maintain an erection.

OTHER FACTORS AFFECTING SEXUALITY

Hormonal changes associated with the climacteric can affect sexual desire and sexual functioning in some women. Body image can also play a major role in women's sexuality. When body build was analyzed among postmenopausal women, it was determined that reduced sexual interest was associated with a kind of body type (fatty tissue in various areas of the body) that did not correspond to the culture-specific idea of beauty.[89] Lack of education about the normal physiologic changes associated with the climacteric and aging can also have a negative impact on the sexual life of the woman.

Sexual development depends on a range of factors that directly affect sexual development, and ultimately affect a woman's sexuality during the climacteric. These range from the messages a person receives from family and religion to those from society at large. All of these messages evolve from a history, some dating back to Biblical times, that was often fraught with extremely negative messages about sexuality in general and about women's sexuality in particular. During the Victorian era, Dr. William Acton, a prominent physician and spokesperson for the Victorian view of sexuality, stated the following:

> The majority of women [happily for society] are not much troubled with sexual feelings of any kind. What men are habitually, women are only exceptionally. It is too true, I admit as the Divorce Court shows, that there are some few women who have sexual desires so strong that they surpass those of men, and shock public feeling by their consequence. I admit, of course, the existence of sexual excitement terminating even in nymphomania, a form of insanity that those accustomed to visit lunatic asylums must be fully conversant with; but with these sad exceptions, there can be no doubt that sexual feeling in the female is in the majority of cases in abeyance, and that it requires positive and considerable excitement to be aroused at all; moderate compared with that of the male ... love of home, of children, and of domestic duties are the only passions they [females] feel.[90]

We would like to think that what is going on sexually today is much different from the sexual behavior of past generations, but contemporary feelings about sexuality are still based on the remnants of an antisexual history, and as a result, our society is still in a state of sexual confusion. Sex feels great, but because it is pleasure of the body, it is generally regarded as somehow less a virtue than activities of the mind. Many still worry about the rightness or wrongness of masturbation and oral-genital sex, even if they want to experience these activities.

In general, society is convinced of the benefits of contraception and sexuality education but still has difficulty in making them available to teenagers. Sexual activity is viewed as a special, important, and loving means of communication between two persons, but it is often not seen as acceptable among the disabled and the aging. Too many have inaccurate information about sexuality and are not comfortable with their own sexuality. Sexual concerns and problems of couples remain commonplace. This is evidenced by the thousands who communicate with the Kinsey Institute each year, asking sexually related questions and expressing confusion about sexual issues, including concerns about whether their own bodies, sexual feelings, and sexual activities are "normal." This confusion has also been demonstrated in the results of the Kinsey Institute's national survey, conducted in 1989, which included a statistically representative group of 1974 adults.[91] The results revealed that most respondents could answer correctly only one half of the questions regarding basic sexuality-related issues, and only 4.5% could answer most of the questions. As reported in the study, "It is clear that the American public is not getting accurate sexual information. Whether in campaigns for preventing AIDS, guidelines for avoiding pregnancy, discussions of intimate sexual problems, or information about sex and aging, the facts are not reaching the majority of Americans."[91]

Remnants of an antisexual history were also demonstrated by the actions of the Bush administration and Congress that withheld funding for any large-scale study of American sexual behavior.[91] This decision did not change even when, in 1989, federal authorities were urged by an expert panel of the National Academy of Science's National Research Council investigating AIDS prevention to sponsor more research on sexual behavior. They were also urged to sponsor this research as a result of the alarming rise in sexually transmitted diseases, teen pregnancies, and sexual abuse of children. There are still many persons in positions of power in the United States who maintain a Victorian attitude toward sexuality.

Research in the field of sexuality remains limited, especially in the area of healthy female sexuality. In 1993, the National Institutes of Health spent $1 million on male erectile dysfunction but not a penny on a similar category for women or on any other sex research on women.[92]

Midlife events and a person's attitude toward aging and sexuality affect sexual life. This is also the case with other lifestyle factors, including stressors associated with a preoccupation with career, family, and financial issues. Alcohol and drug intake, poor diet, and lack of exercise can affect a person's sexual functioning. As persons age, the likelihood of physical problems arises, ranging from arthritis to heart disease to cancer. The medical problem and treatment can have a direct impact on a woman's feelings as a sexual person and her ability to engage in sexual activity, particularly if movement is painful. However, erotic activity, particularly orgasm, may stimulate the body's release of endorphins, producing an analgesic affect similar to that of taking a mild narcotic. This has lead some physicians to "prescribe" sex for persons with various health problems such as arthritis. Sex can be a physical distraction and a pain reliever.

Medical problems and medications and their effects on sexuality comprise an area that is still inadequately addressed by the medical community. Many commonly used drugs can interfere with sexual functioning in women and men. They can cause a decrease or loss of libido, interfere with erection or ejaculation, and delay or prevent orgasm in women. Because patients are often reluctant to discuss sexual difficulties, it is important for the health care provider to know whether a drug that she or he is prescribing can affect the patient's sexuality and discuss this with the patient. Some of the more commonly prescribed drugs that can affect sexuality include antihypertensive agents, Tagamet, antipsychotic and antianxiety drugs, tricyclic antidepressants, high doses of central nervous system depressants, and anticancer drugs.

Unfortunately, not all health care providers take the time to discuss sexuality-related issues with the woman, man, or couple before and after surgery directly related to sexuality, such as hysterectomy or mastectomy. This is also often the case for surgical procedures indirectly related to sexual life, such as coronary bypass surgery. If the health care provider is not knowledgeable about or comfortable with discussing sexuality-related issues, he or she should refer the patient to someone who can provide sexuality education and counseling during this physically and emotionally trying time. By doing this, the provider is giving the patient permission to acknowledge her or his sexuality, the knowledge that a medical problem and treatment can affect a sexual relationship, and the importance of education and counseling in this area.

In addition to the effects of illness, medication, surgery, and a decline in hormones on a woman's sexuality, other factors impinge significantly on the way in which a woman perceives herself as a sexual person during the climacteric. These include her feelings toward her own sexuality, how she feels about being in a relationship, and whether she is in a relationship. If she enters this time burdened by negative sexual experiences, a history of sexual abuse that is unresolved, or general negativity because of familial, religious, and other societal influences, the climacteric may be used as a way to escape from having or maintaining an intimate relationship.

For women in a relationship, the dynamics of the couple's relationship greatly affect her sexuality and the quality of the sexual relationship. Couples who enter the woman's climacteric in a loving, supportive, and sexually satisfying relationship in which they can openly communicate their sexual feelings and experiences have the greatest probability of experiencing fewer or no psychologic problems associated with aging.

Sex is more a matter of the mind and heart than genital organs. To set an age limit on sexuality is unrealistic and unjust. Even with a physical disability, the need for sensual and sexual expression remains. An older couple who is able to function sexually in old age is extremely fortunate. The partners should not be made to feel self-conscious about their desire for each other, but rather should take advantage of it to the fullest. If they understand and accept the unique characteristics of sex in the later years, they may be surprised to find their sexual relationship becoming more sensitive, sharing, tender, and enjoyable than it was in their younger years.

CONTRACEPTIVE ISSUES DURING THE CLIMACTERIC

My periods were so infrequent and the bleeding so scant that I never gave a second thought to the possibility of being able to conceive. And then one day my husband and I faced the fact that I was pregnant at the age of fifty-one. I wish we never had to face that dilemma.[93]

A discussion about sexuality would be incomplete without addressing the issue of pregnancy prevention. Among women 40 years of age or older, the rate of unplanned pregnancies is second only to the unplanned pregnancy rate among teenagers. Health care providers should take an aggressive approach to contraceptive education and counseling for women in this age group.

The perimenopausal woman has available to her the same contraceptive options as a premenopausal woman. These are the barrier methods (ie, female and male condom, cervical cap, and diaphragm), different forms of spermicides (ie, foam, gel, and vaginal contraceptive film suppositories), and natural methods of family planning. Hormonal methods (ie, oral contraceptives, implants, and injectables) and sterilization are other choices available to the perimenopausal woman.

Issues involved in choosing a method of contraception include comfort with one's body, medical contraindications, side effects, previous contraceptive experiences, factors that contribute to contraceptive-related pregnancies, sexual lifestyle, effectiveness rates, and the ability to comply with the method selected. Whether a woman chooses to use a barrier method, an intrauterine device, or a hormonal method or she elects to have a tubal ligation depends on careful consideration of all factors.

The factor that may be more influential for the perimenopausal woman than many others is her need and desire to prevent pregnancy. It is usually greater than that of the premenopausal woman. A contraceptive-related pregnancy experienced by a premenopausal woman may eventually be welcomed because she was planning to have a baby at some point in the not-to-distant future. However, for a perimenopausal woman, giving birth in her forties or fifties may be a less acceptable option. The perimenopausal woman may feel that her contraceptive options are only those that are associated with the highest effectiveness rates. These methods are sterilization, oral contraceptives, injectables, implants, and the intrauterine device. There are some medical issues associated with some of these methods that are unique to perimenopausal women.

Irregular bleeding patterns typically occur with Depo-Provera (DMPA) and Norplant. With DMPA, these often subside by the end of the first year of use. Norplant users may experience irregular bleeding patterns well after the first year, even if they were not experienced initially. However, because the rates of cervical and endometrial cancer increase with age and because irregular bleeding may be one sign of these cancers, the woman cannot be absolutely sure that the irregular bleeding is caused by the contraceptive method rather than a pathologic process. Some health care providers suggest that an endometrial biopsy be taken before initiating use of DMPA or Norplant if the woman is 40 years of age or older. Others feel that this is unnecessary and that performing an endometrial biopsy if irregular bleeding occurs, although not absolutely necessary, is a reasonable choice. If the woman became a DMPA or Norplant user before the age of 40, any irregular bleeding experienced after this age should be evaluated. Amenorrhea is experienced in about 50% of DMPA users within the first year. It is also experienced by Norplant users, but at a much lower rate. A woman who has entered her climacteric must be informed that amenorrhea may result and that she should not assume that she is menopausal and can stop using her method of contraception.

Because some women find that their weight increases with age and have yet to embark on an exercise and nutritional program to deal with this issue, the 4- to 5-pound annual weight gain with DMPA is not usually welcomed. Although this weight gain stabilizes after about 3 years, DMPA may not be the best choice because of the importance of maintaining a healthy body weight. Weight gain may also be experienced among some Norplant users.

A decrease in libido, premenstrual-like symptoms, headaches, depression, and other side effects are possible with DMPA and Norplant. Because estrogen levels are lower compared with a normal menstrual cycle, loss of bone density associated with DMPA may also be an issue and is under investigation. The results of one study showed that bone density measurements were, on average, 7.5% lower in the lumbar spine and 6.5% lower in the femoral neck in women who had used DMPA for at least 5 years compared with the control group.[94] The women's pre-DMPA bone density was unknown, and more women using DMPA were smokers—two issues to consider in assessing the results of this study.

One case history of interest is that of a 39-year-old woman who was on DMPA for 17 years and who developed multiple fractures after falling from a stationary horse. Densitometry revealed significant osteopenia. Although the reported patient was a thin, Caucasian woman, she did not have any other significant risk factors for osteoporosis except for a possible state of partial estrogen deficiency induced by the use of DMPA.[95] The author of this case history observed

> Studies have shown that the estradiol levels of pre-menopausal women who have received this hormonal contraceptive for more than 1 year never reach those seen in the mid-cycle or luteal phase of the normal menstrual cycle. The estradiol levels are comparable only with those found in the early follicular phase. Women who use depot medroxyprogesterone acetate are in a state of partial estrogen deficiency, which may be associated with increased bone loss.[95]

Climacteric-related symptoms of mood changes may also be exacerbated by progestin-only contraceptive methods.

DMPA users may experience a lowering of their high-density lipoprotein levels and rises in total cholesterol and low-density lipoprotein levels.[96,97] Until this issue is resolved, it is wise to monitor lipid profiles on an annual basis.

Oral contraceptives offer a reasonable contraceptive choice for nonsmoking women older than 35 who are not at an increased risk for cardiovascular disease. The minipill is the oral contraceptive option for the smoking woman or the woman with contraindications for estrogen. In general, oral contraceptives appear to have less dramatic side effects than Norplant or DMPA and, unlike these methods, serve as a preventive measure against irregular, heavy, or anovulatory bleeding. They also protect against endometrial hyperplasia and neoplasia.

When should a woman discontinue use of these methods? A study consisting of three groups of women was conducted to establish the optimal way in which the end of a woman's fertility should be established.[98] One group was composed of postmenopausal women who had been on a long-term regimen of low-dose oral contraceptives consisting of three back-to-back packages of oral contraceptives, giving them 63 days on and 7 days off the pill. With this regimen, they had four to five menstrual periods each year. The other two groups consisted of premenopausal and perimenopausal women, all of whom took oral contraceptives as generally prescribed. The recommendations as a result of the findings of this study are to measure follicle-stimulating hormone (FSH) and estradiol during the week that the woman is off the oral contraceptives and again 2 weeks after the oral contraceptives have been discontinued. If estradiol levels are low and FSH levels are above 30 IU/L, it can be assumed that the woman is no longer fertile.

Because the average age of menopause is 51 years, it is reasonable for a woman to continue with oral contraception until 50 to 55 years of age. FSH, luteinizing hormone (LH), and estradiol levels should be tested approximately 3 months after discontinuing DMPA. If these levels are not in the menopausal range, a barrier or spermicidal contraceptive method should be used, and the tests should be repeated 6 to 12 months later.

Users of the minipill, Norplant, and DMPA should also consider discontinuing these methods between the ages of 50 and 55. It has not yet been determined at what point after discontinuing these methods a hormonal evaluation should be made. The best "guess estimate" is about 3 months after the methods have been discontinued.

During the time between discontinuation of the contraceptive method and determination of the end of fertility, a barrier and/or spermicidal or natural family planning method should be used. Although it is unlikely that ovulation will occur after initial results have revealed an elevation of FSH and LH, it has happened. It is prudent for a woman to use contraception until the second hormonal evaluation definitely confirms the end of fertility.

IMPORTANCE OF THE SEXUAL HISTORY AND SEXUALITY EDUCATION

DISCUSSING SEXUALITY

By taking a sexual history and educating your patients about issues related to sexuality and aging, you are acknowledging their sexuality and letting them know that you understand the importance of the emotional aspects of an intimate relationship. You are also showing support for their needs for closeness, love, companionship, and touching. You are confirming that affection, as it is expressed on an intimate level, may be extremely important to them.

Absence of a sexual partner can have a great impact on a woman's feelings about her sexuality. As a response to not having a sexual relationship, a woman may repress her sexual feelings because she feels that it is her only choice. Taking a sexual history and providing sexuality education can help a woman in this situation. It can validate her feelings and provide her the choice of pleasuring herself sexually—an option that some women may not explore without the "permission" of their health care provider.

> I am a 74-year-old widow and have this problem of touching myself, especially my breasts and nipples. I do this until I have an orgasm. I'm too ashamed to speak of this to anyone. Is there any way to stop?"[99]

> After reading about an older lady who masturbated, I got the courage to write for help. I'm too embarrassed to talk to my doctor about this. I'm in my late seventies and have been masturbating since my husband died nine years ago. Just lately, my body feels sore and there's a pressure there that feels as though I am going to urinate. After two days without masturbating, I feel fine. Am I hurting my body?"[99]

Discussing sexuality also provides an opportunity to address risk factors associated with sexually transmitted infections (STI) and to determine whether the woman is concerned about contracting an STI. Research in the area about how the rise in STIs and increased information in the media about human immunodeficiency virus (HIV) infections and women affects the sexual life of women over 40 is limited. However, it may be an area of great concern for some patients. It may also be the only reason some of your patients are abstinent.

A small survey of 268 obstetrician-gynecologists in the Washington, D.C., area revealed that they did not consistently assess patients' risk for HIV infection. They did not counsel patients on how to reduce this risk.[100] Felicia Guest, Deputy Director for Training at the Emory University AIDS Training Network in Atlanta, recommends that health care providers determine the questions to be asked during sexual history taking based on the population being served.[101] Health care providers should also recognize that their assumptions about their patients' sexual lives are not always correct and that discussing HIV during a sexual history may save the patient's life. Recommendations of questions to be asked while taking a sexual history are included in the Guidelines section of this book.

The sexual history interview, even if it involves asking only two or three primary questions, gives a woman permission to discuss sexual issues. This is particularly true if it is prefaced by an explanation abut why the questions are being asked: "It is common for persons to have questions or concerns about sexuality or experience a sexual problem. If this is true for you, I would like us to take some time to discuss these, so that I can be of help to you."

THE PLISSIT MODEL

The PLISSIT model of sexual counseling, developed by Anon and associates at the University of Hawaii, has been used for many years by health care professionals. It provides a framework by which to determine the appropriate intervention when addressing issues of sexuality with their patients.[102]

Permission giving (P) is the first component of the PLISSIT model. It assists health care professionals to respond to patients and to evaluate the levels at which they are able to assist their patients. Permission giving requires that the health care provider be at least somewhat comfortable with his or her own sexuality and have tolerance and understanding for the sexuality of others. It is the first level of therapeutic intervention in which the health care professional gives the patient permission to ask questions about sexuality, discuss sexual issues with partners and others close to them, and engage in or not engage in specific sexual behaviors. Because some persons need only to know that they are "okay," reassurance and permission from a source of authority for specific behaviors may all that the patient needs.

The second component of the PLISSIT model is limited information (LI), which includes providing facts and correcting misinformation. It requires that a health care provider maintain a current level of knowledge about sexual issues. It is also the component in which patients receive a list of materials or actual materials that provide information and reassurance about the concern or problem of the patient.

These first two components are usually the only two that are used by health care providers, because of lack of training in the field of sexuality or time constraints. These components are usually all that are needed to assist most patients.

If a patient is experiencing a more complex problem, the third component of PLISSIT, specific suggestions (SS), should be used. It is a way to provide an individualized response to a specific situation. It includes providing reference to written materials and referrals to other health care providers specifically trained to deal with sexual or other personal problems. Treatment for problems such as premature ejaculation, vaginismus, or orgasmic disorders is initiated by a therapist under this component of the PLISSIT model.

Through taking a sexual history and discussing issues with a patient, it may become evident that severe emotional or psychologic issues underlie the sexual problem. In this case, the patient is referred to a therapist who can provide intensive therapy (IT), which is the last component of the PLISSIT model.

TAKING A PSYCHOSOCIAL HISTORY

Exploration of the woman's attitude toward aging and menopause and her current life situation is as important as exploring sexual issues with her. It can provide invaluable information that may enable you and the woman to determine whether significant stressors exist in her life that are contributing to her symptoms. If this is the case, you can be instrumental in validating her feelings and suggesting that she talk with a counselor, social worker, or religious leader or join a support group. Often, just having other women to talk with, spiritual or professional guidance can be the best "medicine" a woman can receive at this time in her life.

The psychosocial and sexuality aspects associated with midlife and menopause are as important to address as the lifestyle factors of nutrition, exercise, and stress management. Each woman is unique and enters the perimenopausal and postmenopausal periods of her life with her own set of issues and perhaps problems that affect the way in which she views aging and the physiologic and psychologic changes that can result from a decline in hormone levels. A woman may enter her midlife years physically compromised from years of an abusive lifestyle and from familial and relationship problems. Perhaps she was sexually abused and has yet to deal with the trauma associated with the abuse. Women who enter the perimenopausal or postmenopausal time of their lives burdened with various issues that negatively affect their lives are more vulnerable than others to the physiologic and psychologic symptoms associated with menopause. Whatever a woman's health status and other issues are, the health care professional must explore them and be able to provide adequate support and referrals. It is only through a comprehensive approach to the health care of women that the greatest and most positive impact can be made on their physiologic and psychologic experience of the climacteric.

REFERENCES

1. Dennerstien L. Psychologic changes. In: Mishell D, ed. Menopause: physiology and pharmacology, 115. Chicago: Year Book Medical Publishers; 1987:115.
2. Davis P. A change for the better: a woman's guide through the menopause. Essex, UK: CW Daniel; 1993:3.
3. Utian WH. Pieter van Keep Memorial Lecture: menopause—a modern perspective from a controversial history. Maturitas 1997;26:73–82.
4. Millette B. Menopause: a survey of attitudes and knowledge. Issues Health Care Women 1982;3:263–276.
5. Deutch II. The psychology of women: motherhood. New York: Grune & Stratton; 1945:456–485.
6. Rhoades FP. Minimizing the menopause. Am Geriatr Soc 1967;15:346.
7. Severne L. Psychosocial aspects of the menopause. In: Haspels AA, Musap H, eds. Psychosomatics in peri-menopause. Lancaster, England: MTP Press; 1979:101.
8. Flint MP. Sociology and anthropology of the menopause. In: van Keep PA, Serr DM, eds. Female and male climacteric. Lancaster, UK: MTP Press; 1979:1–8.
9. Martin MC, et al. Menopause without symptoms: the endocrinology of menopause among rural Mayan Indians. Am J Obstet Gynecol 1993;6:1839–1845.
10. Greene JG. The cross-sectional legacy: an introduction to longitudinal studies of the climacteric. Maturitas 1992;14:95–101.
11. Neugarten B, Kraines R. Menopausal symptoms in women of various ages. Psychosom Med 1965;27:266–277.
12. Jaszmann L, et al. The perimenopausal symptoms: The statistical analysis of a survey. Med Gynaecol Soc 1969;4:268–277.

13. Rybo G, Westerberg H. Symptoms in the postmenopause: a population study. Acta Obstet Gynecol Scand 1972;9:25–26.

14. Thompson B, et al. Menopausal age and symptomatology in general practice. J Biosoc Sci 1973;5:71–82.

15. McKinlay S, Jefferys M. The menopause syndrome. Br J Prev Soc Med 1974;28:108–115.

16. Van Keep PA, Kellerhals J. The aging woman: about the influence of some social and cultural factors on the change in attitudes and behavior that occur during and after menopause. Acta Obstet Gynecol Scand Suppl 1975;51:17–27.

17. Ballinger CB. Psychiatric morbidity and the menopause: survey of a gynaecological outpatient clinic. Br J Psychol 1977;131:83–89.

18. Wood C. Menopausal myths. Med J Aust 1979;1:496–499.

19. Bungay G, et al. Study of symptoms in middle life with special reference to the menopause. BMJ 1980;281:181–183.

20. Greene JG, Cooke DJ. Life stress and symptoms at the climacteric. Br J Psychol 1980;136:486–491.

21. Kaufert P, Syrotuik U. Symptom reporting at the menopause. Soc Sci Med 1981;4:181–193.

22. Sharma VK, Saxena MSL. Climacteric symptoms: a study in the Indian context. Maturitas 1981;3:11–20.

23. Mikkelsen A, Holte A. A factor analytic study of climacteric symptoms. Psychiatry Soc Sci 1982;2:35–39.

24. Hunter M, et al. Relationships between psychological symptoms, somatic complaints and menopausal status. Maturitas 1986;8:217–228.

25. Oldenhave A. Hot flushes and their relation to other symptoms: results from the third Ede Study in the Netherlands. In: Abstracts of the Sixth International Congress on the Menopause; Bangkok, 1990. Carnforth: Parthenon; 1990:97.

26. Greene JG, Cooke DJ. Life stress and symptoms at the climacteric. Br J Psychol 1980;136:486–491.

27. Prill HJ. A study of the socio-medical relationships at the climacteric in 2,232 women. Curr Med Res Opin 1977;4:46–51.

28. Poli D, Larrocco S. Social and psychological correlates of menopausal symptoms. Psychosom Med 1980;42:335–345.

29. Campagnoli C, et al. Climacteric symptoms according to body weight in women of different socio-economic groups. Maturitas 1981;3:279–287.

30. Holte A, Mikkelsen A. Menstrual coping style social background and climacteric symptoms. Psychiatry Soc Sci 1982;2:41–45.

31. Abe T, Moritsuka T. A case-controlled study on climacteric symptoms and complaints of Japanese women by symptomatic type for psychological variables. Maturitas 1986;8:255–265.

32. Notman Malkah T. Psychiatric disorders of menopause. Psychiatric Ann 1984;14:448–453.

33. Lowenthal MF, et al. Four stages of life. San Francisco: Jossey-Bass; 1975.

34. Nicol-Smith L. Causality, menopause, and depression: a critical review of the literature. Clin Res Educ 1996;313:1229–1232.

35. Dennerstein L. Well-being, symptoms and the menopausal transition. Maturitas 1996;23:147–157.

36. Woods NF, Mitchell ES. Pathways to depressed mood for midlife women: observations from the Seattle Midlife Women's Health Study. Res Nurs Health 1997;20:207–213.

37. Bromberger JT, Mathews KA. A longitudinal study of the effects of pessimism, trait anxiety, and life stress on depressive symptoms in middle aged women. Psychol Aging 1996;11:207–213.

38. Bromberger JT, Mathews KA. A "feminine" model of vulnerability to depressive symptoms: a longitudinal investigation of middle-aged women. J Pers Soc Psychol 1996;70:591–598.

39. Hunter MS, Liao KL. A psychological analysis of menopausal hot flushes. Br J Clin Psychol 1995;34(Pt 4):589–599.

40. McEwen BS. Ovarian steroids have diverse effects on brain structure and functions. In: The modern management of the menopause: a perspective for the 21st century. Proceedings of the VII International Congress on the Menopause; Stockholm, 1993. New York: Parthenon; 1993.

41. MacLuskey NJ, McEwen BS. Progestin receptors in rat brain distribution and properties of cytoplasmic progestin-binding sites. Endocrinology 1980;106:192–202.

42. Pfaff D, Keiner D. Atlas of estradiol-concentrating cells in the central nervous system of the female rat. J Comp Neurol 1973;151:121–158.

43. Simerly RB, et al. Distribution of androgen and estrogen receptor mRNA-containing cells in the rat brain: an in situ hybridization study. J Comp Neurol 1990;294:76–95.

44. Heritage AS, et al. ³H-estradiol in catecholamine neurons or rat brainstem: combined localization by autoradiography and formaldehyde-induced fluorescence. J Comp Neurol 1978;176:607–630.

45. Tischkau SA, Ramirez VD. A specific membrane-binding protein for progesterone in rat brain: sex differences and induction by estrogen. Proc Natl Acad Sci USA 1993;90:1285–1289.

46. Smith SS. Hormones, mood and neurobiology: a summary. In: The modern management of the menopause: a perspective for the 21st century. Proceedings of the VII International Congress on the Menopause; Stockholm, 1993. New York: Parthenon; 1994.

47. Friedman RC. Behavior and the menstrual cycle. New York: Marcel Dekker; 1982.

48. Klaiber EL, et al. Estrogen therapy for severe persistent depression in women. Arch Gen Psychiatry 1979;36:550.

49. Zimmerman E, Parlee MB. Behavioral changes associated with the menstrual cycle: an experimental investigation. J Appl Soc Psychol 1973;3:335–344.

50. Seyle H. Correlations between the chemical structure and pharmacological actions of the steroids. Endocrinology 1942;30:437–453.

51. Holzbauer M. Physiological aspects of steroids with anesthetic properties. Med Biol 1976;54:227–242.

52. Bixo M, Backstrom T. Regional distribution of progesterone and 5-alpha-pregnane-3,20-dione in rat brain during progesterone-induced "anesthesia." Psychoneuroendocrinology 1990;15:159–162.

53. Carl P, et al. Pregnenolone emulsion: a preliminary pharmacokinetic and pharmacodynamic study of a new intravenous anesthetic agent. Anaesthesia 1990;45:189–197.

54. Backstrom T, Corstensen H. Estrogen and progesterone in plasma in relation to premenstrual tension. J Steroid Biochem 1974;5:257–260.

55. Coppen A, Shaw DM. Potentiation of the antidepressive effect of a monoamine oxidase inhibitor by tryptophan. Lancet 1963;1:79.

56. Geller E, et al. Preliminary observations on the effect of fenfluramine on blood serotonin and symptoms in three autistic boys. N Engl J Med 1982;307:165.
57. Hollander W, et al. Serotonin and antiserotonins. Circulation 1957;26:246.
58. Pollin W, et al. Effects of amino acid feedings in schizophrenic patients treated with iproniazid. Science 1961;133:104.
59. Schilldkraut JJ, Keet SS. Biogenic amines and emotions. Science 1961;133:104.
60. Smith B, Prockop DJ. Central-nervous-system effects of ingestion of L-tryptophan by normal subjects. N Engl J Med 1962;267:1338.
61. Stewart D, et al. Psychologic distress during menopause: associations across the reproductive life cycle. Int J Psychiatry Med 1993;23:157–162.
62. Abraham S, et al. Changes in Australian women's perception of the menopause and menopausal symptoms before and after the climacteric. Maturitas 1994;20:121–128.
63. Abraham GE. Nutritional factors in the etiology of the premenstrual tension syndromes. J Reprod Med 1983;29:446–464.
64. Boshes B, Arbit J. A controlled study of the effect of L-dopa on selected cognitive and behavioral functions. Trans Am Neurol Assoc 1970;55:59.
65. Olavson B, Jackson J. Psychosom Med 1987;49:65–78.
66. Lobo R, et al. Psychological stress and increases in urinary norepinephrine metabolites, platelet serotonin, and adrenal androgens in women with polycystic ovarian syndrome. Am J Obstet Gynecol 1983;15:496–503.
67. Woods NR, et al. J Hum Stress 1982;8:23–31.
68. Ballinger S. Stress as a factor in lowered estrogen levels in the early postmenopause. Ann N Y Acad Sci 1990;592:95–113.
69. Goleman D, Gurin J. Mind-body medicine. New York: Consumer Reports Books; 1993.
70. Weg RB. The physiological perspective. In: Weg RB, ed. Sexuality in the later years: roles and behavior. New York: Academic Press; 1983:4–80.
71. Edelman D. Sex in the golden years. New York: Donald I Fine; 1992:23.
72. Masters W, Johnson V. Human sexual response. Boston: Little, Brown; 1966.
73. Verwoerdt A, et al. Sexual behavior in senescence. In: Palmore E, ed. Normal aging: reports from Duke Longitudinal Study 1955–1969. Durham, NC: Duke University Press; 1970:282–299.
74. Janus S, Janus C. The Janus report on sexual behavior. New York: Wiley; 1993.
75. Dennerstein L, et al. Sexuality, hormones and the menopausal transition. Maturitas 1997;26:83–93.
76. Leiblum S, et al. Vaginal atrophy in the postmenopausal woman: the importance of sexual activity and hormones. JAMA 1983;249:2195–2198.
76a. Masters WH, Johnson VE. Human sexual response. Boston: Little, Brown; 1966.
77. Tsai CC, et al. Vaginal physiology in postmenopausal women: pH value transvaginal electropotential difference and estimated blood flow. South Med J 1987;80:987–990.
78. Barbach L. The pause. New York: Penguin Books; 1993.
79. Calhoun, et al. Sexual anxiety and female sexual arousal: a comparison of arousal during sexual anxiety stimuli and sexual pleasure stimuli. Arch Sex Behav 1987;16:311–319.
80. Burger HG, et al. The management of persistent menopausal symptoms with oestradiol-testosterone implants: clinical lipid and hormonal results. Maturitas 1984;6:351–358.

81. Cardozo L, et al. The effects of subcutaneous hormone implants during the climacteric. Maturitas 1984;5:177–184.

82. Zussman L, et al. Sexual response after hysterectomy-oophorectomy: recent studies and reconsideration of psychogenesis. Am J Obstet Gynecol 1981;140:725–729.

83. Kilkku P, et al. Supravaginal uterine amputation vs hysterectomy: effects on libido and orgasm. Acta Obstet Gynecol Scand 1986;62:147–152.

84. Sloan D. The emotional and psychosexual aspects of hysterectomy. Am J Obstet Gynecol 1978;1312:598–605.

85. Craig GA, Jackson P. Sexual life after vaginal hysterectomy. BMJ 1975;3:97.

86. Francis WJ, Jeffsoate TN. Dyspareunia following vaginal operations. J Obstet Gynaecol Br Commun 1961;68:1–10.

87. Amias AG. Sexual life gynaecological operations–II. BMJ 1975;2:680–681.

88. Parker W. A gynecologist's second opinion. New York: Plume Book; 1996.

89. Kirchengast S, et al. Decreased sexual interest ant its relationship to body build in postmenopausal women. Maturitas 1996;23:63–71.

90. Murstein BI. Love, sex, and marriage. New York: Springer; 1974:253.

91. Reinisch J, Beasley MLS. The Kinsey Institute new report on sex. New York: St Martin's Press; 1991.

92. Herman R. Why sex research ignores women. Glamour 1994;June:202.

93. Synderman N. Dr. Nancy Synderman's guide to good health. New York: William Morrow; 1996:217.

94. Cundy T, et al. Bone density in women receiving depot medroxyprogesterone acetate for contraception. BMJ 1991;308:247.

95. Mark S. Premenopausal bone loss and depot medroxyprogesterone acetate administration. Int J Gynecol Obstet 1994;47:260–272.

96. Fahmy K, et al. Effect of long-acting progestogen-only injectable contraceptives on carbohydrate metabolism and its hormonal profile. Contraception 1991;44:419.

97. Enk L, et al. A prospective one-year study on the effects of two long acting injectable contraceptives (depo medroxyprogesterone acetate and norethisterone oenanthate) on serum and lipoprotein lipids. Horm Metab Res 1992;24:85.

98. Castracane DV, et al. When it is safe to switch from oral contraceptives to hormonal replacement therapy? Contraception 1995;52:371–376.

99. Reinisch J. The Kinsey Institute new report on sex. New York: St. Martin's Press; 1990:228–229.

100. Boekloo BO, et al. Knowledge, attitudes, and practices of obstetrician/gynecologists regarding the prevention of human immunodeficiency virus infection. Obstet Gynecol 1993;81:131–136.

101. Contraceptive technology update. STD Q 1993;Dec:181.

102. Anon JS. The behavorial treatment of sexual problems: brief therapy. New York: Harper & Row; 1976.

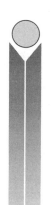

CHAPTER 6

A Total Wellness Program for Women

Chapter 5 discussed the psychosocial and sexual issues related to the climacteric, emphasized the relationship between stressors and symptoms, and discussed some of the potential effects of stressors on the immune and endocrine systems and on steroid secretion. Chapters 3 and 4 focused on some of the research that has demonstrated the vital role that the three lifestyle factors—proper nutrition, adequate exercise, and stress reduction—play in the prevention and treatment of osteoporosis, coronary artery disease, and other chronic diseases. This chapter provides specific recommendations about nutrition, exercise, and stress reduction for women 30 years of age and older. These recommendations form the foundation for a total wellness program for women and are summarized in the Guidelines section.

These recommendations are essential for women's health for two reasons. First, dietary habits of Americans have strongly been implicated in contributing a health care crisis in which 75% of American deaths are caused by chronic diseases.[1] Research continues to demonstrate that most disease is a consequence of environmental and lifestyle factors, including poor nutrition, chemical pollution, smoking, excessive drinking, chronic depression, stressful working conditions, drug use, lack of exercise, and overeating. Second, there is no form of hormone replacement therapy (HRT), medication, or nutrient that can compensate for a disease-promoting lifestyle. You may have already experienced the situation in which a patient has been using HRT for several years but still experiences an osteoporotic fracture, or you may have a patient who has been on HRT for several years and experiences a heart attack.

No single treatment or particular lifestyle change can guarantee a 100% recovery from or prevention of disease, but we can help patients to maximize the possibility that they will not fall victim to debilitating osteoporosis, heart disease, or other chronic degenerative diseases. We do this by educating them about the absolute necessity of following specific lifestyle recommendations.

Based on a review of data from numerous studies, the following estimates have been made of the causes of death and disease in the United States[2]:

- Stress level and attitude: 25%
- Nutrition related: 25%
- Pollution: 11%
- Poor hygiene and poor medical care: 10%
- Sedentary lifestyle: 10%
- Infectious diseases: 3%
- Genetics: 3%
- Accidents: 2%
- Other factors: 11%

NUTRITION

Nutrition is essential to life, and good nutrition is essential to good health.[1] About 20 years after President Lincoln formed the United States Department of Agriculture (USDA), it began to develop nutritional standards for the American public.[3] The USDA released the first tables of food composition and dietary standards, as developed by W. O. Atwater, a pioneer nutrition investigator and first director of the Office of Experiment Stations in the USDA.[3] In 1902, he stated,

> Unless care is exercised in selecting food, a diet may result which is one-sided or badly balanced—that is, one in which either protein or fuel ingredients (carbohydrate and fat) are provided in excess.... The evils of overeating may not be felt at once, but sooner or later they are sure to appear—perhaps in an excessive amount of fatty tissue, perhaps in general disability, perhaps in actual disease.[4]

Atwater was progressive in his thinking, and since his time, the USDA has continued to modify its dietary recommendations, published as food guides. These have taken the form of the "Basic Seven" food guide issued as a leaflet, "National Wartime Nutrition Guide," the "Basic Four," and the "Basic Five" food guide. They all focused on recommending a minimum number of servings from different food groups, and they were the standards for nutritional intake in the United States for many years.

It became obvious that the food guides were inadequate as research began to document the association between nutritional intake and the rise in chronic degenerative diseases in the United States, other Western nations, and areas of other countries in which nutritional patterns changed to ones similar to the Western diet. From the 1970s through the 1980s, various surveys revealed that the nutritional status of Americans continued to be inadequate.[5-7] In one of the studies, only 3% of the 20,749 study subjects were free of the 48 most common symptoms of malnutrition.[8] Americans of all income groups were found to be deficient in several nutrients[2]:

- Vitamins: A, E, D, C, thiamine, riboflavin, pyridoxine, and folic and pantothenic acids
- Minerals: calcium, potassium, magnesium, zinc, iron, copper, chromium, fluoride, and selenium
- Macronutrients: protein, complex carbohydrates, fiber, polyunsaturated fats, and clean water
- Quasinutrients: bioflavonoids, carnitine, eicosapentaenoic acid (EPA), taurine, coenzyme Q10, and lipoic acid

American diets commonly contained excessive amounts of several items:

- Calories, usually from excess carbohydrates, fat, protein, or alcohol
- Fats: saturated, hydrogenated, and cholesterol
- Phosphorus from meats, soft drinks, and processed foods
- Sodium
- Sugar
- Alcohol
- Caffeine

Research findings of this unacceptable nutritional status of Americans, combined with the rise in chronic diseases, forced the scrutiny of dietary recommendations. The Senate Committee on Nutrition and Human Needs issued its 1977 report, "Dietary Goals for the United States."[9] It proposed specific recommendations for consumption of all foods that were significantly different from the "Basic

Five" food guide. For example, emphasis was placed on decreasing intake of protein (particularly in the form of red meat) and milk products and increasing intake of grains, fruits, and vegetables.

Since the release of this report, the National Institutes of Health, the Food and Drug Administration (FDA), the Centers for Disease Control, and the Department of Health and Human Services undertook the task of comprehensively reviewing scientific studies related to diet and health. In 1990, they initiated a vigorous national crusade for health promotion and disease prevention along with the publication of *Healthy People 2000: National Health Promotion and Disease Prevention Objectives*. *Healthy People 2000* is a statement of national opportunities, emphasizing individual control over one's own health destiny. "Personal responsibility, which is to say, responsible and enlightened behavior by each and every individual, truly is the key to good health."[9]

The objectives of *Healthy People 2000* set the stage for establishment of a national strategy for the improvement of the health status and quality of life for Americans. Emphasis has been placed on behavioral and environmental changes needed to reduce risks of chronic diseases, and nutrition, diet, and physical activity have been addressed as some of the priorities for this national health agenda.

AGGRESSIVE APPROACH TO PROPER NUTRITION

Over the years, the media have supplied the public many of the updated recommendations (eg, reduction of fat and cholesterol-laden foods) that are a part of the Surgeon General's *Healthy People 2000* objectives. Educational materials supplied by health care professionals, programs in hospitals, and health management organizations have offered recommendations in the areas of nutrition, exercise, and stress reduction. However, a more aggressive approach is needed for women to understand that it is not through hormones or drugs but through *actions related to their lifestyles* that the greatest impact can be made on prevention and treatment of the diseases and symptoms about which they are most concerned.

Various sources, including the National Center for Health Statistics, Centers for Disease Control and Prevention, the FDA's Food Label and Package Survey, the National Restaurant Association's Survey of Chain Operators, and the U.S. Department of Agriculture's food consumption surveys, provide the good health information. However, even though dietary information is being discussed more today, Americans are still not doing a good job of integrating changes essential to their health.

The number of overweight persons is increasing, and the number engaging in appropriate weight loss practices is decreasing.[10] The prevalence of overweight among adults has increased from 26% to 34%, suggesting that 1 of 3 adults is overweight. More women between the ages of 20 and 54, compared with men in this age group, are overweight. However, the reverse is true for women between the ages of 55 to 74. It also appears from preliminary data that the incidence of overweight adolescents is on the rise.

These estimates translate into approximately 26 million overweight men and 32 million overweight women. This is of great concern because excessive body fat is a major contributor to coronary artery disease and other health problems. There has been only a slight reduction in the average intake of total fat and saturated fat as a percentage of calories for persons 2 years of age and older compared with the baseline established using data from the late 1970s. Only about 1 of 5 persons 2 years or older consumed 30% or fewer calories from total fat. The same proportion consumed less than 10% of calories from saturated fat. More than two thirds of Americans 20 years of age or older and most children and adolescents do not consume five or more servings of fruits and vegetables each day.

Nutritional deficiencies are recognized as a major health care problem in the United States. A few definitions associated with any significant deviation from the proper intake and use of nutrients (forms of malnutrition) is useful in discussing these problems.[1] The deviations are divided into the following categories:

- Critical: threat of death from extreme malnutrition (eg, kwashiorkor in children, arrhythmias from zinc or essential fatty acid deficiencies)
- Clinical: deficiency in which observable symptoms result
- Subclinical: long-term deterioration resulting from insufficient intake in one or more nutrients that is not immediately observable during an examination
- Marginal: lack of well-being or behavioral changes (eg, tiredness, anxiety, depression) caused by an imbalance of nutrients but that may not be observable except in controlled conditions

MALNUTRITION OF PATIENTS

Given what is now known about the nutritional habits of most Americans and the nutritional factors that contribute to coronary artery disease, osteoporosis, diabetes, and other chronic degenerative diseases, you should consider that many of the women for whom you provide care enter their climacteric transition vulnerable to osteoporosis and coronary artery and other diseases in part because they are marginally, subclinically, or even clinically deficient in a few or many nutrients. This vulnerability may be increased more in women than in men because women are more likely to spend years following various weight reduction diets that are typically deficient in nutrients. When this vulnerability is combined with the vulnerability that results from a decline in steroids, it is clear that a health program for women must have as its foundation a strong, comprehensive nutritional component.

Homocysteine is a major factor in coronary artery disease (see Chapter 3), and it can be easily and inexpensively managed through adequate diet and supplementation of folic acid and other B vitamins. If a woman approaches menopause deficient in these vitamins, her homocysteine level may be such that some damage to her coronary arteries has already taken place. Because some research has suggested that estrogen helps keep homocysteine levels in check, her vulnerability to developing coronary artery disease after menopause can be a result of the decline in estrogen levels and of specific nutritional deficiencies and excesses.

NUTRITIONAL GUIDELINES FOR WOMEN OLDER THAN 30 YEARS

In 1990, the USDA developed new guidelines that integrated the findings of two major reviews of the scientific literature on diet and health, the *Surgeon General's Report on Nutrition and Health* and *Diet and Health Implications for Reducing Chronic Disease Risk* from the National Research Council of the National Academy of Sciences.[11] These guidelines, called the *Eating Right Food Guide Pyramid,* focus on preventing disease caused by nutritional imbalances (Fig. 6-1). The Pyramid was developed to be followed by healthy men, women, and children.

The Pyramid was published in the *Washington Post* on April 13, 1992, but 12 days after the release of the article, the Secretary of Agri-

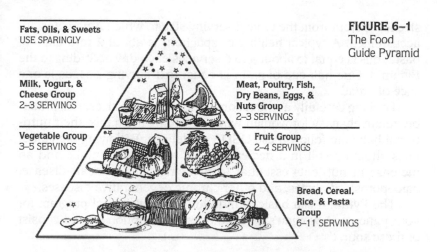

FIGURE 6-1
The Food
Guide Pyramid

Fats, Oils, & Sweets
USE SPARINGLY

Milk, Yogurt, &
Cheese Group
2–3 SERVINGS

Meat, Poultry, Fish,
Dry Beans, Eggs, &
Nuts Group
2–3 SERVINGS

Vegetable Group
3–5 SERVINGS

Fruit Group
2–4 SERVINGS

Bread, Cereal,
Rice, & Pasta
Group
6–11 SERVINGS

culture stopped distribution of the Pyramid. Some think this was a direct result of pressure by the cattle and milk lobbies. However, given the increasing numbers of Americans suffering from diseases directly linked to obesity, excessive fat intake, and inadequate intake of essential vitamins and minerals, the health of Americans took precedence, and the USDA later reaffirmed the value and necessity of its Pyramid.

The top tier of the Pyramid includes only a narrow space relegated to meat and dairy products, because the new guidelines include a minimal intake of meats, cream sauces, and cheese. The lower and larger tiers are relegated to grains, vegetables, and fruit groups in numbers of servings significantly greater than what had appeared in the earlier "Basic 5 Food Group." Many grains, vegetables, and fruits contain *phytohormones*, compounds whose effects are only beginning to be appreciated in the prevention and treatment of heart disease, cancer, osteoporosis, and symptoms associated with the climacteric.

The revised USDA guidelines place more emphasis on the grains, vegetables, and fruits groups, and they recommend sizes and number of servings, which translates into a decrease in the number and size of portions, resulting in decreased caloric intake. The guidelines direct consumers to eat less of the foods with little nutritional value and to eat more of the foods with great nutritional value.

If one of your patients looked at the number of serving sizes recommended by the USDA, her reaction might be, "I could never eat that amount of food in 1 day!" However, the recommended serving size is different from the typical serving size to which Americans are accustomed. A typical helping of spaghetti is about 2 to 3 cups of pasta; this is equal to about 4 to 6 servings each day according to the Pyramid. One-half cup of grain is equal to 1 serving size, as is one slice of bread.

Looking carefully at the recommended serving sizes, it is probably relatively easy for women who are willing to change their nutritional habits to follow these USDA guidelines. Following the guidelines should result in a decrease in fat and caloric intake and an increase in nutrients essential to reducing obesity, heart disease, osteoporosis, diabetes, and other chronic degenerative diseases.

The Pyramid is a basic foundation of a nutritional program for your patients. A woman's daily calorie consumption should consist of these sources:

- Between 50% and 60% from complex carbohydrates such as grains, beans, vegetables, and fruits, consumed for nutrients and fiber (fiber intake should be 20 to 30 g/day)
- Between 20% and 30% from protein
- Between 20% and 30% from total fats; less than 10% from saturated fats, and less than 300 mg cholesterol

These recommendations translate into the following nutritional program:

- Between 6 and 11 daily servings of bread, cereal, rice, and pasta (1 serving is one slice of bread or 0.5 cup of grain or pasta)
- Between 2 and 3 servings (1 to 1.5 cups) of vegetables, preferably fresh
- Between 3 and 5 servings of fruit, preferably fresh; (1 serving is one medium piece of fruit, 0.5 cup of cut fruit, or 0.75 cup of unsweetened fruit juice)
- Between 2 and 4 servings from milk, yogurt, cheese group (1 cup of milk, 8 ounces of yogurt, or 1 to 2 ounces of cheese; low-fat varieties should be used)
- Between 2 and 3 servings of lean meat, poultry (without the skin), fish, legumes, eggs and nuts; some nutritionists recommend that an easy way to deal with these servings is to recommend 7 to 8 ounces of protein over the course of each day (ie, a serving of lean meat is about 2 to 3 ounces, and a 0.5 cup of cooked beans is about 1 ounce; an egg or 10 nuts constitute 1 serving)
- Fats, oils, and sugars should be used sparingly

A woman who is overweight may consider reducing her carbohydrate intake to 40% to 50% of her total dietary intake. A woman who is physically active on a regular basis should probably increase her protein intake to 30% of her total dietary intake each day while maintaining a carbohydrate intake of 40%.

Protein consumption through the intake of red meats should be limited for several reasons. Red meat has 20 times more phosphorus than calcium, which results in an imbalance in the calcium-phosphorus ratio. Red meats also cause calcium excretion to be promoted by stimulating release of the parathyroid hormone, and they contribute to a rise in the homocysteine level.

The Pyramid does not include recommendations for daily caloric intake. However, if an individual carefully follows the recommended number of daily servings and serving sizes, which means a substantial reduction in fat intake for most persons, excessive caloric intake is avoided, and total body fat is reduced.

The recommendations of the Pyramid include 30% of all calories from fat. However, a woman who has heart disease, hypertension, elevated cholesterol and triglyceride levels, or abnormal ratio of low-density and high-density lipoproteins (LDL-HDL ratio) or who has lived a lifestyle or has a family history that puts her into a high-risk category for heart disease should consider decreasing her fat intake to 15% to 20% of her daily calories.[12] There is debate about whether reducing fat intake below 15% is healthy for most, because it may not provide an adequate amount of the essential fatty acids.[13]

These basic nutritional guidelines are compatible with the American Heart Association's Step I Diet for those who do not have heart disease. The Association's recommendations are

- A cholesterol intake of less than 300 mg each day
- A total fat intake not to exceed 30% of total calories, with approximately 10% each contributed by saturated, monounsaturated, and polyunsaturated fats

A basic nutritional program must also maintain a low intake of caffeine, sugar, sodium (not to exceed 2500 mg per day or the equivalent of 1 to 1.5 teaspoons)[14] and phosphorus-laden beverages and foods, and alcoholic beverages. Some women find significant to total relief from hot flushes just by eliminating caffeine and alcohol from their diet; the elimination of spicy and hot (temperature) foods and beverages can also help to reduce hot flushes. The intake of *trans*-fatty acids must be kept low. These compounds are found in margarines, shortenings, convenience foods, and oils made from partially hydrogenated vegetable oils.

Trans-fatty acids have been implicated in increasing levels of cholesterol, LDL, lipoprotein (a), and triglycerides (see Chapter 3) and in decreasing levels LDL; therefore, *trans*-fatty acids has been associated with coronary heart disease. Because Americans ingest approximately 4 to 7 g of these fatty acids through margarine and processed foods containing partially hydrogenated vegetable oils, it is believed that the number of deaths attributable to the consumption of these food products is probably substantial.[13]

Oils should be monounsaturated and unrefined oils, such as canola and olive oils. Virgin unrefined olive oil is a good choice for several reasons; it contains beta-carotene, vitamin E, magnesium, and phytosterols. These and several other components have been linked to stimulation of the flow of bile, protection against peroxidation of fatty acids and cholesterol, and stimulation of fat-digesting enzymes in the pancreas.[13]

Women should be encouraged to consume eight 8-ounce glasses of water each day to maximize transport of nutrients, hormones, and oxygen to the cells and prevent kidney stones, particularly because high levels of dietary and supplemental calcium are encouraged. An adequate intake of water is necessary to maintain the high urine volume needed to minimize development of kidney stones.

Foods should be eaten in as close to their natural state as possible to minimize loss of nutrients. This means consuming fresh vegetables, raw or lightly steamed, and whole fresh fruits (eg, an apple instead of applesauce). This also means avoiding canned and frozen foods, because they contain fewer nutrients than fresh sources and contain food additives such as salt, sugar, fat, and preservatives.

A variety of foods should be eaten to maximize nutrient intake. Small, frequent meals may be a better way to eat to maintain blood glucose levels, which can contribute to a relatively constant state of mental and physical levels of energy. Maintenance of blood glucose levels can also decrease cravings and assist in appetite control.

PHYTOESTROGENS

"Phytoestrogens are not like vitamins—something you can buy in pill form and take in measured quantities. They remain mysterious for the moment—part of the emerging and encouraging picture of how plant foods can prolong life and fight disease."[15] A woman would be well advised to add *soy products* to her diet. For many centuries, soybeans have played an integral part in Asian diets and medicine. They are best known for their protein content in the West, but increasingly foods made from soy are becoming known for their potential roles in the prevention and treatment of chronic disease, most notably cancer and heart disease. Soy foods also may help prevent osteoporosis and kidney disease and thereby have a significant beneficial impact on public health.[16] Soy foods can be incorporated into the diet through the use of soy flour or soy milk or through modern soy protein products such as soy isolates and concentrates.

The database on soy products and the effects of soy intake has been expanding. Since 1994, *The International Symposium on the Role of Soy in Preventing and Treating Chronic Disease* has been convened annually by members of scientific communities throughout the world.

Two of the many compounds found in abundance in soy and flax seed (and to a lesser degree in many fruits, vegetables, and grains) that have generated interest in the medical community are phytoestrogens, isoflavones and lignans. These estrogen-like compounds are structurally similar to estrogen. They appear to have antiestrogenic effects through competitively binding to estrogen receptors, thereby diminishing the binding of stronger endogenous estrogens.[17] Soy may work in the same way as tamoxifen.[18]

This effect may explain why Japanese women, whose diets contain substantial amounts of soy, have a decreased incidence of breast cancer and hot flushes compared with women whose diets are not rich in soy products. Japanese women tend to have 15 to 20 times more circulating phytoestrogens than American women. A group of American women who ate soy rarely or never were compared with those who ate soy sometimes or often.[19] The women who consumed the most soy were nearly 1.5 times more likely to be in the low-symptom group.

Genistein, a form of isoflavone, appears to be a powerful antioxidant. The National Cancer Institute is studying the potential of purified genistein as an anticancer drug. Investigation of the effects of genistein and several other food and herb-derived plant estrogens has shown that high concentrations of genistein markedly inhibits cell proliferation without blocking induction of estrogen-specific gene products.[20] This supports the view that genistein acts as a surrogate estrogen to prevent common diseases and symptoms associated with estrogen deficiency among Asian women who consume a high-soy and low-fat diet. It also suggests that high concentrations of genistein can act as an estrogen agonist, without the harmful side effects of promoting the growth of estrogen-sensitive tumors. Mark Messina, a former program director in the Diet and Cancer branch of the National Cancer Institute, said, "I'd bet good money soy protein will become a widely accepted alternative to estrogen replacement therapy within the next few years."[21]

In 1946, the sheep industry in Southwest Australia was nearly decimated as a result of a mysterious outbreak in infertility among the sheep. It was discovered that the cause of the infertility was the phytoestrogen-rich clover on which the sheep grazed.

A few decades later, a new phytoestrogen, *equol,* was identified in the urine of persons who ate soy foods. This phytoestrogen was of particular interest to researchers because it was found to be structurally similar to estradiol.[22] In a later study, low levels of equol were found in women with breast cancer compared with the levels in cancer-free women.[23] Women who consume a diet rich in phytoestrogens have been shown to have circulating concentrations of these compounds that exceed the range of endogenous estrogens by 100-fold to 1000-fold.[24] Research at Tufts is underway to investigate the effects of soy on vaginal cells and whether eating soy can reduce postmenopausal hot flushes and night sweats.

Much evidence suggests that diets containing large amounts of soybean products are associated with overall low cancer mortality rates, particularly for cancers of the colon, breast, and prostate. A diet rich in soy may slow the growth of malignant prostatic cancers.[25] It appears that genistein converts malignant cells into nonmalignant cells and inhibits key tumor-producing enzymes. Other components of soy may inhibit growth of blood vessels that nourish tumors. Some of the soy-derived compounds, in addition to the ones mentioned, that may reduce cancer mortality rates include a protease inhibitor, phytic acid; the sterol beta-sitosterol; saponins; and soybean trypsin inhibitor.[26]

Soy may decrease the atherosclerotic process.[27] Eighty-eight postmenopausal monkeys with diet-induced coronary artery arteriosclerosis were followed for 30 months. During this time, some of the monkeys were treated with conjugated equine estrogen and a soy-rich and effective lipid-lowering diet; others were treated with estrogen, medroxyprogesterone acetate, and the same diet; still others were treated only through diet. The results showed that, although preexisting coronary artery plaques were not affected by any of the therapies, the lumen of the coronary arteries increased with all three forms of intervention. The magnitude of the change in the group receiving dietary management alone was as great as that in the group receiving hormones in combination with the same dietary management. In the group of monkeys treated by diet alone, total plasma cholesterol concentrations decreased and HDL levels increased. Studies to determine the value of dietary estrogens in the prevention of postmenopausal coronary artery disease in humans are underway.

Subjects with elevated cholesterol who replaced animal protein with soy protein showed an average of 21% reduction in total cholesterol after following this dietary program for 3 weeks.[28] Subjects consuming 50 g of soy protein in combination with a low-fat (less than 30%/day) and low-cholesterol (less than 300 mg/day) diet had a 12% drop in cholesterol and an 11.5% drop in LDL levels.[29] This group found that, of all the dietary protocols, the isolated soy protein worked the best. The researchers concluded, "Based on this study, the fact that a significant reduction was obtained by consuming only 50 g of soy protein each day sets a practical and achievable goal that would be beneficial in the treatment and prevention of high blood cholesterol and coronary artery disease." A meta-analysis of 38 studies indicated that consumption of soy protein is associated with significant decrease in serum cholesterol, LDL, and triglyceride levels and a nonsignificant increase in HDL.[30]

Soy has also been studied for its effect on the menstrual cycle. When 60 g of soy protein containing 45 mg of isoflavones was taken for 1 month by six premenopausal women with regular ovulatory cycles, the follicular phase length was significantly increased, and cholesterol concentrations decreased 9.6%.[31]

Women who had a hysterectomy and were using transdermal estrogen replacement therapy were asked to ingest 50 g of textured soy protein each day. Maximum peaks of luteinizing hormone were mildly suppressed, suggesting an antiestrogenic effect of the phytoestrogens in soy.[32]

Soy contains phytoestrogens, which can have estrogenic or antiestrogen activity, and contains several other vital nutrients. Just 1 cup of boiled soybeans contains 28 g of protein, adequate zinc and B vitamins, and one half of a day's supply of iron plus 6 g of fiber. Four ounces of firm tofu made with calcium sulfate contains 258 mg of calcium. The fat in soy does not contain cholesterol and is very low in saturated fat.

How much soy should a woman consume on a daily basis? It appears that about 13 mg per day, or the amount in a glass of soy milk or 0.5 cup of firm tofu may be enough to substantially lessen the risk for cancer. About 25 mg of soy protein could significantly lower cholesterol. The amount to be taken as a substitute for HRT (if this proves to be a viable alternative) is unknown.

In a yet unpublished study at Bowman Gray School of Medicine, 43 women between the ages of 45 and 55 who were experiencing hot flushes or night sweats on a regular basis were recruited to consume 20 g of soy protein powder each day for 6 weeks. Frequency of the symptoms remained the same, although the severity significantly decreased. In a conversation with Dr. Burke, investigator of the study, he pointed out that the amount of soy a woman should take to decrease her symptoms is unclear, as is the duration of time she should take it. A 2-year study of a larger sample is being initiated to determine if soy protein offers the same benefits of HRT.

Women who are research volunteers at the University of Illinois agreed to add 40 g of soy protein each day to their diet for 6 months by consuming soy-laced meals, soy beverages, and soy snacks.[21,33] One study veteran's cholesterol decreased from 255 to 205 over 6 months. Bone density increased by 2.2%. This is a substantial increase, considering women loose 2% to 3% of total bone in the first few years after menopause without any form of intervention. The increase in bone density is also similar to that found in some studies published about increases in bone density with HRT. Forty grams of soy protein may be a reasonable recommendation. There are numerous soy products on the market, and patients can purchase one of the many flavorless isolated soy protein powders (2 tablespoons usually provides 13 g of soy protein) which can be mixed in a variety of foods, juice, or soup.

It is important that women who increase their soy intake know that they are consuming a major source of protein and make the necessary dietary changes so that their diet does not include an excess amount of protein. The nice thing about soy protein is that calcium excretion is about one half that occurring in animal protein—one more reason for women to consider incorporating soy into their total wellness program.

QUALITY COUNTS

There are soy burgers, hot dogs, shakes, ice cream, protein powders, milks, and tofu, to mention only a few of the soy-based products that have entered the market. Many of these contain some genistein and other isoflavones, but they may not contain equal or even adequate amounts of isoflavones. When some brands of tofu were compared with a commercially available soy drink, tofu contained 10 times the amount of genestein as the soy drink.[33]

If women want to use soy protein powder, it is probably best if they contact the companies that produce soy protein powders used by investigators conducting research on the effects of soy. In a conversation with one of the investigators, the issue of the quality of soy products was discussed. He stated that to ensure quality control, a company was identified for their research whose soy beans were grown under acceptable conditions, processed well, and contained an adequate amount of genistein. The number of this company and other ones used by different investigators is included in the Resource section of the book.

EXPANDING THE BASIC NUTRITIONAL GUIDELINES

A woman following the Pyramid recommendations is not guaranteed an adequate amount of the nutrients needed to ward of osteoporosis and other chronic degenerative diseases. The food she is eating needs to be grown in nutrient-rich soil and be unprocessed. The soil in which nonorganically grown foods are raised is often mineral deficient (see Chapter 4). For the past several decades, farm land in America has been fertilized with only three or four nutrients. This is considered to be one of the causes of inadequate nutritional intake and the need for supplementation.[2] Food grown in nutrient-rich soil and pesticide-free conditions (ie, organically grown) is not always conveniently available and often not affordable for many.

The woman also needs to minimize loss of nutrients through appropriate preparation and cooking methods. Chopping, dicing, slicing, and frying are forms of processing that deplete nutrients in food. Her body would have to be able to absorb most nutrients from the foods she eats—often a problem for women as they become older or because a history of a poor diet can compromise the functioning of the gastrointestinal tract, resulting in the inability to fully absorb and use nutrients. She would have to be in an environment that is free of chronic, negative stressors so that her need for nutrients, beyond what can be guaranteed through the Pyramid, would not be increased. She would have to be free of illness or disease and not be using any form of medication and not having undergone a surgical procedure—factors that increase the body's needs for different nutrients.

An undetermined number of persons are born with metabolic errors that cause their nutritional needs to be expanded. Because of this and other factors, women vary in their nutrient needs throughout their lifetimes (eg, in times of stress, illness, or surgery). Because of all these factors, it is important to address the issue of nutritional supplementation.

RECOMMENDED DIETARY ALLOWANCES

The basis for development of the recommended dietary allowances (RDAs) was concern about the adequacy of food supplies during World War II, and their use today as a guide for an individual's nutritional needs has been widely criticized:

> It is time scientists, nutritionists, and food manufacturers stopped all the silliness about the RDAs. They have nothing to do with the nutritional status of an individual. They are intended for use in estimating the adequacy of food supplies for the whole population as a unit, to prevent the occurrence of certain deficiency diseases.[34]

Members of the Food and Nutrition Board of the National Academy of Sciences[1] develop RDAs by extrapolating data from animal studies on single-nutrient deficiencies and through research conducted on average healthy persons who are deprived of a nutrient and experience deficiency symptoms. These persons are then given the nutrient until a minimum is reached at which the clinical signs of the deficiency are no longer experienced. After this step, an average requirement of each nutrient is estimated, which is then calibrated across sex groups and 17 different age and weight groups. The end result is the RDA per day for each nutrient about which sufficient information is available. According to the Food and Nutrition Board,[35]

- RDAs should not be confused with requirements for a specific individual.
- Special needs for nutrients are not covered by the RDAs.
- RDAs should be applied to population groups rather than individuals.

Alfred E. Harper, Chairman of the Food and Nutrition Board, writes that the RDAs "are not guidelines for formulating diets nor for assessing the nutritional status of individuals."[36] The RDAs do not take into account all factors that affect the amount of nutrients found in foods, an individual's ability to absorb nutrients from foods, or the factors that increase a individual needs for nutrients. They do not take into account that, for many, a highly nutritious diet of fresh whole foods, prepared in a manner that reduces loss of nutrients, is not feasible because of factors such as availability of various foods in different areas of the country, cost, and cultural factors that may determine dietary habits.

The need for increased intake of some of the B vitamins and antioxidants essential for prevention and reduction of the arteriosclerotic process has not been factored into the RDAs, nor have variations in lifestyle. The RDAs do not address the levels of certain nutrients that can decrease hot flushes, fatigue, breast tenderness, and other symptoms associated with the climacteric. A strong case can be made for the necessity of nutrient supplementation for restoring and maintaining health; preventing osteoporosis, coronary artery disease, and other chronic diseases; and treating specific climacteric-related symptoms.

NUTRITIONAL SUPPLEMENTATION

Nutrients work as a team in all functions, including digestion, absorption, and use of other nutrients. It is almost impossible for a person to lack one nutrient with all of the others being adequately supplied. For example, an excess of calcium or phosphorus interferes with the absorption of both minerals, and excretion of the lesser mineral is increased.[36] An excess of magnesium upsets calcium metabolism, and a deficiency in magnesium inhibits calcium absorption. Zinc deficiency prevents transport of vitamin A to the cells.[37] Therefore, recommendations for supplements must reflect the interdependency of nutrients and must minimize the possibility of contributing to a nutrient imbalance.

MINERAL SUPPLEMENTATION

Chewing on Tums or taking a calcium-only supplement at night is not going to do it! Recommendations regarding supplementation of calcium and other minerals are highly controversial. Should a peri-menopausal woman supplement with 1000 mg of calcium and a postmenopausal women supplement with 1500 mg? What about magnesium? Should the ratio of calcium to magnesium be 2:1 or 1:1?

The National Institutes of Health recommends that the amounts of calcium previously given should be a person's total daily intake, ideally obtained through foods. If these daily requirements are not met through diet, supplementation is necessary to maintain bone health and prevent osteoporosis.[37]

The median intake of calcium among American women is only about 600 mg per day, and 25% of women consume less than 400 mg per day.[38] The median intake of magnesium among American women is only about 300 mg per day, compared with the optimal intake of 600 mg suggested by some researchers.[39-42] A group of post-menopausal women who took 250 to 750 mg of magnesium (without calcium supplementation) over a 2-year period had an increase in bone density.[43] This study demonstrates that some women may not be deficient in calcium, but instead are deficient in magnesium.

As discussed in Chapter 4, research findings related to calcium supplementation and increase in bone density vary substantially. The efficacy of calcium supplementation alone, frequently at an average dose of 1000 mg, has yielded somewhat mixed results and conclusions. Some research has demonstrated an increase in bone density from calcium alone; others have not, and the magnitude of the effect has varied by skeletal site. Bone integrity requires many minerals, including zinc, copper, and magnesium. A preliminary study demonstrated that, when the trace minerals zinc, manganese, and copper were combined with calcium supplementation, bone loss was halted, whereas calcium supplementation alone only slowed the process.[44] Additional benefits are derived when vitamin K, boron, folic acid, and other nutrients are added to a woman's nutritional program.

Ingestion of substances such as caffeine, salt, and phosphorus can cause a negative calcium imbalance. Excessive intake of calcium may cause soft tissue calcification.[45] Calcium may be deposited in areas outside of bone, resulting in problems such as kidney stones, calcification of the aorta (as in atherosclerosis), or arthritic symptoms in joints. Some studies of populations in other countries in which calcium intake was 400 mg or less per day show a lower incidence of osteoporosis than in the United States and other countries with similar dietary patterns.[46] Excess calcium intake may interfere with the absorption or use of other essential nutrients such as iron and may lead to magnesium deficiency, already a clinically significant nutritional problem in the United States. "You can't just throw calcium at the system and expect it to form the proper matrix and proper architecture. I think we have to stop looking for the 'magic bullet' situation, and recognize bone as living tissue with multiple nutritional needs."[47]

Additional research is needed, but in the meantime, dosing with large amounts of supplemental calcium is probably not a good idea and could cause more harm than good. The recommendation to avoid an "excessive intake" of calcium is not a simple one. A woman should be advised to take a close look at her typical nutritional intake to determine her approximate daily dose, not only of calcium but of magnesium and the trace minerals as well. This can be done by providing resources that include listings of food sources of nutrients and the amounts of the nutrients they contain (see References section). If possible, a woman should consult with a nutritionist to assist her in this process. She also needs to factor in her intake of foods and substances that contribute to nutritional deficiencies (eg, sugar, excessive protein) and excess excretion of calcium (eg, phosphorus, caffeine, and alcoholic beverages).

If a postmenopausal woman includes an adequate intake of grains, vegetables and fruits, protein, and calcium- and magnesium-rich foods that provide a daily calcium intake of 800 mg to 1000 mg and a daily magnesium intake of 600 mg and if the diet does not include substances that contribute to excessive loss of calcium and she is postmenopausal, she may be advised to supplement with a product containing 500 mg of calcium, trace minerals, and 250 to 500 mg of magnesium. If this woman were to add more than 500 mg of supplemental calcium to her nutritional program, she would probably have an "excessive intake" of calcium. A woman with the same diet as described above who is perimenopausal probably would need to take only a low-dose multimineral complex containing no more than 250 mg of calcium. An opposite example is a postmenopausal woman whose diet consists primarily of meat, sugar, and caffeine, with a daily calcium intake of only 400 mg. You can be sure that she is deficient in several nutrients. She is consuming substances that increase her excretion of calcium. Until her diet improves, she is best advised to add a supplement that also provides a complement of trace minerals, magnesium, and calcium (with about 1000 mg of calcium and 500 to 1000 mg of magnesium). If this woman did not add the magnesium to her nutritional supplementation program, she also would be consuming "excessive amounts" of calcium. In other words, she has not added one of the major minerals essential for adequate calcium absorption.

Although it appears to the woman that her intake of calcium and other nutrients is sufficient, the nutrient content of foods varies. A woman's needs for nutrients also depend on lifestyle factors such as stressors and level of physical activity. By supplementing, she is providing "nutritional insurance."

The recommended ratio of calcium to magnesium considered to maintain equilibrium is 2:1.[48] However, it has also been recommended that a more appropriate ratio of 1:1 can minimize the possibility of magnesium deficiency and is probably more appropriate for prevention and treatment of osteoporosis.[49] This may be a more reasonable approach, because magnesium is depleted through many of the same substances as is calcium and by stress. Women are not as likely to eat magnesium-rich foods, such as green vegetables, as they are to increase their calcium intake, particularly through diary products, and much more calcium than magnesium may be ingested, well beyond the 2:1 ratio. Absorption of calcium may then be inhibited and the demand for magnesium increased, and magnesium deficiency can result.

If a woman's calcium intake is 1500 mg and her magnesium intake remains at the average of 300 mg per day, the calcium-magnesium ratio is 5:1. In Finland, the prevalence of osteoporosis is high, and the calcium-magnesium ratio is 4:1. This ratio has also been associated with the highest death rate in the world from heart disease among young to middle-aged men.[50]

Depending on the various factors that determine a woman's need for supplementation, certain ranges have been recommended for reducing the risk for osteoporosis. A dose of 250 to 1000 mg of calcium is needed during the perimenopause, and a dose of 500 to 1500 mg is needed after menopause. The citrate form may have optimal bioavailability[51] and has reduced propensity for creating kidney stones.[52] The forms of calcium to be avoided are calcium phosphate (diets are already usually high in phosphorus), calcium carbonate (not easily absorbable if the functioning of the digestive system is comprised in any way), and bone meal and dolomite (may contain high amounts of lead and other toxic metals). Another highly bioavailable source of calcium is the organic calcium matrix hydroxyapatite microcrystalline compound, found in raw bones of young cattle and sheep raised on insecticide-free and pesticide-free pastures. It is not heated in the reduction process nor washed with chemical solvents, as is bone meal.

A dose of 600 to 1000 mg of magnesium is required. The amount taken is based on maintaining a minimum ratio of 2:1 (maximum ratio of 1:1) of calcium to magnesium. Magnesium aspartate is considered a better choice than magnesium oxide because of its greater bioavailability. Recommended doses of other minerals are shown in Table 6-1.

VITAMIN SUPPLEMENTATION

Specific vitamins are recommended as supplements for bone and heart health, for cancer prevention, and for some of the symptoms associated with the climacteric. The ranges provided take into account the issues addressed previously, and the dosages should ultimately be determined based on the woman's assessment of the quality of her nutritional intake, her health status, her level of exercise, and her environmental and personal stressors.

A dose of 50 to 100 mg is needed daily for each of vitamins B_1 (thiamine), B_2 (riboflavin), B_3 (niacin), B_6 (pyridoxine), B_{12} (cobalamin). A daily dose of 300 μg is recommended for biotin. Vitamin B_5 (pantothenic acid), in a dose of 250 to 1000 mg, may relieve hot flushes. An initial dose of 500 mg each day should be taken and increased every 2 weeks by 250 mg until a woman experiences relief. If this does not occur, she should reduce her dosage at the rate at which she increased it. If she experiences relief, she should contin-

TABLE 6-1
Additional Minerals

Zinc	10 to 30 mg
Copper	1 to 3 mg
Manganese	5 to 20 mg
Boron	1 to 3 mg
Silicon	1 to 2 mg
Strontium	0.5 to 3 mg
Selenium	200 mcg
Chromium	200 mcg
Iron	18 mg

ue on this dosage for a month and gradually reduce it, if possible, to a level that continues to be a successful treatment for her. A dose of 400 to 800 μg is recommended for folic acid. Any of several brands of balanced vitamin B complexes can provide the recommended amounts of all the B vitamins and folic acid for antioxidant protection and lowering of homocysteine levels.

The recommended daily dose of vitamin E is 100 to 800 IU. A minimum of 400 IU is recommended for women between the ages of 22 and 50, and 600 IU is recommended for women older than 50 for its cardiovascular effects.[53] Vitamin E has been shown since the mid-1940s to be useful in the treatment of hot flushes and other climacteric-related symptoms. At the end of a 4-week daily regimen of 50 to 100 mg of vitamin E, 75% of the women studied experienced an improvement in hot flushes, and 47% to 86% experienced relief of backaches, joint aches, and headaches.[54] Almost all of the women who complained of dizziness and palpitations experienced relief within 2 weeks. After 8 weeks, 70% of the patients who entered the study complaining of fatigue and 67% of those complaining of nervousness experienced relief of these symptoms. In another study, marked improvement of hot flushes and positive mood changes were experienced among 25 women with intractable hot flushes who were treated with 10 to 30 mg of vitamin E daily for 1 to 6 weeks.[55] In another group of women, 20 to 100 mg of vitamin E taken in divided daily doses for 10 days to 7 months (average of 31 days) experienced fair to excellent results with prompt recurrence of symptoms after discontinuation of the vitamin.[56]

A double-blind, placebo-controlled study of 341 patients with Alzheimer's disease was conducted in which 2000 IU of vitamin E was taken on a daily basis for 2 years. The results showed that, for patients with moderately severe impairment, treatment with the vitamin slowed the progression of the disease.[57]

As with pantothenic acid, the dose of vitamin E should be increased gradually, but not beyond 1200 IU, until relief is experienced (which can take a month or more) and then gradually decreased to the lowest dose possible for cardiovascular protection. It has been suggested that, for the woman with hypertension or diabetes, careful monitoring is needed with supplementation over 50 to 100 IU. Higher doses may increase hypertension and may decrease the need for the prescribed dose of insulin. Although not conclusive, it is advised that natural vitamin E (D-alpha-tocopherol) derived from vegetable oils be used as a supplement instead of synthetic vitamin E, which is partially derived from petroleum or turpentine.

In addition to taking a supplement without petroleum or turpentine, it is also advisable to take a vitamin E product that has on the label "D-alpha-tocopherol, plus other tocopherols" or "mixed natural tocopherols." The reason is that another compound found in vitamin E, gamma-tocopherol, may prove to be even more effect that alpha-tocopherol. Preliminary research on this compound has shown powerful antioxidant protection against nitrogen oxides, the reactive compounds that are known to stimulate destructive cellular changes. Gamma-tocopherol is not found in synthetic forms of vitamin E.[58]

The recommended dose of vitamin D is 100 to 400 IU. Intake depends on the woman's exposure to sunlight; the more sunlight (15 to 30 minutes each day), the less vitamin D supplementation is needed. It also depends on the amount of foods consumed that are rich in vitamin D, such as oily fish, liver, and eggs. Although it is important that a woman attempt to determine her intake of all of the nutrients before deciding on the amount of supplementation she will take, it is particularly important in the case of vitamin D, because excessive intake of vitamin D causes excretion of calcium from the bones.

The recommended daily dose of vitamin A is 10,000 IU, and a dose higher than 10,000 IU should not be taken unless the patient is under medical supervision. Doses above this level have been associated with toxic liver effects, blurred vision, hair loss, birth defects, spleen enlargement, and dry skin.[53]

The recommended daily dose of beta-carotene is 6 to 15 mg. Derived from plants, beta-carotene is a precursor of vitamin A and may be a safer alternative for meeting the body's needs for vitamin A than using vitamin A supplementation.

The recommended daily dose of vitamin K is 100 to 500 μg. This vitamin is not to be taken by women on anticoagulant therapy with Coumadin or warfarin, but it can be taken in combination with heparin therapy.

The recommended daily dose of vitamin C is 200 to 3000 mg. If diarrhea is experienced, more vitamin C than the body requires has been consumed, and the dose should be decreased until a level of tolerance has been reached.

The recommended daily dose of bioflavonoids is 500 to 1000 mg. Bioflavonoids have a chemical structure similar to that of estrogen, and they may lessen symptoms that result from a decline in estrogen. They may also be valuable in reducing the intensity and effects of hot flushes, perhaps because of their action on capillary walls. They may enhance absorption and action of vitamin C[59] and may be effective in prevention and treatment of bacterial, fungal, and viral infections.[60] They have been effective in improving blood lipid profiles in animal studies.[61]

ESSENTIAL FATTY ACIDS

Although the basic nutritional guidelines for fat intake included in the Eating Right Food Guide Pyramid do not distinguish between the essential fatty acids (EFAs), such as omega 3 and omega 6, patients should be encouraged to take an EFA supplement. The typical American diet is usually deficient in the omega-3 and omega-6 EFAs and the health benefits derived from them cannot be underestimated.

A variety of EFAs is available, including flax seed, black currant, and evening primrose and borage oils. In addition to the health benefits of EFAs, they may help alleviate hot flushes. Flax seed, in particular, has also been associated with luteal phase lengthening, fewer anovulatory cycles, and a decreased tendency to ovarian dysfunction.[62] For flax seed and black current oils, the dose is 1 teaspoon to 1 tablespoon per day. For evening primrose and borage oils, the dose is 200 mg per day.

DIGESTIVE ENZYMES

It has been said that a person is not what she eats, but what she absorbs and doesn't eliminate. Constipation, flatulence, diarrhea, and other gastrointestinal disturbances can be a sign of inadequate digestion. In the United States, 60 million cases of digestive disease are reported annually, and the number of persons who rely on antacids is astronomic. If a woman complains of such disturbances, supplementing with a digestive enzyme is essential to aid in absorption and transport of nutrients. Even if she does not experience a disturbance but is older than 50, a digestive enzyme is probably "nutrition insurance," because the ability to absorb nutrients declines with age. Indications for digestive enzyme supplementation include

- Aging
- Digestive disorders
- A high-protein and high-carbohydrate diet
- Intake of dairy foods
- Food allergies
- Improved vitamin and mineral absorption
- Improved protein, carbohydrate, and fat use

Several multidigestive enzyme products are available in health food stores. Ideally, one that contains several enzymes, including pancreatin, bromelain, papain, amylase, cellulase, diastase, and lipase, should be taken as directed on the bottle. A product containing several enzymes is preferred to maximize digestion and assimilation of all nutrients. Each of these enzymes is capable of breaking down only a specific substance (eg, an enzyme capable of breaking down fats cannot break down carbohydrates or proteins).

WHEN AND HOW TO TAKE SUPPLEMENTS

There is limited information about supplementation, but it appears that the total daily dosages should be divided and taken with meals or shortly thereafter, two to three times each day. For some of the vitamins, such as vitamin E, absorption is enhanced when taken with meals. Some persons experience gastrointestinal distress after ingesting vitamins and minerals on an empty stomach. The issue of whether calcium should be taken with food or on an empty stomach is not settled. Some research states that urinary excretion of calcium is highest at bedtime because of inactivity and fasting.[63] When calcium levels fall, the parathyroid hormone compensates by dissolving calcium from bones; therefore, they conclude that calcium is best taken at bedtime.

Until this controversy is settled, perhaps the best recommendation is that calcium dosages be divided throughout the day, with the last dose taken at bedtime. If taking calcium on an empty stomach at night causes nausea, calcium can be taken with food, so long as the food is not high in fiber. High fiber-containing foods appear to inhibit absorption of calcium. Calcium should be taken with a complement of trace minerals and magnesium as previously described (see the Guidelines section). Calcium should also be taken with 8 ounces of water to reduce the possibility of developing kidney stones.

QUALITY OF SUPPLEMENTS

Two hundred fifty-seven vitamin products underwent testing to assess ratios, quality, and amount of nutrients.[64] The results showed that many contained incorrect ratios of some nutrients, others contained too little of the more expensive and better quality nutrients, and others were missing some nutrients altogether. Only 49 of the

257 products were considered adequate. Recommended products are listed in the Guidelines section.

In calcium supplements, the amount of elemental (absorbable) calcium varies. Women must read the label on the bottle to check for the amount of elemental calcium that is listed. A supplement of 1000 mg of calcium may only have 50% elemental calcium and therefore only 500 mg of absorbable calcium in that product.

NUTRITIONAL ISSUES: TIME, SUPPORT, AND EXPENSE

Your patients depend on you to provide information essential to their health. Because your time is limited, you may find yourself frequently attempting to "catch up." You may have so little time to deal with basic health issues that discussing nutrition is at the bottom of the list. However, at least ask your patients to begin to look at their eating habits and to consider ways in which they can modify those habits to maximize their nutrient intake. Even if lack of time is an obstacle to discussing specific recommendations, giving patients a written summary of the information presented here sends a clear message that you believe in the importance of the information. By providing a list of books and newsletters (see the References section), you are offering a specific direction to take. This further reinforces the importance of adequate nutrition in their lives. If you are serving a population that cannot afford to purchase books, ask your local library to offer a selection of books about menopause, nutrition, and healthy cooking.

You can also help your patients by admitting that learning to eat in a healthful way may be very challenging for them. It takes knowledge, patience, and time to learn, to experiment, and to make changes. If a woman lives with others and is the primary cook for them, she will appreciate your encouragement to discuss her nutritional needs with them so that they can support the changes that she needs to make.

Because developing and following a nutritionally sound program can be difficult, consider identifying resources in your community that may be helpful for your patients. Perhaps you can organize a special program for women, using a local nutritionist. You might be able to arrange for a local chapter of the American Heart Association, a women's group, or a hospital to offer a series of sessions about basic nutrition and cooking for health.

It is important to help women learn about nutrition and how to practically integrate the new information into their lives. For many, their diet is the only avenue available for getting the nutrients they need. During conferences, in books for the lay public, and in books such as this, nutritional supplementation is discussed as being an integral aspect of an adequate nutritional program and one that all women should be encouraged to consider. However, this assumes that all women can afford to purchase supplements. Spending $20.00 per month for supplements is out of the question for many persons. Until government-sponsored health programs, insurance companies, and health maintenance organizations recognize that paying for nutritional supplements (beyond ferrous sulfate) is as important as paying for medications, your patients may have the foods they consume as the sole dietary means to assist them in preventing and treating osteoporosis, coronary artery disease, climacteric-related symptoms and other health problems.

EXERCISE

Exercise adds energy to body tissues and to the mind and spirit. It boosts intellectual performance, self-esteem, self-confidence, emotional resilience, resistance to stress, resistance to illness.... It reminds the body of the range of activity it is capable of, from total relaxation to strenuous effort. Too many of us exist in a state of moderate tension most of the time, somewhere in the middle of our potential range, and we maintain that state of tension for so long that it becomes the norm and eventually traps us into illness, or into mental and emotional cul de sacs.[65]

A sedentary lifestyle is epidemic in the United States. With all of the publicity touting the value of exercise, Americans should have heeded the warnings of the consequences of an inactive lifestyle. However, a February 1995 Harris poll documented a steady climb in the number of Americans who are overweight. Despite the billions of dollars spent on weight loss products and the thousands of sugar- and fat-free products lining the grocery store shelves, Americans keep getting fatter (69% in 1994 versus 58% in 1982). This results from poor dietary habits and from inactivity. Fewer than 10% of Americans older than 18 years of age meet the proposed national 1990 exercise activity objectives.[66]

A lack of opportunity for exercise is not the problem. A person can usually exercise at home or take walks without incurring any expense. Participation in sports with family and friends is an option for some. For those who can afford the cost, gyms and health spas are to be found just about everywhere.

The problem is lack of motivation. A person's motivation to change is based on a multitude of factors, some of which health care professionals cannot control or alter. However, education and support are within the domain of health care professionals.

You may assume that your patients truly understand the benefits of exercise. After all, the media have been a force in stressing the health benefits of exercise on the heart, for weight reduction, and as a means to prevent and treat osteoporosis. However, the overall emphasis continues to be on the appearance of an individual instead of the impressive array of physiologic benefits that exercise offers and that greatly contribute to the prevention and treatment of many diseases. The only time many patients are provided adequate guidance and support for an exercise program is during physical therapy after an injury, heart attack, or stroke. There is an excellent possibility that a patient has never had a conversation about exercise that was initiated by her health care provider. Rarely in the course of a routine clinic or office visit is time spent in educating patients about exercise in ways similar to discussing, for example, the patient's need for a particular medication or surgical procedure.

Health care providers frequently provide education about risks and benefits, as in discussing the risks and benefits of HRT to educate the patient and allay the patient's fears about this form of treatment. In contrast, exercise may be discussed for only a few seconds or not at all. Often, it is not a discussion, but a directive, such as "be sure to exercise regularly to strengthen your heart and bones." The patient is then expected to begin exercising. However, for a person who has led a sedentary life, has a health problem that causes her discomfort or pain, or has a disability, exercising may be difficult.

It is also assumed that the patient who appears "fit" is performing the correct exercises that maximize bone mass and cardiovascular fitness. For all of these patients, we suggest that, during a routine visit, at least a few minutes be spent in providing information about a basic exercise program and community resources that offer such programs. Educational materials that can assist the patient in developing her own program should also be offered. The more a patient is advised about exercise by a health care provider to whom she has entrusted her health, the greater is the possibility that she will be motivated to exercise.

EDUCATION ABOUT BENEFITS AND RISKS

Let your patients know about the benefits of exercise:

- Increases muscle mass and strength while decreasing body fat
- Helps to maintain normal blood pressure and resting heart rate
- Decreases vulnerability to cardiac arrhythmias and development of thrombi
- Contributes to maintenance of normal levels of HDL, LDL, and triglycerides
- Increases blood and oxygen to the heart by increasing the size of vessels and number of arteries
- Minimizes reduction in the size of the heart
- Reduces the risk of developing diabetes, in part by triggering the use of more insulin by muscles
- Strengthens the immune system and may decrease development of some cancers such as breast cancer (for some women, this statement will convince them to exercise)
- Facilitates emotional well-being by decreasing anxiety, insomnia, fatigue, depression, and other stress-related disorders
- Helps to maintain mineral content in bone, promoting bone remodeling
- Increases renal function, helping to prevent kidney disease
- Decreases for some women the degree of symptoms associated with the climacteric, such as fatigue and hot flushes; for others, exercise prevents some symptoms

A woman who gradually develops the habit of briskly walking 30 minutes each day for 4 to 5 days each week can reduce her risk of heart disease by about 55%.[67] This is an enormous reduction and does not impose pressure on her to advance to faster and longer workouts.

Another benefit of exercise pertains to relationships. It is not unusual to hear couples and parents and children discuss feelings ranging from frustration to sadness in not having enough time to spend with each other. By the end of the day, everyone is too tired to consider exercising. Remind your patients that the fatigue that they are experiencing is often psychologic, not physiologic, in origin. Working all day, being at school, and studying cause mental fatigue, which often feels like physical fatigue.

If loved ones and friends commit to exercising together 1, 2, or more days a week—even if only for 30 minutes in a walk after dinner—they can enjoy being together and knowing that they are supporting each other in maintaining health. After physical exercise, energy usually returns, contributing to a personal sense of well-being and an enhanced ability to complete the day more alert. Exercise can also contribute to ending the day relaxed, which means experiencing deeper, more nourishing sleep.

Disability and death from all causes, including cancer and heart disease, can be dramatically reduced through exercise. No pill or hormone can accomplish so much and contribute to such profound physiologic and psychologic benefits for a woman, whether she is 30 or 80 years old.

The risks of not exercising are disability and death. Women may experience some bothersome effects of exercise:

- Muscle soreness and stiffness
- Injury, if the program involves performing exercises beyond current capabilities
- Frustration at not being able to move in the way or at a level of endurance that the woman prefers

KEY COMPONENTS OF AN EXERCISE PROGRAM

Unless physical limitations exist, a woman's exercise goals for improving the cardiovascular system should include the following:

- Aerobic training for prevention and treatment of coronary artery disease
- Ten minutes of stretching and warm-up exercises for the upper and lower body to prepare muscles for increased energy demands and to prevent fatigue and injury
- Thirty minutes of cardiovascular exercise every day or an hour every other day that achieves between 45% and 80% percent of maximum heart rate. (The rate is determined by subtracting the person's age from 220 and multiplying the result by 0.45 and

0.80. Ideally, aerobic activity should be increased to at least 60% of maximum heart rate.[68])

⊘ Ten minutes of cool-down and stretching exercises

It has been demonstrated that 20 minutes of moderate-intensity, low-impact exercise 3 days per week is effective in maintaining bone mineral density in early postmenopausal women.[69] This amount of time spent on adequate aerobic activity also produces beneficial cardiovascular changes (so does 10 minutes). However, a 30-minute or longer aerobic session has a greater effect on the reduction of heart disease.

For the prevention and treatment of osteoporosis, the following exercises can have a beneficial effect on bone density:

⊘ Strength training (bone-loading) exercises three times per week (not consecutive days) for 20 minutes
⊘ Warm-up and cool-down exercises, as with cardiovascular exercise
⊘ Exercises to strengthen the abdominal and back muscles for maintenance of pelvic structures, good posture, and prevention of back problems

Bone loading exercises enhance the bone remodeling process by twisting, stretching, bending, and compressing bones. *Bone Loading* explains a complete exercise program developed as an outcome of research conducted at the Hebrew University and Haddasseh Medical Organization in Jerusalem.[65] The focus of this work was to determine whether a set of specifically designed exercises that stressed the bones could increase bone mass. Women between the ages of 33 and 74 who were not physically active before the study took part in the exercise program for 5 months. These women performed bone loading exercises for 20 minutes, 3 days each week. An additional 30 minutes was spent on warm-up, cool-down, and flexibility exercises.

Bone density was measured 1 year before, at the beginning of, and at the end of the study. Bone density decreased 2% to 3% during the year leading up to the beginning of the exercise program. At the end of the program, the control group continued to lose 2% of bone mass, and the group of exercising women had a 4% increase in bone density. This gain effectively restored the radii of these women's bones to their status of 1 to 1.5 years earlier. Those who had back pain before beginning the exercise program experienced relief from this pain. The control group's complaints of back pain remained consistent.

For the woman who has led a sedentary lifestyle or has exercised only occasionally, it is important that she receive "permission" to begin her program in whatever way is most comfortable for her. Her exercise program must be personalized to fit her schedule and must focus on how her body reacts to exercise. Initially, her exercise program may be one of taking five 6-minute walks or three 10-minute walks each day. The most important aspects of beginning an exercise program are consistency and low injury potential. *Duration takes precedence over intensity.* Only when she begins to feel stronger and has developed the new habit of taking time to walk or perform any other type of exercise should the intensity be increased.

All the recommendations listed require that a woman's exercise program eventually evolve to one that lasts for 1.5 hours at least 3 days a week or is divided into segments of 1 hour on each of 6 days a week or any other combination that enables her to spend an adequate amount of time in performing cardiovascular, bone loading, stretching, and abdominal exercises. Spending 1 to 1.5 hours in exercise may not be possible for some, depending on work and home responsibilities. If this is the case, please remind your patient that whatever she can do will help her. Often, after a woman establishes a habit of 10- to 15-minute exercise sessions, she begins to feel so good that she is able to substantially increase the duration of these sessions.

It has been recommended that a woman who has been living a sedentary life or who exercises sporadically begin an exercise program in which her heart rate is at her lowest maximum heart rate, gradually increasing it as her strength and aerobic capacity increase. For these women, for those older than 40, and for those who have had a health problem making aerobic activity difficult (eg, pulmonary or heart disease), a cardiovascular evaluation before initiating an exercise program is considered essential. A graded exercise stress test with a study of maximal oxygen uptake should be performed so that intensity and duration of exercise time are established.[70] As muscular strength and cardiovascular ability increase, the exercise program can be adjusted accordingly.

A woman who has been diagnosed with osteoporosis or has other physical limitations should be encouraged to embark on an exercise program with the assistance of a physical therapist. Too often, a woman may not believe exercise to be of benefit for her because she is unable to engage in vigorous activity or is unable to partially or completely move some areas of her body. However, any form of exercise, even if it involves stretching without major aerobic activity or limited strengthening exercises (eg, performed with one arm or only the legs) has its benefits in muscle strengthening and bone density. The entire musculoskeletal system gains mineral content even if stress is placed on only one area of the body.[71] Exercise has been beneficial in decreasing depressive symptoms in persons with disabilities ranging from stroke to spinal cord injury.[72]

Patients need to hear that it is never too late to begin an exercise program. Elderly persons who embarked on a strength training program for 12 weeks showed tremendous results, some being able to lift more weight than the 25-year-old graduate students working with the research project.[71] Another study with a focus on improving the quality of 87- to 96-year-old men's and women's lives by increasing their functional capacity through improving their strength showed that, after a training period of just 8 weeks, the subjects' muscle strength almost tripled and the size of their thigh muscles grew by more then 10%.[73] Speaking for many of his peers in the study, Sam Semansky, 93 years old, stated, "I feel as though I were 50 again. Now, I get up in the middle of the night and I can get around without using my walker or turning on the light. The program gave me strength I didn't have before. Every day I feel better, more optimistic. Pills won't do for you what exercise does!"[71]

EXERCISING FOR CLIMACTERIC-RELATED SYMPTOMS

A survey conducted by *Prevention Magazine* in collaboration with the Irving Center for Clinical Research, Columbia University, and the Center for Women's Health at Columbia Presbyterian Medical Center suggests that exercise may have an impact on symptoms associated with the climacteric.[19] Responses from 15,000 women revealed that, in the group who exercised three or more times per week (64%), menopause was described as "not bothersome," and these women experienced fewer symptoms than women who exercised two times per week or less.

Another survey revealed that women who exercised on a regular basis had significantly fewer vasomotor symptoms, a lesser degree of negative moods, a lesser degree of decreased sexual desire, and significantly higher well-being scores than women who did not exercise.[74] Similar findings were demonstrated when premenopausal, perimenopausal, and postmenopausal women who exercised were compared with the sedentary control group. Women who exercised scored lower on somatic symptoms and memory concentration difficulties.[75]

Exercise can help a woman feel she is doing something positive for herself. Embarking an on exercise program may be the first time that a woman has taken time for herself. Fitness and energy levels increase, and weight is often kept under control. All of these benefits can have a positive effect on a woman's sense of well-being and self-esteem.

COMMUNITY RESOURCES AND EDUCATIONAL MATERIALS

You can assist your patients in learning about exercise. Providing a summary of exercise recommendations and list of community resources and educational materials is extremely helpful to your patients and reinforces for them the important role that you believe exercise plays in their total wellness program.

STRESS

> Overall, the goal of stress management is not only to help persons withstand short-lived stressful events, but to defuse the effects of chronic stress—a more serious threat because chronic stress may not give the body the respite it needs to recover.[76]

A variety of psychosocial factors, including those specifically related to the midlife, can contribute to the development and severity of some climacteric-related symptoms. Evidence also links stress to deleterious alterations in the cardiovascular, nervous, immune, and endocrine systems.

Stress may influence immunity through many pathways; for example, under certain conditions, the activity of immune system cells can be affected by epinephrine, cortisol, and related hormones.

Stress may play a role in a wide variety of endocrine-related illness-es such as diabetes and hyperthyroidism and in psychiatric-related disorders such as panic attacks and obsessive-compulsive disorder. Proliferation of certain immune system cells (ie, eosinophilia) may be associated with severe heart failure.[76] If psychologic factors prove to influence eosinophilia, it would provide an intriguing link among the cardiovascular, immune, and nervous systems. Animal and human studies have already demonstrated a link between stress and strong emotions and the precipitation of sudden heart attacks and triggering of ischemia.

It makes sense to add stress reduction techniques to the foun-dation of a total wellness program. These techniques decrease the potentially harmful psychologic and physiologic effects of stress, and they can contribute to the development of positive coping behaviors.

The way in which a person responds emotionally to life events is primarily responsible for the impact of stressors.[76] The ways in which persons cope with stressors may be as important as the stressors in determining health or illness. Coping behaviors are determined by factors such as mood, personality characteristics, suppressed anger, a sense of hopelessness, and psychologic vulnerability. If the effects of stressors can be intensified by negative psychologic traits, can the effects of stress be diminished through positive coping behaviors?

Positive coping behaviors cannot increase funds in the bank account of a woman who is struggling to make ends meet, nor can they change objectionable behavior of a boss, child, or spouse. How-ever, if a woman is able to deal with life stressors in a more positive manner, their physiologic and psychologic effects can be greatly less-ened. Positive coping behaviors may also be the impetus for enabling the woman to view stress-causing situations in a new light. The woman may gain confidence to create changes in her life such as seeking new employment or ending an unhappy relationship. Posi-tive coping behaviors can change a negative attitude toward menopause to one that is positive.

The woman who is happy with her life and feels that stress is not an issue may not realize that she still must deal with day-to-day stressors such as the 11 o'clock news of wars and a zillion other dis-asters, traffic jams, and mundane assaults on her. Ideally, a woman should develop a comprehensive stress management program that involves dealing with three elements[77]: stressors, perception of stress, and physical and emotional reactions to stress. To do this, techniques must be used that eliminate, modify, or control stressors; alter the person's perception of stressors; and manage or control the stress response after it occurs.

Techniques that accomplish these three components of a stress management program can result in a woman learning how to manage stress so that it is not detrimental to her happiness, productivity, or health. This program can be developed by the woman herself with the assistance of sources such as those listed in the References section, through the help of a social worker or therapist, or through programs offered (often free of charge) to the community by resources such as a local hospital or YWCA. These programs usually include assistance in areas such as establishing priorities, learning to "let go" of tasks in day-to-day life to make it less stressful, self-monitoring of patterns of stress reactions, relaxation strategies, and coping skills such as exercise.

One of the easiest ways women can begin to modify stress is through informal techniques or ways that contribute to their ability to cope with the problems of daily life. These include a hobby, reading for pleasure, listening to music, writing in a journal, and visiting with friends or family. None of these informal techniques replaces a well-planned stress management approach, but they can supplement it.

Exercise and informal techniques should be encouraged. However, the body and mind need the opportunity to experience true relaxation (ie, the relaxation response), sometimes described as a state of calmness, peacefulness, or serenity. Some of your patients may feel that this is not possible for them. They have coped with stressors in the same ways for so long that the thought of truly relaxing or feeling a sense of total calmness does not seem to be within their grasp. To put themselves into a hypometabolic or restful state in which oxygen consumption and respiration and heart rate decrease while alpha wave activity increases seems to be something only for yogis and Zen monks.

Although it is important for women to hear from their health care providers that any form of meditation can be beneficial, it is probably counterproductive to focus on these as being the only options for stress reduction. Some patients may resist meditation. It may seem like such a foreign concept, or the thought of taking 20 minutes each day to meditate feels like an impossibility, and that could very well be the case.

What women do need to hear is that there are several stress reduction techniques. Although they do not elicit a relaxation response, they can help in coping with stress-evoking situations. They can be performed when a person is experiencing a stressful situation. Some can even be performed "privately," without anyone else noticing they are being used.

Simple, easy-to-manage stress reduction techniques may be so helpful that, at some point, a woman may decide to explore additional ways to deal with stress, perhaps eventually finding a meditative technique that works for her. Eventually, she may end up experiencing the relaxation response on a daily basis. Your recommendation that your patient consider learning ways to decrease stress may be the support that she needs.

EXERCISES FOR STRESS REDUCTION

The following simple relaxation techniques are excellent ways to begin to learn to reduce the effects of stress and to cope with stressful situations. As with making nutritional changes or embarking on an exercise program, it may be more beneficial to start "small" by committing just 5 minutes each day to perform an exercise such as the following examples.

Exercise #1 for stress reduction[78]:

1. Lie or sit in a comfortable place with the eyes closed.
2. Feet should be slightly apart, and one hand should be placed on the abdomen near the navel. The other hand should be placed on the chest.
3. Breath by inhaling through the nose and exhaling through the mouth.
4. Concentrate on breathing, noticing which hand is rising and falling with each breath.
5. Gently exhale most of the air out of the lungs.
6. Slowly inhale while counting to 4, while slightly extending the abdomen so that it rises about 1 inch. While inhaling, the chest and shoulders should not move.
7. Imagine warm air flowing into and throughout the entire body while breathing in.

8. Hold the breath for 1 second, and then slowly exhale to a count of 4, while imagining all tension and stress leaving the body. The abdomen should be moving inward when exhaling.
9. Repeat this exercise for 5 minutes or until a deep sense of relaxation is achieved.

This exercise and others are described in Murray's *Stress, Anxiety, and Insomnia: How You Can Benefit from Diet, Vitamins, Minerals, Herbs and Exercise.*[78]

Exercise #2 for stress reduction:

1. Sit comfortably, but with the spine straight.
2. Rest the hands on the thighs. The eyes should be closed.
3. Take a slow deep breath through the nose while counting to 4. With each breath in, the abdomen should move outward.
4. Hold the breath for a count of 4.
5. Slowly exhale through the nose to the count of 4. With each breath out, the abdomen should move inward.
6. With each exhalation, concentrate on relaxing all the muscles of the body, beginning with the neck, shoulders, and back. The spine should be kept straight.
7. Repeat this breathing exercise for 2 to 5 minutes or longer if possible.

Another effective way to reduce stress is to sit comfortably as previously described, perform deep breathing, and combine this form of breathing with visualizing a relaxing situation, silently repeating a word or words that have a positive influence on mental outlook (eg, " I am feeling relaxed" or "peace"). Prayer is an excellent option for some. Whichever option is chosen, it is essential that the focus be on breathing deeply and fully, maintaining an erect spine, and relaxing the muscles.

These exercises encourage deep breathing and relaxation. The exercises can be performed at work. The working woman who does not have a quiet place to go during the course of her work can still help herself to relieve stress any time by standing or sitting with the spine straight and slowing and deeply inhaling and exhaling through the nose while concentrating on relaxing the neck and shoulders. Persons are often surprised that deeply breathing for even a short period "takes the edge off" the stressful moment. Deep breathing is also useful for relaxing during out-of-work stressors such as standing in line in a store or being stuck in a traffic jam.

These deep breathing exercises can also reduce hot flushes. Post-menopausal women were recruited to participate in a research study of behavioral treatments for hot flushes.[79] Some women used deep breathing exercises, others used a muscle relaxation technique, and a third group used biofeedback. Hot flushes were significantly reduced in the group that received training in slow, deep breathing. This was not the experience of the other groups of women.

Several wonderful books describe many "quickie" relaxation techniques and various forms of meditation (see the References section).

EFFECTS OF STRESS REDUCTION

You should tell your patients that using ways to reduce the effects of stress may help to alleviate or prevent symptoms associated with the climacteric; may help to prevent health problems such as hypertension, which can lead to heart disease; and can assist them in positively coping with stressful life situations. If you do not have the luxury of time to discuss these relaxation techniques in detail, providing some stress reduction recommendations and resources in writing can give much-needed guidance. Your actions serve as reinforcement for them, because you demonstrate that you believe stress reduction is a beneficial aspect of their health care program.

Some health care providers underestimate their influence on the courses of action that their patients follow. This underestimation may occur because patients often do not take their medications, do not perform the monthly breast self-examinations that were thoroughly explained, or do not return for follow-up assessment of an abnormal Pap smear result, no matter how much time and energy has been expended in discussing the necessity for this. For some providers, this results in discouragement: "Why bother to take the time? They're not going to do it anyway." However, remember that there are just as many patients who truly benefit from the education and guidance that you offer them and who act on your recommendations. They know that you are taking the time to discuss these things with them because you care about how they feel. They recognize that you would not be spending your time talking with them about specific health recommendations if you were not concerned about the quality of their lives.

REFERENCES

1. Beasley J, Swift J. The Kellogg Report: the impact of nutrition environment and lifestyle on the health of Americans. Annandale-on-Hudson, NY: The Institute of Health Policy and Practice at the Bard College Center; 1989:169.
2. Quillin P. Healing nutrients. New York: Vintage Books; 1989.
3. Welsh S, et al. A brief history of food guides in the United States. Nutr Today 1992;Nov/Dec:6–10.
4. Atwater WO. Principles of nutrition and nutritive value of food. Farmers bulletin no 142 of the U.S. Department of Agriculture. Washington, DC: Government Printing Office; 1902:48.
5. Centers for Disease Control. Ten-state nutrition survey 1968-70. DHEW publication no. (HSM) 72-8129, 81130, 8131, 8132, 8133. Atlanta: Department of Housing, Education, and Welfare; 1973.
6. National Center for Health Statistics. Caloric and selected nutrient value for persons 1–74 years of age: first Health and Nutrition Examination Survey, United States 1971–1974. Vital and Health Statistics series 11, no. 209. DHEW publication no. (PHS) 9-1657. Hyattsville, MD: U.S. Public Health Service; 1982.
7. Hamilton E, et al. Nutrition: concepts and controversies. St. Paul, MN: West Publishing; 1985:53.
8. Lowenstein FW. Bibl Nutr Dieta 1981;30:1.
9. U.S. Senate Select Committee on Nutrition and Human Needs: Dietary goals for the United States, 2d ed. Washington, DC: U.S. Government Printing Office; 1977.
10. Lewis C, et al. Healthy People 2000: report on the 1994 Nutrition Progress Review. Nutr Today 1994;25(6):6–15.
11. U.S. Department of Agriculture. The food guide pyramid. Home and garden bulletin no. 252. Washington, DC: Government Printing Office; 1990.
12. Ross E, Sachs J. Healing the female heart. New York: Pocket Books; 1996.
13. Eramus U. Fats that heal; fats that kill. Burnaby BC: Alive Books; 1993.
14. Margen S, Editors of University of California at Berkeley Wellness Letter. The wellness encyclopedia of food and nutrition. New York: Rebus; 1992.
15. The promise of phytoestrogens. UC Berkeley Wellness Lett 1996.
16. Messina M. Modern application for an ancient bean: Soybeans and the prevention and treatment of chronic disease. J Nutr 1995;125:567S–569S.
17. Setchell KDR, Aldercreutz H. Mammalian lignans and phytoestrogens: recent studies on their formation, metabolism and biological role in health and disease. In: Rowland IR, ed. Role of the Gut Flora in Toxicity and Cancer, pp 315–345. London: Academic Press; 1988.
18. Special report. Tufts Univers Diet Nutr Lett 1995;12.
19. Triumph over menopause: Prevention survey with the Center for Women's Health at Columbia-Presbyterian Medical Center. Prevention 1994;August.

20. Zava D. The phytoestrogen paradox. Soy Connection 1994;3.
21. Jaret P. The miracle bean. Health 1995;Oct:32.
22. Setchell K, et al. Nonsteroidal estrogens of dietary origin: Possible role in hormone-dependent disease. Am J Clin Nutr 1984;40:568–578.
23. Aldercreutz HH, et al. Excretion of the lignans enterolactone and enterodiol and of equol in omnivorous and vegetarian postmenopausal women and in women with breast cancer. Lancet 1982;1982:1295–1299.
24. Aldercreutz H. Determination of urinary lignans and phytoestrogen metabolites, potential antiestrogens and anticarcinogens in urine of women on various habitual diets. J Steroid Biochem 1986;25:791–797.
25. Aldercreutz, et al. Plasma concentrations of phyto-oestrogens in Japanese men. Lancet 1993;342:1209–1210.
26. Kennedy A. The evidence for soybean products as cancer preventative agents. J Nutr 1995;125:733A–743S.
27. Clarkson TB, et al. Sex steroids and coronary arthrosclerosis of monkeys. Fertil Steril 1994;62(6 suppl):1475–1515.
28. Sirtori CRE, et al. Clinical experience with the soybean protein diet in the treatment of hypercholestesterolemia. Am J Clin Nutr 1979;32:1645–1658.
29. Erdman JW, et al. Soy products and the human diet. Am J Clin Nutr 1989;49:725–737.
30. Anderson J, et al. Meta-analyses of the effects of soy protein intake on serum proteins. N Engl J Med 1995;333:276–282.
31. Cassidy A, et al. Biological effects of a diet of soy protein rich in isoflavones on the menstrual cycle in premenopausal women. Am J Clin Nutr 1994;60:333–340.
32. Nicholls J, et al. Phytoestrogens in soy and changes in pituitary response to GnRH challenge tests in women. Davis, CA: Department of Nutrition and Division of Reproductive Biology and Medicine, School of Medicine; 1996.
33. Dwyer T, et al. Tofu and soy drinks contain phytoestrogens. J Am Diet Assoc 1994;94:739–743.
34. Colgan M. Your personal vitamin profile. New York: William Morrow; 1982:55.
35. National Academy of Sciences. Recommended dietary allowances, 9th ed. Washington, DC: National Academy of Press; 1980.
36. Harper A. Uses and misuses of recommended dietary allowances. N Y St J Med 1979;April 79(5):806–807.
37. Ensminger ME, et al. Food and nutrition encyclopedia. Clovis, CA: Peegus Press; 1983.
38. Office of Medical Applications, Research National Institutes of Health. Osteoporosis. JAMA 1984;252:799.
39. U.S. Department of Agriculture, Human Nutrition Information Service. Nationwide food consumption survey: continuing survey of food intakes by individuals women 19 50 and their children 1–5 years of age. Washington, DC: U.S. Government Printing Office; 1988.
40. Lakshmanan FI., et al. Magnesium intakes balances and blood levels of adults consuming self-selected diets. Am J Clin Nutr 1984;40:1380–1389.
41. Morgan KJ, Stampley GL. Dietary intake levels and foods sources of magnesium and calcium for selected segments of the US population. Magnesium 1988;7:225–233.
42. Spillman DM. Calcium, magnesium and calorie intake and activity levels of healthy adult women. J Am Coll Nutr 1987;6:454.

43. Cohen L, Kitzes R. Infrared spectroscopy and magnesium content of bone mineral in osteoporotic women. Isr J Med Sci 1981;17:1123–1125.
44. Strause L, et al. Spinal bone loss in postmenopausal women supplemented with calcium and trace minerals. J Nutri 1994;124:1060–1064.
45. Mazess RB, et al. Calcium intake and bone. Am J Clin Nutr 1994;42:568–571.
46. Chalmers J. Georgraphical variations in senile osteoporosis. J Bone Joint Surg Br 1970;52:667.
47. Gaby A. Meno times. San Rafael, CA: Spring, 1996.
48. Hathaway ML. Magnesium in human nutrition. Home economics research report #19. Washington, DC: USDA Agricultural Research Service; 1962.
49. Abraham G. A total dietary program emphasizing magnesium instead of calcium. Affect on the mineral density of calcaneous bone in postmenopausal women on hormonal therapy. J Reprod Med 1990;35:503–507.
50. Karppanen HR, et al. Minerals, coronary heart disease, and sudden coronary death. Adv Cardiol 1978;25:9–24.
51. Gaby A. Preventing and reversing osteoporosis. Rocklin, CA: Prima Publishing; 1994.
52. Harvey JA, et al. Calcium citrate: reduced propensity for the crystallization of calcium oxalate in urine resulting from induced hypercalciuria of calcium supplementation. J Clin Endocrinol Metab 1985;61:1223.
53. Cooper K. Dr Kenneth Cooper's antioxidant revolution. Atlanta: Thomas Nelson Publishers; 1994.
54. Gozan HA. The use of vitamin E in treatment of the menopause. N Y State Med J 1952;May:1289–1291.
55. Cristy CJ. Vitamin E in menopause. Am J Obstet Gynecol 1945;50:84.
56. Finkler RS. The effect of vitamin E in the menopause. J Clin Endocrinol Metab 1949;9:89–94.
57. Sano M, et al. A controlled trial of segiline, alpha-tocopherol, or both as treatment for Alzheimer's disease: the Alzheimer's Cooperative Study. N Engl J Med 1997;336:1216–1222.
58. Weil A. The benefits of vitamin E. In: Self-Healing. July, 1997.
59. Bland J. Bioflavonoids. New Canaan: Keats; 1984; 7, 8.
60. Shub T, et al. Antibiotiki 1981;26:268.
61. Rathi A, et al. Acta Vitaminol Enzymol 1983;5:255.
62. Phipps WR. Effect of flax seed ingestion on the menstrual cycle. J Clin Endocrinol Metab 1993;77:1215–1219.
63. Nordin BEC. Clinical significance and pathogenesis of osteoporosis. Br Med J 1971;1:571.
64. Colgan M. The new nutrition medicine for the millennium. Vancouver, BC: Apple; 1995.
65. Simkin A, Ayalon J. Bone loading. London: Prion; 1990:18.
66. U.S. Dept. of Health and Human Services. Centers for Disease Control and Prevention, Physical Activity and Health: A Report of the Surgeon General, 1996. Pittsburgh: Superintendent of Documents.
67. Blair S. Cooper Institute for Aerobics Research. Prevention 1996;April.
68. Hurley B. Aerobic versus strength training for coronary risk factor intervention. Ann Med 1994;26:153–154.
69. Grove K, Londerlee BR. Bone density in postmenopausal women: high impact vs low impact exercise. Med Sci Sports Exerc 1990;24:1990–1994.

70. Notelovitz M. Exercise and health maintenance in menopausal women. Ann N Y Acad Sci 1990;592:204–220.
71. Evans W, Rosenberg I. Biomarkers: the 10 determinants of aging you can control. New York: Simon & Schuster; 1991.
72. Coyle C, Santiago M. Aerobic exercise training and depressive symptomatology in adults with physical disabilities. Arch Phys Med Rehabil 1995;76:647–652.
73. Fiatarone A, et al. High intensity strength training in nonagenarians: effect on skeletal muscle. JAMA 1990;263:3029.
74. Collins A, Landgren BM. Experience of symptoms during transition to menopause: a population-based longitudinal study. In: The Modern Management of Menopause, A Perspective for the 21st Century: proceedings of the VII International Congress on the Menopause; Stockholm, 1993. New York: Parthenon; 1994.
75. Slaven L, Lee C. Mood and symptom reporting among middle-aged women: the relationships between menopausal status, HRT and exercise participation. Health Psychol 1997;16:203–208.
76. Goleman D, Gurin J. Mind-body medicine. New York: Consumer Reports Books; 1993:25.
77. Cottrell R. Stress management. Guilford, CT: Dushkin; 1992.
78. Murray M. Stress, anxiety, and insomnia: how you can benefit from diet, vitamins, minerals, herbs, and exercise. Rocklin, CA: Prima Publishing; 1995.
79. Freedman RR. Mechanisms and behavioral treatment of menopausal hot flushes. In: The modern management of menopause, a perspective for the 21st century: proceedings of the VIIth International Congress on the Menopause; Stockholm, 1993. New York: Parthenon; 1993.

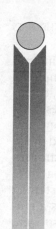
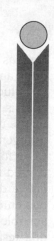

CHAPTER 7

Hormonal and Drug Therapies

This chapter provides an overview of the benefits, side effects, and complications of hormone replacement therapy (HRT) and other selected drug therapies. It also examines why some women choose to use or not to use HRT and ways in which women can be assisted in putting these therapies into perspective. Recommendations for basic HRT regimens are found in the Guidelines section. You can find detailed information about HRT in resources such as Mishell's *Menopause: Physiology and Pharmacology*, Byyny and Speroff's *A Clinical Guide for the Care of Older Women*, *Primary and Preventative Care*, Carr and colleagues' *The Medical Care of Women*, and other sources listed in the References section.

HORMONE REPLACEMENT THERAPIES

GENERAL APPLICATIONS

In the 1960s, conventional medical treatment of climacteric symptoms was simple. Premarin was the estrogen replacement therapy (ERT) available at that time; it was considered the panacea, the "fountain of youth" for women, and that was all there was to it! The focus of ERT was solely on the treatment of symptoms.

As research began to demonstrate additional benefits of HRT and as potential side effects, complications, and contraindications were identified, the types of estrogens and progestins available for use grew, as did their modes of administration. With the research findings came an expansion of the 1960s focus on HRT for relief of symptoms to include the reduction in the risk of cardiovascular disease, osteoporosis, and other health problems. Although the degree of research on the use of natural (plant-based; compounded) progesterone and estrogens, testosterone, dehydroepiandrosterone (DHEA), and melatonin for the climacteric has been considerably less than estrogen-related research, the literature slowly has begun to include a more active discussion of their potential benefits. Natural progesterone has entered the arena as an alternative to progestins and as a reasonable hormonal therapy without the combined use of estrogen, and testosterone is considered beneficial for some women. It also appears that DHEA therapy may prove to be an important component of a treatment program for women during their climacteric.

Increasing numbers of researchers and health care professionals are recognizing that in addition to a decline in estrogen the climacteric is also associated with a decline in the levels of progesterone, DHEA, and in some women, testosterone, and the degree and onset of decline varies. Because of this a multifaceted approach to HRT may prove more beneficial to women than focusing solely on the benefits of estrogen.

There are various schools of thought regarding the kinds of hormones to use. On one end of the spectrum, there are clinicians who believe in prescribing synthetic or conjugated equine estrogens and synthetic progestins. On the other end, there are those who believe that only plant sources of estrogen and progesterone should be prescribed. Some clinicians are open to considering all forms of hormonal therapies.

AVAILABLE THERAPIES

The most commonly prescribed hormonal therapies used in the United States by conventional health care providers include estrogen only, estrogen with testosterone or progestins, progestins or natural progesterone, and testosterone. The estrogen-only formulations are available in several forms:

⊘ Conjugated equine estrogens in oral and vaginal forms (Premarin, Menest, Estratab)

- Micronized (synthetic) estradiol in oral forms (Estrace)
- 17β-estradiol (synthetic) in oral, vaginal (Estrace), and transdermal forms (Estraderm) and in a vaginal ring
- Estropipate (estrone) in oral and vaginal forms (Ogen, Ortho-Est)
- Dienestrol (synthetic) in vaginal form (Ortho Dienestrol cream)

Estrogen is also available with testosterone:

- Esterified estrogen and methyltestosterone (synthetic) in oral form (Estratest)
- Conjugated equine estrogen and methyltestosterone in oral form (Premarin with methyltestosterone)

Estrogen with progestin is available in the form of conjugated equine estrogen and medroxyprogesterone acetate (synthetic) (Prempro-Premarin, Prem-Phase, Cycrin)

Natural progesterone is derived from wild Mexican yam or soybeans and is considered to have a molecular structure similar to the progesterone produced by the ovary. Progestins and natural progesterones are available in several forms:

- Medroxyprogesterone acetate in oral form (synthetic) (Provera, Amen, Cycrin)
- Norethindrone acetate in oral form (synthetic) (Aygestin)
- Natural progesterone in micronized oral, vaginal, and rectal suppositories and sprays; intramuscular and sublingual forms; and skin creams, gels, and oils.

Plant-based, compound hormone therapies for the climacteric include progesterone, DHEA, testosterone, and melatonin. These hormones are sometimes referred to as "natural."[1] However, they are not, as some imply in their marketing, hormones directly extracted from soybeans or a family of the wild Mexican yam. Although they are plant based and not synthetic, they are derived from plant steroids taken from these sources and then converted in the laboratory to reproduce hormones with a molecular structure identical to the human forms. Various forms of estrogens also are compounded from soybeans and the wild Mexican yam family.

Two myths should be dispelled for patients. First, the American yam does not contain the steroid found in the wild Mexican yam that can be converted into a hormone. Second, purchasing products that are advertised as containing wild Mexican yam is misleading.

Women who purchase these products assume they are reaping the benefits of progesterone; however, there exists no enzymatic processes in the body that can transform the progesterone precursor of the yam into progesterone.[2] Women can only reap the benefits of progesterone if the wild Mexican yam product contains a pharmaceutical grade of progesterone.

The amount of progesterone in creams and gels depend on the product. Patients who use a progesterone-based cream or gel probably should obtain a prescription for a pharmacy product. Information about the amount of progesterone in several products can be obtained from Aeron Lifecycle, a biomedical research company that continues to update a list of several progesterone-based products and the amount of progesterone contained in these products (see Appendix C).

Testosterone is available as methyltestosterone (synthetic) in an oral form (Android, Oreton, Testred).

BENEFITS OF HORMONAL THERAPIES

SYMPTOM RELIEF

VASOMOTOR SYMPTOMS

Although the pathophysiology of vasomotor instability is not completely understood, supplementary estrogen in some form (eg, oral, transdermal, vaginal) completely or partially relieves hot flushes for most women within 1 week to 2 months of initiating therapy. Although estrogen has always been the hormonal treatment of choice for relief of hot flushes, progestins and natural progesterone can also be considered for women who cannot or do not want to use ERT and for those who experience intolerable side effects from it.

Progestins and progesterone may relieve hot flushes by mediating hypothalamic activity (ie, vasomotor liability) resulting from low levels of estrogen and progesterone.[1] Rising levels of these hormones creates a negative feedback effect in the pituitary and hypothalamus. Supplementation with progesterone may cause estrogen receptors in these areas to become more sensitive and hot flushes to subside.

An injection of 150 mg of depo-medroxyprogesterone acetate (DMPA) every 3 months was shown to be as effective a treatment for hot flushes as a daily dosage of 0.625 mg of oral conjugated equine estrogens.[3,4] Doses of 50 and 100 mg of DMPA have also been effective in relieving hot flushes.[5] Daily doses of 10 to 20 mg of medrox-yprogesterone acetate (MPA) also have been effective in substantially relieving hot flushes.[6]

Natural progesterone is another treatment for relieving hot flushes. Unlike the progestins, natural progesterone has been shown in some research to cause minimal or no decrease in high-density lipoprotein (HDL) or its subfractions.[7,8] The progesterone is an exact chemical duplicate of the progesterone that is produced in the body, and it appears to have fewer associated side effects than progestins.

Research in the area of DHEA and climacteric-related symptoms is limited. Because DHEA can be converted to estrone or estradiol, progesterone, and testosterone, it may be a reasonable treatment option when used alone or in combination with ERT or HRT. DHEA (5 to 10 mg/day) can relieve hot flushes for some women, and for others, relief is enhanced by the addition of natural progesterone.

UROGENITAL SYMPTOMS

The presence of estrogen receptor cells in the vaginal epithelium makes ERT an excellent choice for the prevention and treatment of symptoms associated with vaginal atrophy, including vaginal dryness, discharge, itching, burning, and bleeding and dyspareunia.[9] ERT is also effective for the treatment of pruritus vulvae.

After uterine prolapse occurs, surgery is usually indicated, but ERT can improve the natural support of the uterus. Although rare, support of the uterus can dramatically improve, obviating surgery.[10]

Because estrogen receptor cells also exist in the urethral mucosa, ERT has been shown in some women to prevent, reduce, or eliminate the symptoms associated with atrophic urethritis: urgency, frequency, dysuria, and suprapubic pain experienced in the absence of a urinary tract infection. Recurrent urinary tract infections in women with atrophic vaginitis may also benefit from ERT, because it promotes recolonization of the vagina by lactobacilli, resulting in a reduction of vaginal pH and the growth of gram-negative fecal pathogens.[1] Some women experience relief of vaginal dryness and atrophy and symptoms associated with atrophic urethritis after 3 to 4 months of natural progesterone therapy.[11]

DECLINE IN LIBIDO

The beneficial effects of ERT on libido are difficult to evaluate because of the anatomic, physiologic, and psychologic changes that often influence how a woman feels about her sexuality as she ages. Research findings on ERT and improvement of libido have been mixed. Some women have experienced an improvement, and others have not.

Research on the relationship of libido and natural progesterone has yet to be conducted. However, some clinicians have reported that some of their patients have noticed an increase in libido when natural progesterone has been used without other forms of hormonal therapy.

The results of studies using testosterone as treatment for a decline in libido are mixed. In two groups of women, one treated with estradiol implants and the other with estradiol and testosterone implants, a significant reduction in severity of many symptoms associated with the climacteric and an improvement in sexual interest, responsiveness, satisfaction, orgasmic capacity, and a lessening of dyspareunia were experienced.[12] A significant difference in improvement between the groups was not demonstrated. However, in another study women treated with estradiol and testosterone implants experienced an improvement in all sexual parameters—sexual activity, satisfaction, orgasm, and relevancy—compared with the group treated only with estradiol.[13] Similar results were demonstrated among women who had had oophorectomies.[14]

Research on the association of DHEA and libido has yet to be conducted. However, because DHEA can be converted into other hormones, including estrogen and testosterone, it is reasonable to consider that supplementation with DHEA may prove beneficial in increasing libido.

MOOD CHANGES, MEMORY PROBLEMS, AND HEADACHES

The effect of ERT on mood is difficult to evaluate for the same reasons a decline in libido is difficult to assess. Research has shown that, if a woman experiences anxiety, irritability, depression, or other mood changes, the symptoms can be related to life situations, attitudes toward menopause, and coping behaviors. These symptoms may also result from other climacteric-related symptoms, such as sleep deprivation resulting from nighttime hot flushes.

Changes in mood may also be a secondary response to the reduction in physical symptoms achieved with HRT. Mood changes may result from the effects of a decline in estrogen on the biochemistry of the brain. ERT has been found to reduce insomnia, anxiety, irritability, memory problems, and headaches independent of hot flushes.[13] Significant increases in ratings of confidence and feelings of elation have been associated with ERT and HRT among women with surgically induced menopause when treated with an injectable form of estrogen.[15]

Research in the area of memory has resulted in conflicting results. Some investigators have demonstrated improvement in verbal memory, short-term memory, and reasoning ability, but others have not.[16,17]

Research has shown that women with Alzheimer's disease were less likely to have used ERT.[18,19] Study of a small sample of elderly women with Alzheimer's disease showed an improvement in memory and mood after treatment with estrogen,[20] and another small sample showed improved scores on a test developed for dementia.[21] A larger study of more than 1000 elderly women demonstrated that the onset of Alzheimer's disease occurred significantly later in women who had taken estrogen than in those who had not. The relative risk of developing the disease was significantly reduced as well. The investigators in this study think estrogen use may delay the onset and decrease the risk of Alzheimer's disease. They also concluded that prospective studies are needed to establish dose and duration of the estrogen necessary to provide these benefits and to assess the safety of the therapy in elderly postmenopausal women.[22]

ERT does not appear to have an effect on true clinical depression.[23] Nevertheless, it may help relieve some of the symptoms of depression when the severity and duration do not meet the diagnostic criteria for major depression.[24]

In addition to the potential effects of steroids, mood is affected by many other factors, such as psychosocial events, the quality of nutritional intake, and adherence to an exercise program. Perhaps a reasonable approach to discussing ERT is to consider discussing the potential benefits but not to "sell" it as the definitive treatment for changes in mood. "By advocating estrogen therapy as a treatment for psychologic problems, the belief that menopause causes them is often, by implication, reinforced. This view of the menopause might encourage the negative stereotypes which have been shown to be predictive of depressed mood at this time of life."[25]

Women 40 to 70 years of age given 50 mg of DHEA each night for 3 months reported an improved sense of well-being.[26] Specific statements of well-being included improved quality of sleep, feeling more relaxed, having more energy, and an improved ability to deal with stress. Improvements of preexisting joint pain and mobility were self-reported. No change in libido was experienced. Within 2 weeks of initiating this dose, DHEA levels were restored to those found in young adults. A twofold increase in serum levels of androstenedione, testosterone, and dihydrotestosterone resulted, with no change in circulating levels of estrone and estradiol. HDL levels declined slightly.

PREVENTION OF CARDIOVASCULAR DISEASE

"More than 30 observational studies and one small randomized, controlled clinical trial have provided evidence that estrogen replacement reduces cardiovascular risk by approximately 50%."[27] Estrogen's protective effect can be experienced by women who have undergone surgical menopause or natural menopause. It has been estimated that, if all eligible women used estrogen, myocardial infarctions could be reduced as much as 45%.[28] This impact is comparable to the effect of elimination of smoking or the prevention of hypertension.

In one large cross-sectional study, postmenopausal women experienced a 56% decrease in the relative risk of coronary artery disease.[29] In the Nurses' Health Study, 620 of the 48,470 postmenopausal women followed developed fatal or nonfatal coronary disease. Current users of estrogen therapy showed the age-adjusted relative risk of coronary disease to be reduced by 50%.[30] A 63% reduction in the relative risk of fatal cardiovascular disease has been demonstrated in current estrogen users, including a protective effect in current and ex-smokers.[31]

The protective effect of estrogen against heart disease is a result of several mechanisms, including effects on lipoprotein levels, particularly decreasing low-density lipoprotein (LDL) and lipoprotein (a)[32] levels and increasing HDL levels.[33] These effects appear to be maintained as long as women remain on estrogen.[34] Estrogen therapy also has a positive effect on the cardiovascular system because of its ability to maintain the antioxidant state.[35]

Estrogen has a direct protective effect on the arterial wall,[36] it functions as an antioxidant,[37–39] and it mediates insulin metabolism. The oral form of conjugated estrogen at a dosage of 0.625 mg has been shown to lower fasting insulin levels and diminish the insulin response to glucose.[34,40,41]

Estrogen in doses of 0.625 mg or less may also have a favorable impact on the clotting mechanism, resulting in protection against thrombosis.[34] However, higher doses can cause thrombosis.[34] Doses of estrogen higher than the equivalent of 0.625 mg of conjugated estrogens should be avoided. A conjugated equine estrogen dosage of 0.625 mg per day or other estrogen therapy equivalent to this dosage appears to be the amount needed for cardiovascular protection.

Dr. Michael Colgan devised a computer model to assess the dosage yielding the greatest overall cardiovascular protection, taking into account that "high doses of estrogen replacement, which often raise HDL cholesterol the most, also raise the triglyceride levels the most."[42] Through this computer model he determined that a dose of conjugated equine estrogen of 0.33 mg per day raised HDL cholesterol as much or more than doses of 1.25 mg. However, the low dose raised triglycerides by only 1.5%, compared with the 33% rise caused by the 1.25 mg dose. He suggested that 0.33 mg per day affords better cardiovascular protection for postmenopausal women than any higher dose.

Concern has been raised regarding combined estrogen and progestin therapy. In some research, progestins have been shown to attenuate the LDL cholesterol-elevating properties of estrogen. Some research has shown that, when medroxyprogesterone was used alone, it reduced HDL by 16%, and when medroxyprogesterone was used with estrogen, HDL was reduced by 8%.[7,43,44] Although it appears that there is an approximately equal reduction in cardiovascular risk with estrogen-only and estrogen plus progestin therapy,[45–47] there is still concern that progestins may not be the optimal choice to use with estrogens. In one study, four estrogen treatment regimens produced significant increases in LDL and decreases in HDL. These lipid profiles were changed less in women using estrogen alone or estrogen with natural (micronized) progesterone.[8] However, all four regimens increased triglyceride levels.

Another study compared the use of conjugated equine estrogen (0.625 mg daily) and MPA (10 mg the first 10 days of each calendar month) and the same dose of estrogen with 200 to 300 mg of progesterone.[48] Women in the progestin group had increases in HDL levels and no change in total cholesterol levels. The natural progesterone group also had increased HDL levels and a decrease in total cholesterol levels. Climacteric-related symptoms were also relieved, minimal side effects were experienced, and endometrial hyperplasia was prevented. One of the investigators in this study, Dr. J. Hargrove, has not found natural progesterone in doses ranging from 300 to 500 mg per day to be associated with negative effects on the cardiovascular system during his 13 years of prescribing these dosages.[48]

Using estimates provided by Dr. Suzanne Oparil, President of the American Heart Association, a woman could lower her risk of heart disease by 12% by using natural progesterone instead of MPA in combination with estrogen.[49]

Although research on the effects of DHEA on cardiovascular health in postmenopausal women is limited, some evidence indicates that DHEA given as the sole form of therapy can increase the cardiovascular risk in postmenopausal women.[50] However, when estrogen levels have been restored to normal ranges in these women, DHEA may increase cardiovascular protection.[31,51] DHEA in a dose of 50 mg per day can enhance insulin sensitivity and lower triglycerides in postmenopausal women.[52]

PREVENTION OF OSTEOPOROSIS

The skeleton is a major target organ for sex steroids. Although the mechanisms are not understood, it appears that estrogens reduce the rate of bone remodeling.[53] ERT increases bone density[54] and prevents bone loss in postmenopausal women compared with placebo,[55-60] and it prevents vertebral fractures. A reduction in the risk of hip and lower forearm fractures[61] and reduction in tooth loss[62] have also been demonstrated.

The positive effects on bone loss are associated with initiation of ERT within 5 years of menopause. Long-term use (10 or more years) of ERT is needed for maximal protection against osteoporosis-related fractures.[34] Rapid bone loss results after estrogen withdrawal, and the protective effects of estrogen cease when discontinued.[63]

The dose determined to reduce the risk of osteoporosis is, as with heart disease, 0.625 mg of conjugated equine estrogen. An analysis of studies conducted by Colgan suggests that doses in the range of 0.2 to 0.6 mg per day, combined with progesterone, nutritional guidelines for osteoporosis prevention, and exercise may be effective in stopping bone loss and increasing the strength of bones.[42]

A combination of ERT's bone resorption effect with that of the bone formation effect of natural progesterone may be considered a better choice than ERT alone. However, if ERT is contraindicated or a woman does not want to use it, progesterone alone may significantly enhance bone density.[64,65]

A study of 100 postmenopausal women using ERT (0.3 to 0.625 mg/day for 3 weeks/month) and natural progesterone showed a progressive rise in bone mineral density of about 10% at 6-month and 1-year intervals and an annual increase of 3% to 5%, until stabilizing at the levels of healthy 35-year-old women.[66] Increased bone mineral density directly correlated with the lowest initial bone mineral densities, and occurrence of osteoporotic fractures dropped to zero. However, in this study, progesterone was given as a 3% cream (equivalent to about 25 to 35 mg/day) and was applied dermally at bedtime during the later 2 weeks of ERT. There is concern that a dose of 200 mg per day, as used by many clinicians and in the Postmenopausal Estrogen/Progestin Intervention (PEPI) study, may exceed the therapeutic window for osteoporosis treatment.[65]

DHEA may enhance bone density by stimulating bone formation and calcium absorption.[68] Women with higher levels of DHEA have been found to have greater bone mass than those with lower levels.[69] Women with osteoporosis had lower levels of DHEA than women of a similar age group who did not have osteoporosis.[70]

Postmenopausal women with Addison's disease have profound reductions in DHEA (94%) compared with healthy postmenopausal women[71] and have a dramatic loss of bone beyond what should be expected among postmenopausal women. They also had reduced levels of estrogen and testosterone. These results suggest that premenopausal women with Addison's disease do not develop osteoporosis because of adequate ovarian secretion of DHEA that compensates for weakened adrenal glands.[72] However, because DHEA production declines during the climacteric, the adrenal glands are unable to take over the function, and a substantial deficiency in DHEA results.

Testosterone may help to prevent osteoporosis. Women receiving implants of estradiol and testosterone showed a more rapid increase in bone mineral density in the hip and lumbar spine than in the estradiol-only treated group.[12]

ORAL HEALTH

Because ERT has been shown to reduce the risk of osteoporosis, it makes sense that it would also help prevent tooth loss and the need for dentures. This was shown to be the case among a large sample of women in the Leisure World Cohort Study.[62] Oral discomfort, burning, bad taste, and dryness may be relieved by ERT,[73] and gingival inflammation and bleeding may be reduced.[74]

OTHER HEALTH BENEFITS OF HORMONE THERAPIES

ERT significantly reduces the death rate from colorectal cancer.[75,76] Increased skin collagen[77] and increased skin thickness[78,79] have occurred with estrogen therapy and with a combination therapy of estrogen and testosterone.[80] Progesterone therapy may stimulate collagen growth,[81] and DHEA may help alleviate specific lupus symptoms and the systemic manifestations of lupus.[82–84]

RISKS AND SIDE EFFECTS OF HORMONE THERAPIES

Excess estrogen or a sensitivity to the form of estrogen being taken can cause several symptoms:

- Breast swelling and tenderness
- Dysmenorrhea
- Menorrhagia
- Elevated blood pressure
- Fluid retention and bloating
- Weight gain
- Migraine headaches
- Nausea and vomiting
- Chloasma
- Mood changes (eg, depression, irritability)
- Decreased libido
- Loss of frontal and crown head hair
- Confusion
- Intolerance of contact lenses

In addition to the potential for experiencing one or more of these side effects, a susceptibility factor for asthma not yet identified may be enhanced by estrogen. In the Nurses' Health Study, postmenopausal women who used estrogen with or without progestin had a 50% greater risk of developing asthma than women who had never used hormones.[85]

Excess progestin or a sensitivity to the form of progestin being taken can cause several symptoms:

- Irregular bleeding
- Abdominal bloating
- Headaches
- Breast tenderness
- Nervousness
- Decreased libido

Although for some women the sedative effects of natural progesterone can have a calming effect, other women experience transient drowsiness and fatigue. Research regarding the side effects of natural progesterone is extremely limited.

DHEA, primarily in higher doses such as 25 mg to 50 mg, is associated with several side effects:

- Irritability
- Aggressiveness
- Increased growth of facial and body hair

Research on the side effects of DHEA is extremely limited. However, conversations with several pharmacists who compound DHEA confirm that they agree that the listed symptoms may occur if the dosage is too high.

Side effects associated with synthetic testosterone include acne and mood changes. The hormone may also reduce the beneficial effects of estrogen on serum lipids. The effects of long-term synthetic testosterone therapy are unknown. Research on the side effects of natural testosterone is extremely limited, although an increase in facial and body hair, acne, and mood changes probably results from excessive intake.

BREAST CANCER

According to general consensus, when HRT is used for less than 5 years, there is no increase in the risk of breast cancer.[86] However, some studies have shown a 30% to 80% increase in breast cancer risk with more than 10 years of estrogen use.[87] Other studies have not shown any association between the two. The bottom line is that there is not enough data to definitively confirm or refute an association between HRT and breast cancer.

ABSOLUTE CONTRAINDICATIONS

Several absolute contraindications[88] apply to ERT:

- ❷ Undiagnosed vaginal bleeding
- ❷ Suspected breast or endometrial cancer
- ❷ History of breast cancer or endometrial cancer
- ❷ Malignant melanoma
- ❷ Active thrombophlebitis or thromboembolic disorders
- ❷ Acute liver disease

Although the use of ERT by women with cancer is being debated, some of these women who strongly wish to use ERT are being treated with it.

OTHER MEDICAL CONSIDERATIONS

Other diseases and disorders affect the recommendations for HRT.[88] The use of progestins or natural progesterone has been recommended for women with a history of endometriosis, even if the uterus has been removed. Though ERT does not usually stimulate the growth of fibroids and endometriosis, women should be carefully monitored. If a woman has not had her uterus removed and is taking a progestin or natural progesterone, she should also be monitored, because these hormones can stimulate the growth of fibroids.

Migraines may be worsened or alleviated by the use of HRT. A thorough history may help to determine whether the patient's migraines are affected by hormones.

A twofold increase in the rate of systemic lupus erythematosus (SLE) was associated with the use of postmenopausal estrogen in the Nurses' Health Study.[89] However, in a follow-up study of postmenopausal women with stable SLE, adverse effects of HRT were not detected.[90]

A dose-related increase in some procoagulants and anticoagulants has occurred with use of oral conjugated equine estrogens. A dose of 0.625 mg or less does not appear to increase the risk of thrombosis. Use of transdermal estrogen is also an option.

Functioning of the liver is affected by estrogens and progestins. These hormones should not be used by patients with acute liver disease or a history of chronically impaired liver function.

An increase in bile saturation of cholesterol can result from the use of oral estrogens. A nonoral estrogen is probably the best choice.

Increased triglyceride levels have not been associated with nonoral estrogen therapy.

Seizure disorders may be worsened by HRT due to the excitatory effect of estradiol on brain activity.

SYNTHETIC OR NATURAL HORMONES?

Debate about the term "natural" continues on. There are those in the health care community who consider conjugated equine estrogen "natural" as it is derived from an animal source. However, others disagree as the hormone product contains some estrogens whose molecular structure is unique to the mare and as a result, may be the cause of some of the side effects associated with this therapy.

Hormones compounded from the wild Mexican yam or soybeans have a molecular structure identical to that of the human and therefore are considered natural by the pharmacists who compound them and others in the health care community. However, there are others who disagree since the hormones must be synthesized in the laboratory from their plant sources.

One of the "natural" or plant-based compounded hormones that has appreciated increasing interest is estriol.

ESTRIOL

Advocates of estriol believe that it will prove to be a healthier choice for women, be associated with fewer side effects and complications, and may offer some protection against breast cancer.

In 1978, the *American Journal of Medicine* published Dr. Follingstad's call for the use of estriol as a safer estrogen.[91] Estriol is commonly used in Europe and Asia and is one form of estrogen being discussed and used more in the United States today. Although research is limited, estriol does not appear to be associated with breast cancer and may have a protective effect. Animal studies have shown that estriol inhibited the potential breast cancer–promoting effects of estradiol.[92–94] Epidemiologic studies have shown that women in countries with high rates of breast cancer have lower rates of estriol than women in countries with a low incidence of breast cancer.[95] Thirty-seven percent of women with metastatic breast cancer treated with 2.5 to 15 mg of estriol experienced a remission or an arrest of cancer.[96]

Estriol has been effective in treating vaginal and urinary tract symptoms,[97–100] and when 0.5 mg was used vaginally every night for 2 weeks followed by twice-weekly applications for 8 months, the incidence of urinary tract infections was significantly reduced in postmenopausal women.[101] A dose of 8 mg of estriol per day was not associated with endometrial hyperplasia and breakthrough bleeding, and 2.0 to 8.0 mg of estriol each day prevented vaginal atrophy and eliminated climacteric-related symptoms.[102] A prospective double-blind study of 136 women who were 0.5 to 21 years postmenopausal was conducted to demonstrate the effects of a long-acting estriol-derivative on bone loss and lipids. The results showed a decrease in LDL levels and an increase in HDL levels without significant changes in triglyceride levels. Loss of bone density of the forearm declined.[103] Another study revealed an increase in bone mineral density in postmenopausal women who received 2 mg of estriol each day combined with 2 mg of calcium lactate each day for 1 year.[72]

Estriol is not converted to estradiol and estrone. As a result, some believe that it may not be the best choice for ERT when used alone and instead should be used with other estrogens. Tri-Est was a product developed with this in mind. It is available in various strengths in the United States by prescription through several pharmacies that compound plant-based hormone therapies. Derived from soybeans, Tri-Est contains 80% estriol and 10% each of estradiol and estrone. Tri-Est was developed by Dr. J. Wright, an American physician who has worked with estriol since the early 1980s.[101] Some women need estriol in high doses of 10 to 15 mg per day to relieve menopausal symptoms that are often not well tolerated in such high doses. Because of this and research that has shown that 12 mg of a standard estriol per day is needed for osteoporosis prevention,[72] Wright concluded that the best way to use estriol was in combination with estrone and estradiol. He believes that risks are minimized and estrogen-related benefits are maximized by combining the plant-derived estrogens.

According to Wright, symptoms associated with the climacteric, such as vaginal atrophy and hot flushes, are usually relieved with the 2.5 mg combination of Tri-Est (therapeutically equivalent to 0.625 mg conjugated equine estrogen), although 5 mg per day (therapeutically equivalent to 1.25 mg conjugated equine estrogen) may be necessary. His treatment regimen uses Tri-Est for 25 days each month in combination with natural progesterone during the last 12 days of the regimen.[72]

For information about the use of natural estrogens and Tri-Est, you can speak with a pharmacist at one of the pharmacies that compounds these hormones. These pharmacies usually have a pharmacist available for consultation with health care providers (see Appendix C).

OTHER TREATMENTS FOR OSTEOPOROSIS

If a woman cannot or does not want to use an estrogen, progestin, or natural progesterone therapy, calcitonin or bisphophonates can be useful as a treatment for osteoporosis. Both of these treatments are initiated during the postmenopausal period.

CALCITONIN

Postmenopausal women with osteoporosis usually exhibit some degree of calcium malabsorption. They also commonly have low serum concentrations of 1,25-dihydroxyvitamin D (calcitriol).[72]

Calcitonin is a calcium-regulating hormone secreted by the thyroid gland. It inhibits osteoclasts, the cells that cause bone resorption. Levels of calcitonin begin to decline as men and women age. In postmenopausal women with osteoporosis, the levels have been found to be lower than in women of the same age who did not have osteoporosis.

Calcimar, a synthetic form of calcitonin given subcutaneously or intramuscularly, and Miacalcin, a calcitonin in nasal spray form, have been approved by the Food and Drug Administration (FDA) for the treatment of postmenopausal osteoporosis. Calcitonin should be given with calcium, magnesium, and other minerals and with vitamin D supplementation. In addition to being used as a treatment for postmenopausal osteoporosis, it may also be helpful in relieving pain caused by osteoporosis.

Some research has shown calcitriol to be beneficial in normalizing calcium absorption in postmenopausal patients with osteoporosis and in decreasing osteoporotic fractures; with long-term use, it may stimulate bone formation.[104] Other research results have not been so favorable. For example, in a comparison of alendronate plus 500 mg of calcium and intranasal salmon calcitonin plus 500 mg calcium, calcitonin failed to demonstrate an increase in bone mineral mass at any site. However, in a study in which women used calcitonin, ERT, or etidronate, the three agents appeared to be equally effective in increasing bone mineral density in the lumbar spine.[105] In another study, one group of postmenopausal women used 50 mg of transdermal beta-estradiol per day and 10 mg of MPA for 10 days; a second group took 1 g of elemental calcium per day; and the third group took 40 IU of eel calcitonin for 10 days each month. total-body bone mineral content increased in all groups.[106] There were significant losses in femoral neck density in the calcitonin and etidronate users but no loss in the ERT users.

Favorable results with calcitonin were observed in women using salmon calcitonin nasal spray plus 500 mg of calcium.[107] They had an 81% reduction in risk of bone loss. Salmon calcitonin nasal spray alone has also been shown to prevent loss of bone in the lumbar spine in women taking corticosteroids.[108] A combined therapy of intravaginal estriol and nasal spray salmon calcitonin taken by postmenopausal women decreased symptoms such as hot flushes (effect of estriol) and inhibited the decline in bone mineral density (effect of calcitonin).[109] Pain caused by osteoporosis has been significantly reduced within 2 weeks of treatment with different modes of calcitonin administration.[110]

BISPHOSPHONATES

Several bisphophonates interfere with the activity of osteoclasts, thereby inhibiting bone resorption. A second-generation bisphophonate, alendronate sodium (Fosamax), has been approved by the FDA for the prevention and treatment of postmenopausal osteoporosis. Studies have demonstrated a greater impact on improvement of bone mineral density than with first-generation bisphophonates, and the drug appears to be well tolerated when the directions for use are carefully followed.

Alendronate reduces the elevated rate of bone turnover observed in postmenopausal women to approximate more closely the turnover rate in premenopausal women. Increased bone mineral density of the spine, femoral neck, trochanter, and total body has resulted from administration of alendronate,[111–114] and the frequency of clinical vertebral fractures among women who already had experienced vertebral fractures was reduced.[115]

Some health care providers have prescribed concomitant use of alendronate and ERT. However, because of a lack of clinical experience, Merck and Company, the pharmaceutical company that manufactures Fosamax, recommends that this combined therapeutic approach not be prescribed.

TILUDRONATE

Tiludronate is a treatment for Paget's disease of bone and is currently being investigated for use in treating osteoporosis.[116]

SELECTIVE ESTROGEN RECEPTOR MODULATORS

Selective estrogen receptor modulators (SERM) is a new class of drugs that attaches to estrogen receptors. An example of a SERM is tamoxifen, the first widely used drug in this class. A newer SERM, raloxifene (Evista), is now available for osteoporosis prevention. SERMs such as tamoxifene and raloxifene have been shown to produce beneficial estrogen-like effects on bone and lipid metabolism while antagonizing estrogen in reproductive tissue.[117]

OTHER TREATMENTS FOR HOT FLUSHES

BELLERGAL

Bellergal is a drug that has been used for years for the relief of many symptoms, including hot flushes, restlessness, and insomnia associated with the menopause; palpitation, tachycardia, and vasomotor disturbances associated with cardiovascular disorders; and hypermotility, hypersecretion, and alternate diarrhea and constipation associated with gastrointestinal disturbances. It is also used as a treatment for recurrent, throbbing headaches. One of Bellergal's main components is phenobarbital; it therefore helps in relieving symptoms that respond to a therapy that exerts a sedative or calming effect.

It can be habit forming, and there are other precautions and potential side effects associated with its use. Although the side effects are not common, they include palpitations, urinary retention, gastrointestinal motility, tachycardia, flushing, and drowsiness. The *Physician's Desk Reference* can provide more information about this drug and the others discussed in this section.

BROMOCRIPTINE

Bromocriptine is a dopamine receptor agonist used for the treatment of hyperprolactinemia and acromegaly and for prevention of physiologic lactation. The effectiveness of this drug in alleviating hot flushes is unknown, although it appears to be helpful for some women. Low doses of this drug should be used to minimize the possibility of side effects such as drowsiness, dizziness, faintness, nausea, and headaches.

CLONIDINE

Clonidine is a hypertensive agent that can be taken orally or used transdermally. The transdermal route is recommended, because it appears to be associated with fewer side effects. The sedative effect seems to help some relieve hot flushes for some women.

Several potential side effects can aggravate other climacteric symptoms. Although these side effects may not be experienced by some women who may be candidates for clonidine, they are important to consider:

- Gastrointestinal effects: nausea, constipation, and change in taste
- Central nervous system effects: fatigue, headaches, lethargy, sedation, insomnia, dizziness, and nervousness
- Genitourinary effects: sexual dysfunction

PUTTING HORMONE REPLACEMENT AND DRUG THERAPIES INTO PERSPECTIVE

As with all forms of medical treatments, the risks and benefits of hormonal and drug therapies must be weighed by the patient in making a decision that is most comfortable for her. Too many women do not have adequate information about the various therapies available to make an informed choice. This may be a consequence of having a health care provider who does not offer this information or does so in a biased manner. Women may also have difficulty in making a comfortable decision about using ERT or HRT because of confusion and fears that may result from the media's often inadequate or incorrect discussion of research findings and the biases of some of the authors of books about menopause.

Fear is the most profound feeling that influences a woman's decision not to use hormonal therapy. More often than not, women have learned about the side effects and complications of a drug or hormone (eg, diethylstilbestrol, unopposed estrogen therapy, high-dose oral contraceptives) that has had a direct impact on the health of some women. They are aware that the problems associated with these became known after their use was commonplace and that many women bore the consequences of a serious side effect or complication. It is not surprising that some women do not want to consider any form of HRT.

What can health care professionals do to alleviate this fear? Being honest is probably the best course of action. For example, women should be told that prolonged use of ERT or HRT may increase the risk of breast cancer, although increasing numbers of studies have shown that this may not be the case. They also should be informed that the risk of disability and death from cardiovascular disease and the complications associated with osteoporosis are far greater than those resulting from a possible increased risk of breast cancer. The data support improvements in morbidity and mortality rates among women with coronary heart disease, myocardial infarction, congestive heart failure, hypertension, peripheral vascular disease, diabetes, stroke, and thromboembolic disorders.

One study showed that, of the women who had never taken HRT, one half had concerns about such treatment, and few wanted it at menopause. However, 96% (about 150) of these women said that, if their bone scan suggested an increased risk of osteoporosis, they would consider HRT.[118] Another study revealed that, of the 80 45-year-old women who expressed an opinion about HRT, about 44% thought that they might use HRT, and 42% said that they did not want to use it.[25] Thirteen percent expressed a lack of knowledge on which to base a decision. Reasons for intending to use HRT included general hopes to "feel better"; in this group, a significant number reported lower self-esteem and higher levels of depressed mood, anxiety, and negative attitudes toward menopause than the nonintenders. They also expressed stronger beliefs in their doctor's ability, compared with their own, to control their menopause experience. The nonintender group did not want to use HRT because they preferred not to use drugs, did not want to interfere with what they considered a normal process, or were concerned about possible side effects.

Another study showed that the main reasons women discontinued HRT were the belief that they did not need it and the undesirable side effects they experienced (bleeding was most common). Women who never initiated HRT felt they did not need it.[119]

Higher noncompliance rates were found among older women, those who used a progestin or experienced side effects, and those received care from a gynecologist or male physician. Women who were compliant were those who experienced menopausal symptoms, who used transdermal estrogen, or who had cardiovascular problems.[120]

Information obtained from the Healthy Women Study[121] showed that women who had ever used HRT were more reflective (ie, aware of private feelings and symptoms) and more aggressive and competitive than women who had never used HRT. They were also more educated than women who had never used HRT.

Among women who had breast cancer, the severity of their climacteric-related symptoms, particularly feelings of depression and sleep disturbance, was the deciding factor for those who were willing to use ERT, rather than their awareness that ERT decreased the risk of heart disease and osteoporosis. Those women unwilling to use ERT believed that the risk of recurrent breast and uterine cancer would be increased.[122]

When women reporting hot flushes once a week or more frequently were asked to choose between no treatment, HRT, or psychologic therapy (ie, cognitive-relaxation therapy), 75% wanted no treatment, 60% wanted relaxation therapy, and 40% wanted HRT. No significant difference was found between those preferring one or the other treatment; however, those seeking treatment for hot flushes were found to be significantly more anxious, did not cope well with stress, had lower internal focus of control scores, and had lower self-esteem than those not wanting treatment.[123]

The results of these studies can be useful in considering various approaches to discussing hormonal therapies with patients. You could suggest to patients, for example, that results from their bone scans should be considered an important factor in their decision-making process and your formulation of an opinion about their need to initiate HRT. It could prove beneficial to explore patients' attitudes about menopause and how they feel about themselves. If a patient's attitude toward menopause and her level of self-esteem are positive, you could approach discussion of HRT differently from the approach to be used with woman for whom this is not the case, particularly if she believes that HRT is the only solution for her negative feelings.

The next step is to help women to assess their risks for cardio-vascular disease and osteoporosis by discussing several factors, including the following:

- Current health status
- Family history
- Personal risk based on past and current lifestyle
- Ability and willingness to make the lifestyle changes that influence prevention and treatment of these health problems

In addition to assessing risks for cardiovascular disease and osteoporosis, other possible symptoms and health problems that may result from a decline in steroids should be discussed. Some women may be concerned about experiencing side effects that may be even more disruptive in their lives than their climacteric-related symptoms. Every woman probably has at least one friend or relative who has complained of hormone-related side effects. The possibility of side effects should be discussed, and the woman should be assured that, if side effects are experienced, various types of hormones and modes of administration can be used to alleviate or minimize the side effects. She also should be assured that, if any side effects are experienced, you will work closely with her to determine the best choice of therapy for her. Your willingness to experiment with different dosages, products, and regimens and to listen to how she is feeling can greatly contribute to her willingness to persevere.

Financial issues may override medical concerns. Some women cannot afford hormonal therapy.

Ideally, the woman should be encouraged to make a decision only after she has taken the time to consider the facts presented and to study some of the educational materials available on the subject. How long it takes to make this decision is not as important as arriving at the one with which she is most comfortable. A decision that has been made after careful thought is also probably the best one in terms of compliance. Many women leave the office or clinic with a prescription for a hormonal therapy in hand, only to leave it unfilled or to discontinue use after a few months.

REFERENCES

1. Lee J. Natural progesterone the multiple roles of a remarkable hormone. Sebastopol, CA: BLL Publishing; 1993.
2. Dentali S. Hormones and yams: what's the connection? Am Heart Assoc 1994;10:4.
3. Lobo RA, et al. Depo-medroxyprogesterone for the treatment of post-menopausal women. Obstet Gynecol 1984;63:1.
4. Erlik Y, et al. Effect of megestrol acetate on flushing and bone metabolism in postmenopausal women. Maturitas 1981;3:167.
5. Schiff I, et al. Oral medroxyprogesterone in the treatment of postmenopausal women. JAMA 1980;244;1443.
6. Loprinski CL, et al. Megestrol acetate for the prevention of hot flashes. N Engl J Med 1994;331:347.
7. Ottosson UB, et al. Subfractions of high-density lipoprotein cholesterol during estrogen replacement therapy: a comparison between progestogens and natural progesterone. Am J Obstet Gynecol 1985;151:746–750.
8. The Writing Group for the PEPI. Trial effects of estrogen or estrogen/progestin regimens on heart disease risk factors in postmenopausal women: the post-menopausal estrogen/progestin intervention (PEPI) trial. JAMA 1995;273:199–208.
9. Bergman A, Brenner P. Beneficial effects of pharmacologic agents—genitourinary. In: Mishell D, ed. Menopause: physiology and pharmacology. Chicago: Year Book Publishers, Chicago; 1987.
10. Cardozo L, Kelleher C. Estrogen deficiency and urinary incontinence. In: The modern management of the menopause: a perspective for the 21st century: proceedings of the VII International Congress on the Menopause; Stockholm, 1993. New York: Parthenon; 1994.
11. Dow MGT, Hart DM. Hormonal treatments of sexual unresponsiveness in postmenopausal women: a comparative study. Br J Obstet Gynecol 1983;90:361–366.
12. Davis SR, et al. Testosterone enhances estradiol's effects on postmenopausal bone density and sexuality. Maturitas 1995;21:227–236.
13. Bellerose SB, Binik YM. Body image and sexuality in oophorectomized women. Arch Sex Behav 1993;22:435–459.
14. Campbell S, Whitehead M. Oestrogen therapy and the menopausal syndrome. Clin Obstet Gynecol 1977;4:31–37.
15. Sherwin BB. Affective changes in estrogen and androgen replacement therapy in surgically menopausal women. J Affect Discord 1988;14:177–187.
16. Fedor-Freyergh P. The influence of oestrogen on the well-being and mental performance in climacteric and postmenopausal women. Acta Obstet Gynecol Scand 1977;64:5–69.
17. Rauramo L, et al. The effect of castration and personal estrogen therapy on some psychological functions. Front Horm Res 1975;8:133–151.

18. Henderson VW, et al. Estrogen replacement therapy in older women. Arch Neurol 1994;51:896–900.

19. Henderson VW. The epidemiology of estrogen replacement therapy and Alzheimer's disease. Neurology 1997;48(Suppl 7):S27–35.

20. Fillit H, et al. Observations in a preliminary open trial of estradiol therapy for senile dementia—Alzheimer's type. Psychoneuroendocrinology 1986;11:337–345.

21. Honjo HJ, et al. In vivo effects by estrone sulphate on the central nervous system-senile dementia (Alzheimer's type). J Steroid Biochem 1989;34:521–525.

22. Tang MX, et al. Effect of oestrogen during menopause on risk and age at onset of Alzheimer's disease. Lancet 1996;348:429–432.

23. Schneider MA, et al. The effects of exogenous oestrogens on depression in menopausal women. J Affect Discord 1988;14:177–187.

24. Sherwin B. Hormones, mood, and cognitive functioning in postmenopausal women. Obstet Gynecol 1996;87(Suppl 2):205–265.

25. Hunter MS, Liao KL. Intentions to use hormone replacement therapy in a community sample of 45-year-old women. Maturitas 1994;20:13–23.

26. Morales A, et al. Effects of replacement dose of dehydroepiandrosterone in men and women of advancing age. J Clin Endocrinol Metab 1994;78:1360–1367.

27. Sullivan J, Fowlkes L. The clinical aspects of estrogen and the cardiovascular system. Obstet Gynecol 1996;87(Suppl 2):36S.

28. Beard CM, et al. The Rochester Coronary Artery Heart Disease Project: effect of cigarette smoking, hypertension, diabetes and steroidal estrogen use on coronary heart disease among 40- to 59-year-old women, 1960 through 1982. Mayo Clin Proc 1989;64:1471.

29. Sullivan JM, et al. Postmenopausal estrogen use and coronary arthrosclerosis. Ann Intern Med 1988;108:358.

30. Stampfer MJ, et al. Postmenopausal estrogen therapy and cardiovascular disease: ten-year follow-up from the Nurse's Health Study. N Engl J Med 1991;325-756.

31. Bush TL, et al. Cardiovascular mortality and noncontraceptive use of estrogen in women: results from the Lipid Research Clinics Program Follow-up Study. Circulation 1987;75:1102.

32. Taskinen MR, et al. Hormone replacement therapy lowers plasma Lp(a) concentrations, comparison of cyclic transdermal and continuous estrogen-progestin regimens. Arterioscler Thromb Vasc Biol 1996;16:1215–1221.

33. Manolio TA, et al. Associations of postmenopausal estrogen use with cardiovascular disease and its risk factors in older women. Circulation 1993;88(Part I):2163.

34. Byyny R, Speroff L. A clinical guide for the care of older women: primary and preventative care, 2d ed. Baltimore: Williams & Wilkins; 1996.

35. Clemente C, et al. Alpha-tocopherol and beta-carotene serum levels in postmenopausal women treated with transdermal estradiol and oral medroxyprogesterone acetate. Horm Metab Res 1996;28:558–561.

36. Ingegno MD, et al. Progesterone receptors in the human heart and great vessels. Lab Invest 1988;59:353.

37. Rifici VA, Khachadurian AK. The inhibition of low-density lipoprotein oxidation by 17-beta-estradiol. Metabolism 1992;41:1110.

38. Knopp RH, et al. Effects of estrogens on lipoprotein metabolism and cardiovascular disease in women. Atherosclerosis 1994;110(Suppl 1):S83.

39. Lindheim SR, et al. The independent effects of exercise and estrogen and lipoproteins of postmenopausal women. Obstet Gynecol 1994;83:167.
40. Cagnacci A, et al. Effects of low doses of transdermal 17-beta-estradiol on carbohydrate metabolism in postmenopausal women. J Clin Endocrinol Metab 1992;74:1396.
41. Lobo R, et al. The Menopause Study Group: metabolic impact of adding medroxyprogesterone acetate to conjugated estrogen therapy in postmenopausal women. Obstet Gynecol 1994;84:987.
42. Colgan M. Hormonal health. Vancouver, BC: Apple; 1996:140.
43. Silfverstolpe G, et al. Lipid metabolic studies in oophorectomized women: effects on serum lipids and lipoproteins of three synthetic progestogens. Maturitus 1982;4:103–111.
44. Hirvonen E, et al. Effects of different progestogens on lipoproteins during postmenopausal replacement therapy. N Engl J Med 1981;304:560–563.
45. Barrett-Connor E, et al. Postmenopausal estrogen use and heart disease risk factors in the 1980's Rancho Bernardo California, revised. JAMA 1989;267:2095–2100.
46. Nabulsi AA, et al. Association of hormone-replacement therapy with various cardiovascular risk factors in postmenopausal women. N Engl J Med 1993;328:1069–1075.
47. Falkeborn M, et al. The risk of acute myocardial infarction after oestrogen and oestrogen-progestogen. Br J Obstet Gynecol 1992:Oct:821–828.
48. Hargrove J, et al. Menopausal hormone replacement therapy with continuous daily oral micronized estradiol and progesterone. Obstet Gynecol 1989;73:606–612.
49. News Conference at the American Heart Association Annual Meeting; Dallas; November 17, 1994. Womens Health Forum 1994;4.
50. Barrett-Connor E, Khaw KT. Absence of an inverse relation of dehydroepiandrosterone sulfate with cardiovascular mortality in postmenopausal women. N Engl J Med 1987;317:711.
51. Casson PR, et al. Lipoprotein lipase regulation by insulin and glucocorticoid in subcutaneous and omental adipose tissues of obese women and men. J Clin Invest 1993;92:2191–2198.
52. Casson PR, et al. Replacement of dehydro-epiandrosterone enhances T-lymphocyte insulin binding in postmenopausal women. Fertil Steril 1995;63:1027–1031.
53. Lindsay R. The menopause and osteoporosis. Obstet Gynecol 1996;87(Suppl 2):165–195.
54. The Writing Group for the PEPI. Effects of hormone therapy on bone mineral density: results from the postmenopausal estrogen/progestin intervention (PEPI) trial. JAMA 1996;276:1389–1389.
55. Lindsay R, et al. Long-term prevention of postmenopausal osteoporosis by estrogens. Lancet 1976;1:1038–1041.
56. Atkens JM, et al. Oestrogen replacement therapy for prevention of osteoporosis after oophorectomy. BMJ 1973;3:515–518.
57. Christiansen C, et al. Bone mass in postmenopausal women after withdrawal of oestrogen/gestagen replacement therapy. Lancet 1981;1:459–461.
58. Natchtigall LE, et al. Estrogen replacement therapy: a 10-year prospective study in the relationship to osteoporosis. Obstet Gynecol 1979;53:277–281.

59. Reese W. A better way to screen for osteoporosis. Contemp Obstet Gynecol 1983;November.

60. Tohme J, et al. Osteoporosis. In: Becker KL, ed. Principles and practices of endocrinology and metabolism, 2d ed. Philadelphia: JB Lippincott; 1995:567–585.

61. Weiss NS, et al. Decreased risk of fractures of the hip and lower forearm with postmenopausal use of estrogen. N Engl J Med 1980;303:1195.

62. Paganini-Hill A. The benefits of estrogen replacement therapy on oral health. Arch Intern Med 1995;155:2325–2329.

63. Lindsay R, et al. Bone response to termination of oestrogen treatment. Lancet 1978;1:1325–1327.

64. Ren Y, Zhu G. The effects of progestin on the bone metabolism in post-menopausal women. Chung Hua Fu Chan Ko Tsa Chih [Chin J Obstet Gynecol] 1995;30:135–137.

65. Prior JC, et al. Cyclic medroxyprogesterone treatment increases bone density: a controlled trial in active women with menstrual cycle disturbances. Am J Med 1994;96:521–530.

66. Lee J. Osteoporosis reversal: positive effects of progesterone supplementation to standard therapy. Int Clin Nutr Rev 1990;10(3).

67. Gaby A. An interview with Alan Gaby. Meno Times 1996;Spring.

68. Taelman P, et al. Persistence of increased bone resorption and possible role of dehydroepiandrosterone as a bone metabolism determinant in osteoporotic women in late post-menopause. Maturitas 1989;11:65–73.

69. Wild RA, et al. Declining adrenal androgens: an association with bone loss in aging women. Proc Soc Exp Biol Med 1987;186:355–360.

70. Nordin BCE, et al. The relation between calcium absorption serum dehy-droepiandrosterone and vertebral mineral density in postmenopausal women. J Clin Endocrinol Metab 1985;60:651–657.

71. Devogelaer JP, et al. Bone mineral density in Addison's disease: evidence for an effect of adrenal androgens on bone mass. BMJ 1987;294:798–800.

72. Gaby A. Preventing and reversing osteoporosis. Rocklin, CA: Prima Publishing; 1994.

73. Volpe A, et al. Oral discomfort and hormone replacement therapy in the post-menopause. Maturitas 1990;13:1.

74. Norderyd OM, et al. Periodontal status of women taking postmenopausal estro-gen supplementation. J Periodontol 1993;64:957.

75. Potter JD, et al. Hormone replacement therapy is associated with lower risk of adenomatous polyps of the large bowel: the Minnesota cancer prevention research unit case-controlled study. Cancer Epidemiol Biomark Prev 1996;5:779–784.

76. Calle EE, et al. Estrogen replacement therapy and risk of fatal colon cancer in a prospective cohort of postmenopausal women. J Natl Cancer Inst 1995;87:517–523.

77. Brincat M, et al. Sex hormones and skin collagen content in postmenopausal women. BMJ 1983;287:1337–1338.

78. Brincat M, et al. Skin thickness and skin collagen mimic an index of osteo-porosis in the postmenopausal woman. In: Christiansen C et al, eds. Osteo-porosis: proceedings of the Copenhagen International Symposium on Osteo-porosis, 1984:353–355.

79. Vaillant L, Callens A. Hormone replacement treatment: a skin aging therapy. 1996;51:67–70.

80. Savvas M, et al. Type III collagen content in the skin of postmenopausal women receiving oestradiol and testosterone implants. Br J Obstet Gynecol 1993;100:154–156.

81. Pieerard GE, et al. Effect of hormone replacement therapy for menopause on the mechanical properties of skin. Am Geriatr Soc 1995;43:662–665.

82. Robinson T, Neuwelt CM. Neuropsychiatric lupus and hormones. Ann Med 1996;147:276–280.

83. Van Vollenhoven RF, McGuire JL. Studies of dehydroepiandrosterone (DHEA) as a therapeutic agent in systemic lupus erythematosus. Ann Med Interne 1996;147:290–296.

84. Van Vollenhoven RF, et al. Dehydroepiandrosterone in systemic lupus erythematosus: results of a double-blind, placebo-controlled, randomized clinical trial. Arthritis Rheum 1995;38:1826–1831.

85. Mann D. Asthma: long-term estrogen may double risk of developing disease. Med Tribune 1995;Nov 23.

86. Ewertz M. Hormonal replacement therapy and incidence of breast cancer. In: The modern management of the menopause: a perspective for the 21st century: proceedings of the VIIth International Congress on the Menopause; Stockholm, 1993. New York: Parthenon; 1994.

87. Brinton LA, Schairer C. Estrogen replacement therapy and breast cancer risk. Epidemiol Rev 1993.

88. Greendale GA, Judd HL. Hormone therapy in the menopause. In: Carr P et al, eds. The medical care of women. Philadelphia: WB Saunders; 1995.

89. Sanchez G, et al. Postmenopausal estrogen therapy and the risk for developing systemic lupus erythematosus. Ann Intern Med 1995;122:430.

90. Arden NK, et al. Safety of hormone replacement therapy (HRT) in systemic lupus erythematosus (SLE). Lupus 1994;3:11.

91. Follingstad A. Estriol: the forgotten hormone. JAMA 1978;239:29–30.

92. Henry Lemon, et al. Reduced estriol excretion in patients with breast cancer before endocrine therapy. JAMA 1966;196:1128–1136.

93. Wotiz H, et al. Effects of estrogens on DMBA-induced breast tumors. J Steroid Biochem 1984;20:1065–1075.

94. Lemon HM. Estriol prevention of mammary carcinoma induced by 7,12-dimethylbenzanthracene and procarbazine. Cancer Res 1975;35:1341–1353.

95. Speroff L. The breast as an endocrine target organ. Contemp Obstet Gynecol 1977;9:69–72.

96. Lemon H. Pathophysiologic considerations in the treatment of menopausal patients with oestrogens: the role of oestriol in the prevention of mammary carcinoma. Acta Endocrinol 1980;233:S17–S27.

97. Kirkengen P, et al. Oestriol in the prophylactic treatment of recurrent urinary tract infections in postmenopausal women. Scand J Prim Health Care 1992;10:139–142.

98. Heimer GM, Englund DE. Effects of vaginally administered oestriol on postmenopausal urogenital disorders: a cytohormonal study. Maturitas 1992;3:171–179.

99. Raz R, Stamm WA. Controlled trial of intravaginal estriol in postmenopausal women with recurrent urinary tract infections. N Engl J Med 1993;329:753–736.

100. Di Stefano L, et al. Transvaginal administration of estriol in postmenopausal urogynecological disorders. Minerva Ginecol 1993;4591:551–556.
101. Tzingounis VA, et al. Estriol in the management of the menopause. JAMA 1978;239:1638–1641.
102. Lauritzen C. Results of a five-year prospective study of estriol succinate treatment in patients with climacteric complaints. Horm Metab Res 1987;19:579–584.
103. Guo-jun C, et al. Prospective double-blind study of CEE3 in peri- and postmenopausal women: effects on bone loss and lipoprotein levels. Chin Med J 1994;103:929–933.
104. Adami S, et al. Effects of oral alendronate and intranasal salmon calcitonin on bone mass and biochemical markers in postmenopausal women with osteoporosis. Bone 1995;17:383–390.
105. Cosman F, et al. Postmenopausal osteoporosis: patient choices and outcome. Maturitas 1995;22:137–143.
106. Perez-Jaraiz, et al. Prophylaxis of osteoporosis with calcium, estrogens, and/or eel calcitonin: comparative longitudinal study of bone mass. Maturitas 1996;23:327–332.
107. Overgaard K, et al. Patient responsiveness to calcitonin salmon nasal spray: a subanalysis of a 2-year study. Clin Ther 1995;17:680–685.
108. Adachi JD, et al. Salmon calcitonin nasal spray in the prevention of corticosteroid-induced osteoporosis. Br J Rheum 1997;36:255–259.
109. Melis GB, et al. Salmon calcitonin plus intravaginal estriol: an effective treatment of the menopause. Maturitas 1996;34:83–90.
110. Pontiroli AE, et al. Analgesic effect of intranasal and intramuscular salmon calcitonin in postmenopausal osteoporosis: a double-blind, double placebo study. Aging 1994;6:459–463.
111. Harris, et al. Four-year study of intermittent cyclic etidronate treatment of postmenopausal osteoporosis: three years of blinded therapy followed by one year of open therapy. Am J Med 1993;95:557.
112. Weinstein R. Alendronate: treatment of osteoporosis in elderly women. J Bone Miner Res 1994;9(Suppl).S144.
113. Adami S, et al. Treatment of postmenopausal osteoporosis with continuous daily oral alendronate in comparison with either placebo or intranasal salmon calcitonin. Osteoporos Int 1993;3:S21–S27.
114. Devogelaer, JP, et al. Oral alendronate induces progressive increases in bone mass of the spine, hip, and total body over 3 years in postmenopausal women with osteoporosis. Bone 1996;18:141–150.
115. Black D, et al. Randomised trial of effect of alendronate on rest of fracture in women with external fractures. Lancet 1996;348:1535–1541.
116. Chestnut CH. Tiludronate: development as an osteoporosis therapy. Bone 1995;17:517S–519S.
117. Hu B, Dere WH. Selective estrogen receptive modulators: an alternative to hormone replacement therapy. Pro Soc Exp Biol Med 1998;217:45–52.
118. Garton M, et al. The climacteric osteoporosis and hormone replacement: views of women aged 45–49. Maturitas 1995;21:7–15.
119. Salamone LM, et al. Estrogen replacement therapy: a survey of older women's attitudes. Arch Intern Med 1996;156:1293–1297.

120. Berman RS, et al. Risk factors associated with women's compliance with estrogen replacement therapy. J Womens Health 1997;6:219–226.
121. Matthews KA, et al. Educational attainment and behavioral and biologic risk factors for coronary heart disease in middle-aged women. Am J Epidemiol 1989;129:1132–1144.
122. Rozenberg S, et al. Compliance to hormone replacement therapy. Int J Fertil Menopausal Stud 1995;40:S23–S32.
123. Ghali W, et al. Determinants of treatment choice for menopausal hot flushes: hormonal versus psychological versus no treatment. J Psychosom Obstet Gynaecol 1995;16:101–108.

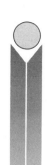

CHAPTER 8

Complementary Therapies and Holistic Medicine

Len Duhl, Professor at the School of Public Health of the University of California at Berkeley, said, "The joining together of conventional and alternative traditions may well permit us to have a more balanced quality of life. At least it has helped to bring the concept of health back to medicine."[1] Bezold, Carlson, and Peck, in their book *The Future of Work and Health,* predicted that, although 21st-century medicine will have a highly technologic component, it will also have an equally strong "high touch" component. Technologic advances in diagnostic and therapeutic measures will be combined with greater reliance on self-care practices, wellness programs, therapeutic nutritional and fitness regimens, and alternative or complementary health care practices. These investigators also predict that various spiritual practices for health and healing will be integrated into Western medicine.[2]

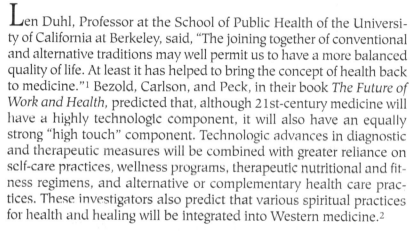

> When one looks at the history of health care, conventional Western medicine has been practiced for less than a blip on civilization's time line. Therapies such as Chinese medicine, herbal medicine, and acupuncture; indigenous practices such as shamanism and curanderismo; and other approaches such as prayer and healing touch have been practiced since the earliest times of recorded history. In Europe holistic practices such as homeopathy and herbal use are the norm rather than the exception.[3]

Between 70% and 90% of health care throughout the world is delivered through an organized health care system that is based on complementary traditions or practices and self-care according to folk principles.[4] Only 10% to 30% is delivered by conventional, biomedically oriented practitioners.

Although practiced and accepted much more in other countries, complementary therapies are gaining ground in the United States. A survey conducted by Eisenberg and colleagues in 1990 revealed that 425 million visits were made to practitioners of complementary therapies, exceeding the 388 million visits to general and family practitioners, pediatricians, and internal medicine specialists.[5] The list of complementary therapies used for this survey included relaxation techniques, chiropractic, lifestyle diets (eg, macrobiotics), herbal medicine, megavitamin therapy, hypnosis, homeopathy, and acupuncture.

The research showed that complementary therapies were used as an adjunct to, rather than a replacement for, conventional therapies. The researchers reported, "It is likely that virtually all medical doctors see patients who routinely use unconventional therapies. For medical doctors currently caring for patients with back problems, anxiety, depression, or chronic pain, the odds are greater than one in three that a patient is simultaneously using unconventional therapy for these problems without disclosing this fact."[5]

The researchers estimated that at least 70% of patients using unconventional (ie, complementary) therapies do not reveal to their physicians that they are doing so. They said that the results of the survey "suggest a deficiency in current doctor-patient relations. Perhaps medical doctors do not discuss the use of unconventional therapies because they lack adequate knowledge of these techniques."[5] They recommended that clinicians ask their patients about their possible use of complementary therapies and that the clinicians also enhance their understanding of such therapies. Because complementary health is based on a foundation of prevention of health care problems and treatment that focuses on providing the body with what it needs to heal itself, it is the foundation that may prove to have great impact on the prevention and treatment of the chronic debilitating diseases that effect millions of women as they pass through menopause and enter the last several decades of their lives.

Limited information is available on U.S. physicians' attitudes and practice regarding complementary therapies. However, a study conducted in 1995 yielded promising results. Analysis of 572 responses from board-certified primary care physicians revealed that 92% were comfortable in referring patients to at least one form of therapy and that 57% were willing to refer patients to six or more complementary therapies. More than one third of the respondents directly provided treatment through at least one complementary therapy.[6] However, a 1993 Gallup survey of menopausal women revealed that only 2% of their doctors had discussed any of the various complementary therapies, with the focus being entirely on hormone replacement therapy (HRT).

The findings from these studies, combined with the fact that complementary practices have a significant and growing presence in the United States health care system, are two of the reasons that this chapter is devoted to complementary therapies. Another is that increasing numbers of conventionally (Western) trained health care professionals are searching for ways in which they can better meet the health care needs of their patients, as evidenced by the growing trend of medical centers offering programs in complementary therapies and establishing departments in complementary medicine. Government-funded research in complementary therapies is increasing, more medical schools are integrating many of these therapies into their curricula, and some health insurance companies are reimbursing for selected therapies.

Health care professionals are becoming more open to supplementing their conventional medical knowledge base with a greater array of health "tools." Conventional medicine is extremely effective in treating traumatic injuries, infectious diseases, and some other health care problems. However, conventional medicine is often ill equipped to handle the complex, chronic conditions affecting an enormous number of Americans, particularly because of emphasis on the single "magic bullet" solution for each condition or disease.[7] Such one-dimensional solutions are not sufficient to treat many chronic conditions such as osteoporosis and cardiovascular disease, and multifaceted approaches are more appropriate treatment interventions. Some health care professionals do not want to practice complementary therapies themselves but are open to learn more about them so they can support their patients who wish to explore the possibility of using these therapies.

A complementary medical approach may be the only option for some women when it comes to symptoms and health problems associated with the climacteric. As stated in an article in *Clinical Obstetrics and Gynecology,*

> Despite the many advantages of estrogen replacement therapy, it is not appropriate for all women. Cultural, personal, and

medical considerations may eliminate the use of estrogen, in which case it is important to offer alternative medical advise and direction to minimize bothersome symptoms of menopause and enhance the quality of life.[8]

Chapter 7 highlighted some of the reasons why women do not want to use HRT or why they often discontinue the treatment program within months of initiating it. These women and those who are medically unable to use hormonal therapies must have other treatment options available to them. An estimated 43 million women are experiencing the climacteric. Assuming, for example, 50% are willing to use a hormonal therapy, will continue it indefinitely, and do not have any medical contraindications, 21.5 million other women will not be using HRT, and 75% of these women will experience bothersome symptoms. Consequently, at least 16 million women will be in need of some type of treatment to relieve their symptoms, setting the stage for the use of complementary therapies.

THE HOLISTIC HEALTH MODEL

All complementary therapies are based on a holistic health model of self-care and personal responsibility for wellness. This model has also become the foundation for increasing numbers of conventionally trained health care professionals. Holistically oriented practitioners believe in the integration of several forms of conventional and complementary therapies—whatever aids in the healing of the patient's body, mind, and spirit. The emphasis is on the "wholeness" of a person, prevention of disease, and maintenance of health.

A gynecologic oncologist can be "holistic," while a massage therapist may not be. It is the approach to healing that treats the whole person, instead of primarily focusing on the treatment of the symptoms, that separates a holistically oriented health care professional from a nonholistically oriented one. For example, if a woman is diagnosed with breast cancer, a holistically oriented physician would perform the necessary surgical procedure and recommend irradiation or chemotherapy, as appropriate. The clinician would also include, as a vital component of the woman's treatment program, specific nutritional and exercise recommendations, stress reduction, and perhaps herbs or other complementary health care practices. The physician may also advise the woman to use a technique such as guided imagery to aid in her recovery and to strengthen her immune system and would stress that all of these components of her treatment program are essential to healing and maintenance of her health. If the physician was not able to directly offer the education and guidance for the lifestyle recommendations and complementary therapies, the patient would be referred to practitioners who could.

PRINCIPLES OF HOLISTIC AND COMPLEMENTARY HEALTH CARE

Regardless of the therapy or system, all holistic or complementary practices share several basic principles[9]:

- The individual is empowered to play an integral role in her or his recovery and future health maintenance.
- Balanced lifestyle and appropriate rest, sleep, exercise, nutrition, and emotional tranquility are recognized prerequisites for health.
- The individual, rather than the symptoms, is treated.
- Health depends on balance or harmony among the physical, emotional, and spiritual aspects of a person.

These therapies view health, the causes of illness, and the ways in which healing takes place quite differently from conventional medicine. Even the terminology is different and sounds nonmedical to the Western ear. An example is the word *energy*. You have heard patients who are recovering from some illness say, "I feel my energy returning" or " I don't have any energy today." It is a word that in some way conveys a force within us that enables us to do what we need and want to do in our lives.

In complementary therapies such as traditional Chinese and Ayurvedic medicines, the word *energy* is translated into a *vital life force* that activates every function and drives every voluntary and involuntary process in the body. This vital life force is considered the key to life. It moves throughout the body in specific ways and is altered by the foods we eat, our activities, our emotions, and our spiritual thoughts.

Because the concept of the vital life force is the foundation for many complementary therapies, the diagnostic process includes evaluating the flow of energy (ie, life force) and determining areas of weaknesses and strengths in this flow in the corresponding physiologic systems to determine areas in which an imbalance of energy exists. The focus of the treatment is one of correcting imbalances. The diagnosis of a particular disease or illness is not of primary importance; instead, it is the diagnosis of the source of the imbalance in the flow of energy.

Even if not understood or accepted, this concept is important for conventionally trained health care professionals to acknowledge, because it is not unusual to hear some ask, for example, "What herbs should I use for hot flushes?" A practitioner of Asian medicine might respond that, although there are herbs for the treatment of this symptom, the herbs that a woman should use are ideally based on the organs or systems in which the imbalance of the vital life force exists for her. If, through the diagnostic process, it is determined for one woman that an imbalance exists in her thyroid or adrenal glands, specific herbs and other forms of treatment would be prescribed. Another woman may have hot flushes but may have an imbalance in her liver or kidneys, and her treatment would be different from that of the first woman. The ultimate goal is dealing with the cause of the imbalance that is unique to her. However, it may also be appropriate to prescribe the same herbs for both women to assist in treating their hot flushes.

The focus of treatment in these examples is based on alleviating symptoms and correcting imbalances in the flow of energy that contributed to the symptoms. Treatment is integrated to correct imbalances that are being or may be experienced as a disease or illness in the future. In this respect, treatment focuses on addressing the immediate problem and on preventing future health problems.

Complementary therapies share the same principles listed previously as well as the principle of the vital life force and some of the same initial evaluation processes. An initial consultation by a practitioner of a complementary health care method usually requires a 1- to 2-hour visit, during which time extensive information is obtained from the patient regarding her medical and family history and lifestyle, such as diet, physical activities, and stressors (eg, family, work, exposure to environmental and occupational toxins). The way in which an individual deals with stressors is explored. The symptoms that the individual may be experiencing and a diagnosis made by a conventionally trained health care professional are also discussed with the patient. The extensive information obtained from the patient, combined with specific diagnostic practices of the complementary therapy being used, results in the development of a multi-faceted treatment program that addresses the physiologic, emotional, and spiritual needs of the patient.

COMPLEMENTARY THERAPIES

Numerous beneficial therapies are practiced throughout the United States. However, I have chosen to discuss those that are reimbursed by some U.S. health insurance companies, that are approved by some health maintenance organizations and medical centers, and that appear to be most commonly accepted and used for the treatment of climacteric-related symptoms:

- Traditional Chinese medicine
- Acupuncture
- Ayurvedic medicine
- Naturopathic medicine
- Homeopathy
- Herbal medicine
- Osteopathic medicine
- Chiropractic
- Stress reduction techniques, guided imagery, and massage

TRADITIONAL CHINESE MEDICINE

When looking through the stacks of books at the UCLA Biomedical Library, it was surprising to find at least 20 books, some more than 40 years old, written for physicians about Traditional Chinese medicine (TCM). One of the books published in 1962 included a Foreword by Aldous Huxley:

> That a needle stuck into one's foot should improve the functioning of one's liver is obviously incredible. It can't be believed because, in terms of currently accepted physiologic theory "it makes no sense." Within our system of explanation there is no reason why the needle-prick should be followed by an improvement of liver function. Therefore, we say it can't happen. The only trouble with this argument is that, as matter of empirical fact, it does happen. Inserted at precisely the right point, the needle in the foot regularly affects the function

of the liver. The fact remains that there are many pathologic symptoms on which the old Chinese methods work very well. For the patient whose only wish is to get well as quickly as possible, this is all that matters.[10]

Chinese medicine is a system of healing that is more than 3000 years old. It has as its foundation the philosophical and metaphysical world views of Taoism, Confucianism, and Buddhism. It has always emphasized moderation in all aspects of life for the maintenance of health and prevention of illness. Chinese physicians have always taught their patients how to live a moderate and balanced lifestyle and ways in which they could create harmony among the emotional, physical, and spiritual aspects of life. Historically, Chinese physicians were paid only if their patients remained healthy.[11]

HISTORICAL PERSPECTIVE

Over the centuries, many styles of Chinese medical practices developed. However, the one with which Westerners are most familiar is TCM. This form has been supported by the People's Republic of China since the 1949 Communist Revolution. With this support came organized training of practitioners with a curriculum that included herbal medicine, acupuncture, oriental massage, and pharmacology.

Physicians trained in Chinese medicine in France introduced it in the United States in the 1700s, and in the 1800s, practitioners from Asia began to practice Chinese medicine in the United States.[12] The 1901 edition of *Gray's Anatomy* and the 1892 through 1947 editions of *Osler's Principles and Practice of Medicine* referred to the successful treatment of sciatica and lumbago through acupuncture therapy, which contributed to some acceptance of Chinese medicine.[12] This statement was deleted from subsequent editions. It was not until the 1970s that the practice of Chinese medicine began to be accepted in the United States by conventional health care practitioners and the public.

James Reston, a *New York Times* correspondent, has been credited with contributing to this acceptance through the publication of an article in which he described his own experience with TCM. While in China in the early 1970s, Reston underwent an emergency appendectomy that was performed with local anesthesia and acupuncture. Acupuncture was also performed postoperatively. His article described his experiences with TCM and the effects of acupuncture in preventing pain during surgery and for relief of pain after surgery.[12]

Since the 1970s, at least 35 TCM schools have opened in the United States, and a national accrediting body has been formed. Increasing acceptance of acupuncture, combined with the number of schools that exist, has resulted in more than 3000 physicians attending courses in acupuncture and 9 to 12 million patient visits to acupuncturists in 1994.[13] There are several thousand acupuncturists in the United States today. TCM is practiced by more than one fourth of the world's population and has been selected by the World Health Organization for worldwide propagation to meet the health needs of the 21st century.[14]

PRINCIPLES OF TRADITIONAL CHINESE MEDICINE

When people turn to Chinese medicine, they find one person who understands how their back problem is connected to their abdominal distention, which is connected to the dryness in their eyes, which is connected to their sometimes aggressive and sometimes passive feelings. All the symptoms the person may experience become integrated, which enables her to feel like one whole person who is seeking guidance from another for help with all the parts of herself.[15]

It is not an unusual sight to see persons sporting T-shirts or wearing pendants and earrings portraying the yin-yang symbol, yet some may not realize that this symbol represents one of the basic principles on which TCM is based. The symbol is composed of two colors (ie, black and white or red and green), with each color forming a specific shape. At first glance, these colors and shapes appear to be extreme opposites of each other, but on closer examination of the symbol, it becomes obvious that these opposites form a complete circle. This symbol—the joining of opposites to form a whole, complementary unit—represents a duality of opposing forces: yin and yang. Practitioners of TCM believe that these energy flows affect everything in life, animate and inanimate. When yin and yang are in balance, harmony and good health exist. When they are unbalanced, discord and illness result.

How persons respond during the seasons is a typical example of the principles of yin and yang. During the summer, a person usually eats a more yin (cooling) diet of fruit, vegetables, and more liquids. If a person has been out in the sun (yang, or hot and stimulating) for a while, that person will at some point seek a cooler, darker, and more passive environment (yin) to create a balance between yin and yang.

Yin is sometimes described as the feminine principle and yang as the masculine principle. Each has qualities associated with it. For example, yin energy is passive, nurturing, dark, cool, and contractive; yang energy is active, stimulating, light, warm, and expansive. The interplay of yin and yang is expressed in every aspect of life, including the physiologic processes. Organs are yin or yang, and symptoms can be analyzed in terms of these energy flows. The ultimate goal of TCM is to facilitate the body's ability to create a balance of the opposite energies of yin and yang so that healing and maintenance of health can occur.

Another basic principle is that all forces that operate in the universe also operate in human beings, and there is an energy force in man and all living things that we call *ch'i* or *qi*[16] (pronounced *chee*), in which yin and yang are complementary. Qi circulates throughout the body, and its amount, quality, and balance determine the state of a person's health.

Everything in life can affect qi: weather, diet, exercise, and emotional state. If there is an inadequate amount of qi or it is unable to freely flow throughout the body, an imbalance or disharmony results. The greater the imbalance of qi, the more likely that disease will arise.

Qi moves throughout the body through pathways known as meridians. Twelve of the many meridians carry qi. Meridians run from head to toe throughout the extremities and organs and are named after the organ through which they pass, such as the liver meridian. The network of all meridians forms a circuit through which qi travels. If energy is moving too quickly, too slowly, or not at all, one of the goals of TCM is to stimulate the affected meridians to correct the imbalance. This is accomplished through herbs, acupressure massage, or acupuncture.

ACUPUNCTURE

Acupuncture is one of the most thoroughly researched and documented of the so-called alternative medical practices.... The diversity of clinical applications and supporting basic physiology studies points to acupuncture having a therapeutic effect that exceeds a purely placebo or culturally dependent action.[17]

During an acupuncture treatment, specifically designed needles are inserted into acupoints located just beneath the skin. More than 1000 of these points can be stimulated to aid in healing by correcting the flow of qi through the meridians. Do meridians actually exist? The research appears to demonstrate that they do. Microdissection techniques used by researchers in Korea revealed an independent flow of ductlike tubes through which a fluid flowed.[18] These corresponded to the meridian pathways. It was observed that the fluid sometimes traveled in the same direction as the blood and lymphatic fluids, and at other times, it flowed in the opposite direction.

Further research conducted in France involved injection of radioactive isotopes into acupoints. The movement of the isotopes was tracked as they traveled along the meridians. When isotopes were injected in blood vessels, they did not travel in the same manner, indicating that there existed separate pathways within the body: the meridians.[19]

Galvanic skin responses of meridians and acupuncture points have been measured to reveal a specific relation between them and electrical currents of the body. Further research funded by the National Institutes of Health has shown that electrical currents flow along the meridians.[20]

Through a series of controlled experiments, acupuncture has been shown to be effective in the treatment of numerous health problems, including osteoarthritis, chemotherapy-induced nausea, asthma, back pain, and dysmenorrhea. Trigeminal neuralgia, tonsillitis, asthma, duodenal ulcers and other gastrointestinal disorders, sciatica, and osteoarthritis are among the 104 specific health care problems that the World Health Organization has cited as treatable through acupuncture.[21]

The frequency and severity of muscle tension, migraine headaches, and chronic pain appear to respond well to acupuncture,[22] as do addictions to alcohol, tobacco, and heroin.[23] This may be in part a result of the ability of acupuncture to stimulate the release of endorphins and enkephalins.

Six weeks of acupuncture produced an increase in alpha and a decrease in delta waves, which successfully treated depression in 90% of the 20 patients treated.[24] Average pain scores of 83% of the 50 patients treated through acupuncture because of chronic back pain were reduced by one half, and 58% of these continued to show improvement 40 weeks after the treatment had ended.[25]

Women undergoing gynecologic surgery and who received electroacupuncture while still under anesthesia used only one half as much medication for pain as the control group.[26] Among 16 male patients with liver cancer, herbs and ear acupuncture minimized abdominal distention and urinary retention postoperatively, but the other treatment, epidural morphine, prolonged them.[27]

Acupuncture has also been shown to be beneficial in the treatment of paralysis from stroke. Margaret Naser, Associate Professor of Neurology at the Boston University School of Medicine and Veteran Affairs Medical Center, found that acupuncture treatments enhanced recovery of patients who had strokes.[28] She provided an example of the way in which complementary and conventional medical practices can be used together. By using computed tomographic scans of these patients' brains, Dr. Naser could predicts which patients would benefit from acupuncture. These benefits may result from the increase in blood flow created through acupuncture, which may affect neurons or possibly create alternative neuronal connections. Acupuncture increases blood cortisol levels that may mediate the improvement in paralysis after acupuncture treatment. An increase in cortisol levels through acupuncture may also have a positive effect on reducing brain swelling.

CHINESE HERBS

Herbs are used to assist in the correction of imbalances in the flow of qi. More than 3000 herbs are used in Chinese medicine. Complex mixtures of these herbs create several effects, including correcting an imbalance, preventing potential side effects, and acting as therapeutic agents for a specific area or a physical process in body. Applications of Chinese herbal medicine include treatment of various cancers in which a combination of herbs with radiation therapy demonstrated significantly higher survival rates and an increase in patients' tolerance to chemotherapy.[29–33] Use of Chinese herbs has demonstrated a reduction in high blood pressure, relief from angina-related pain, improved cardiac function, reduction in blood lipid levels, and improvement in electrocardiographic indices.[34–36] They are also commonly used for the treatment of reproductive disorders and climacteric-related symptoms.

DIAGNOSIS AND TREATMENT

Diagnosis begins by assessing the appearance of an individual, including posture, complexion, eyes, and facial expression. The tongue, voice, breath, and pulses at the radial arteries of both wrists are also evaluated. There are six positions (pulses) on each wrist used in this diagnostic process at which differences in the frequency, intensity, and quality of the pulse beats are assessed. The qualities of these pulses are used to determine energy conditions of the corresponding internal organs systems. Pulses located in femoral, posterior-tibial, and dorsalis pedis sites may also be evaluated.

After a diagnosis is made, a course of acupuncture treatments usually is initiated, and recommendations for a nutrition and exercise program are discussed with the patient. Often, it is recommended that a patient consider learning the ancient practice of t'ai chi or ch'i kong, each of which integrates specific movements and breathing techniques to promote the flow of qi, increase strength, and relieve stress.

Herbs are prescribed, and vitamin and mineral supplementation may also be recommended. Because herbs and foods are yin or yang, the ones recommended are based on the diagnosis of the imbalance of yin and yang in the body. Asian massage therapy may be advised to improve circulation, for relaxation, and to harmonize energy and balance the body.

HERBS AND THE CLIMACTERIC

Ideally, a woman should be evaluated by a practitioner of TCM to determine the source of the imbalance of energy unique to her and analyze various facets of her lifestyle. However, this may be unaffordable, or the resources may not be geographically available to many women. When a TCM diagnosis cannot be made and specific herbs cannot be prescribed, prepared formulas are the compromise. Many health food stores and herbal or homeopathic pharmacies carry such formulas.

Several herbs are used in the treatment of climacteric-related symptoms, including Angelica sinensis (dong quai) and ginseng. Dong quai is used to treat hot flushes, anxiety, depression, and insomnia related to the climacteric. This herb is considered to be a blood nourisher and is rich in B vitamins and minerals. It is also used to help relieve vaginal dryness, headaches, and fluid retention and to enhance liver function. Dong quai is used in combination with other herbs during the climacteric[37] and is one of the major herbs increasingly discussed in conventional medical circles. A double-blind study of the effects of dong quai (and other herbs) is underway at Columbia Presbyterian Hospital's Division of Alternative Medicine.

Ginseng is one of the best known of all herbal medicines. It is considered an energy tonic, rich in B vitamins, essential fatty acids, and minerals. It may contain phytohormones, which are precursors of estrogen, progesterone, and testosterone. Depending on the results of TCM diagnosis, it may be used for the treatment of hot flushes, decreased libido, depression, and anxiety and to counteract the effects of stress. It is also used to regulate endocrine activity, improve energy level, improve memory and concentration, and reduce cholesterol and blood pressure.[37] There are different types of ginseng, but the one that is often recommended for climacteric-related symptoms is Chinese ginseng.

Other herbs used for climacteric-related symptoms include *Schizandra* (wu wei zi) for hot flushes and *Polygonum multiflorunlaulis* (he shou wu) for relief of insomnia and stimulation of hormone production.[37]

If a woman has not had the benefit of a TCM diagnosis, she is best advised not to purchase a single herb product but to purchase a Chinese herbal product specifically developed for the climacteric (as is stated on the packaging) that contains several herbs. The multiherbal combinations contain a few or several primary agent herbs that are part of the blend for specific purposes. Although a TCM practitioner has not made a diagnosis and therefore the specific imbalances unique to the woman are unknown, multiherbal combinations may be effective in providing substantial or complete relief for some of the symptoms she may be experiencing. Because some of the herbs are phytohormones, the probability that her symptoms will be successfully treated is enhanced. The names of some of these products are listed in the Guidelines section.

AYURVEDIC MEDICINE

Traditional Ayurveda is a sophisticated system of Indian medicine, and the designation roughly means the science or knowledge of life. As with other forms of complementary medicine, its focus is "on the whole organism and its relation to the external world, in order to reestablish and maintain the harmonious balance that exists within the body and between the body and its environment."[38]

Ayurvedic medicine is one of the four main branches of ancient Hindu philosophic and spiritual teachings based on texts compiled more than 5000 years ago. The teachings from these texts spread to many countries, including China. Consequently, Chinese medicine and Ayurvedic medicine share similarities such as the major principle of the vital life force or energy. In Ayurvedic medicine, this force is called *prana*. As with TCM, pulse diagnosis is used, and the maintenance of a balance of various energy forces within one's own body and environment is the primary goal. Ayurvedic medicine and TCM also share integrated approaches to preventing and treating illness through natural therapies and lifestyle interventions.

Although Ayurvedic medicine has been practiced in the United States for years, it has primarily been the work of Dr. Deepak Chopra, a conventionally trained physician with a specialty in endocrinology, that has been instrumental in increasing Americans' understanding and knowledge about the principles of Ayurveda and the mind-body connection.

The growth in the practice of Ayurvedic medicine has resulted in the treatment of more than 25,000 patients in the United States and the establishment of many freestanding clinics and some training centers for health care professionals.[39] Through the perseverance of Chopra, Sharp Medical Center in La Jolla, California, opened the first hospital-based Ayurvedic center in the United States. Through the research efforts of this center and others in the United States, we can expect to see a rise in the number of scientific publications about the benefits of Ayurvedic medicine.

PRINCIPLES OF AYURVEDIC MEDICINE

The foundation of Ayurvedic medicine is prana, or the vital life force. It is also based on the balance of three basic principles or *doshas* that "govern all the biologic, psychologic, and physiopathologic functions of the body, mind, and consciousness. They act as basic constituents and protective barriers for the body in its normal physiologic condition: when out of balance, they contribute to disease processes."[40] Doshas are linked with specific energies present in every life form, and it is through a balance of them that health is maintained. Together the doshas determine our personal metabolism and mind-body type. Three of the major mind-body types are *vata, pitta,* and *kapha*. Each person is born with a unique ratio of body types, with one usually predominating. Each body type has associated with it specific physical, emotional, and spiritual qualities.

It is through the identification of the correct body type that an appropriate nutritional and exercise plan that integrates other

Ayurvedic therapies can be developed. An imbalance in the doshas is believed to increase susceptibility to outside stressors, such as bacterial and viral infections, and to create a vulnerability to disease. If a person understands her body type and the lifestyle factors associated with it, she will know what is needed to prevent illness and to restore and maintain health.

According to Chopra, drinking coffee in the morning may be okay for a kapha diet but not so for a pitta type. An individual with a predominantly pitta-type build may need a vegetarian diet with a focus on raw foods, but someone with a predominantly vata body-type may need to eat these only occasionally and instead consume heartier foods.

Doshas also characterize the world around us—the time of day, seasons, and foods. There are specific nutritional regimens, exercises, and activities and a daily routine for each type of dosha. Individuals can follow these to maintain balance in every aspect of their lives.

If illness occurs, Ayurvedic medicine uses several methods for treatment. Toxins are considered the core of a disease and are often attributed to foods that are not adequately digested, absorbed, or assimilated. It is believed that the initiation of any form of treatment without eliminating the toxins responsible for the disease will only worsen the problem. Practitioners of Ayurvedic medicine believe that, by treating only the symptoms, the fundamental cause of the illness cannot be addressed, and the problem will recur or will be experienced at some point as a different health care problem.

The first stage of a treatment program is initiation of techniques for detoxifying the body. This process may begin with a special type of herbal massage, followed by herbal steam or sauna and herbs and enemas to aid in elimination of toxins.

The spiritual dimension of healing is attended to through the use of various therapies, including herbs, yoga, and meditation. Yoga and meditation are also advised for healthy persons to practice to maintain their state of health. *Rejuvenation* is another important aspect of the healing program, in which herbs and exercises, particularly various yoga positions, are used.

Research in the areas of Ayurvedic herbs and other therapies have demonstrated beneficial effects for preventing and treating infectious diseases, promoting health, and reducing rates of tumor growth. Basic animal research on specific Ayurvedic herbal therapies has demonstrated reduction and elimination of tumors.[41] Reduced mortality from the chemotherapeutic drug doxorubicin (Adriamycin) has been demonstrated,[42] as has increased lymphocyte proliferation[43] and inhibition of the formation of cancer cells in human lung tumor cells.[44]

Some Ayurvedic herbs are more effective as antioxidants than vitamins E and C and the cholesterol-lowering drug probucol.[45] A herbal program, Maharishi-4 (MAK-4), has been shown to reduce the incidence of breast cancer in rats.[46] MAK-5 prevented human platelet aggregation in vivo.[47]

The multidimensional approach of Ayurvedic medicine toward chronic illnesses such as chronic headaches, constipation, and sinusitis, eczema, hypertension, and bronchial asthma was investigated in the Netherlands.[44] Of the 126 subjects who participated in a 3-month program of treatments, 79% experienced significant improvement, and 10% experienced complete resolution of illness.

Ayurvedic compounds have been included on the list of the National Cancer Institute's (NCI) potential chemopreventive agents. The NCI has funded a series of in vitro studies of these compounds that have shown significantly inhibited cancer cell growth in human tumor and rat tracheal epithelial systems.[41] The National Institutes of Health Division of Alternative medicine has funded studies in Ayurvedic medicine and yoga, including one that will investigate the use of Ayurvedic herbs for the treatment of Parkinson's disease and hatha yoga as a treatment for heroin addiction.

DIAGNOSIS AND TREATMENT

In addition to obtaining information about many aspects of the person's life, diagnostic techniques include evaluation of the pulses and palpation of various areas of the body. The tongue, eyes, urine, and stool are also evaluated.

Several Ayurvedic herbal formulas for the climacteric are available in health foods stores and pharmacies. However, as with TCM, the ideal situation is one in which a woman can receive a complete evaluation by an Ayurvedic practitioner, ensuring that she would receive the appropriate information about necessary lifestyle changes and treatments.

For the woman wanting to explore Ayurvedic medicine herself, books can assist her in identifying her body type and the specific dietary and other lifestyle changes that should be made. Some of these books are listed in Appendix C.

NATUROPATHIC MEDICINE

Naturopathic medicine traces its roots to many systems of healing such as Ayurvedic, TCM, Native-American medicine, and the Greek medicine of Hippocrates. It is based on a belief that our bodies are designed to maintain health, overcome disease, and restore optimal functioning. All of the healing approaches used are based on the body's intrinsic healing processes.

HISTORICAL PERSPECTIVE

The birth of naturopathic medicine in the United States occurred around 1900, when physicians and other interested persons with diverse medical interests and expertise in various healing therapies established a coalition to integrate many forms of natural healing into one discipline.[11] These forms included hydrotherapy, herbal remedies, homeopathy, nutritional and exercise therapies, massage, manual manipulation therapies, and stress reduction techniques. The term *naturopathy* was adopted by this coalition, and the first training program was established in New York City.[11]

During this time, others in the United States, such as Seventh-Day Adventists, were attempting to popularize healthy eating. Dr. Kellogg and his brother were Seventh-Day Adventists. They did not smoke nor drink coffee or alcoholic beverages. Kellogg gained a national reputation for his work as the superintendent of a sanitarium in Battle Creek, Michigan. Persons came to the sanitarium to learn to stay healthy. His program included a vegetarian diet, correct posture, regular exercise, and fresh air and sunshine. It excluded all refined sugar and dairy products.

Kellogg's brother established a business to mass produce corn flakes, and C. W. Post, at one time a patient at the sanitarium, marketed a wheat flake cereal and a coffee substitute. Their cereals were made from organically grown whole grains without additives and sugar, quite unlike most of the cereals that bear their names today.

The naturopathic movement grew rapidly in the early 1900s. More than 20 naturopathic colleges were established in the United States. However, by the 1950s, conventional medicine, pharmaceutical companies, and the American Medical Association (AMA) had become extremely powerful and overshadowed naturopathic medicine. The AMA included naturopathy on its list of "forbidden" complementary systems and succeeded in suppressing it for several decades.[12]

There are two accredited national naturopathic medical schools in the United States. These schools offer a rigorous curriculum that includes some of the same courses as conventional medical schools. They also offer training in body work techniques, spinal manipulation, herbal and nutritional sciences, homeopathy, various forms of hydrotherapy, and stress reduction techniques.

In Great Britain and Europe, naturopaths are often the primary care physicians and refer patients to conventionally trained physicians as needed. In the United States, there is renewed interest in naturopathy, which has resulted in granting licenses to practice naturopathic medicine in several states and a growing movement of collaboration between conventional and naturopathic physicians.

PRINCIPLES OF NATUROPATHY

Drawing from the healing wisdom of many cultures, naturopathic medicine is based on six principles[12]:

- Use the healing power of nature. The role of the naturopathic physician is to aid the body in its natural ability to heal with natural, nontoxic therapies.
- Treat the cause rather than the effect. An attempt is made to determine the underlying cause of a disease instead of suppressing symptoms.
- First, do no harm. This tenet is accomplished through using safe and effective natural therapies.
- Treat the whole person. No disease is viewed automatically as incurable, and a multifactorial approach to healing is employed to respond to the complex interaction of physical, mental, emotional, spiritual, social, and other factors.
- The physician is a teacher. The naturopathic physician is one who educates, empowers, and motivates patients to assume personal responsibility for health, such as through adopting a healthy attitude, diet, and lifestyle.
- Prevention is the best cure. Naturopathic physicians are preventive medicine specialists. Education about a lifestyle that supports health is a primary goal.

As with TCM and Ayurvedic medicine, naturopathy does not separate the mind and body. Since the beginning of this health care system, it has advocated a high-fiber, low-fat, primarily vegetarian diet of organically grown, unprocessed foods. Herbal treatments, including Chinese, Ayurvedic, and homeopathic remedies, are used by the naturopathic physician. Treatment programs also include stress reduction techniques and psychologic counseling, hydrotherapy, and therapeutic manipulation of the muscles, bones, and spines.

Hydrotherapy originated with the Egyptians, Persians, Greeks, Hebrews, Hindus, Chinese, Native Americans, and Eastern Europeans. It involves using various temperatures of water (ie, hot, cold, steam, ice) with various methods of applications (ie, sitz baths, steam, sauna, whirlpools, colonic irrigation). Other forms of therapy recommended by naturopathic physicians include exercise, massage, and use of physiotherapy techniques such as ultrasound.

A series of clinical research studies using a naturopathic treatment protocol for cervical dysplasia resulted in 38 of the 43 women having normal tissue biopsies and Pap smears at the conclusion of the treatment.[49] Clinical and endocrine effects of a naturopathic botanical formula revealed a 100% reduction in the total number of menopausal symptoms, compared with 17% in the placebo group.[50]

An abbreviated list of research underway in the United States to investigate naturopathic principles includes[12] an antioxidant vitamin and cancer study at the University of Colorado Health Sciences Center and a macrobiotic and cancer study at the University of Minnesota School of Public Health. Bastyr University in Seattle has received funding from the National Institutes of Health Division of Alternative Medicine to study alternative treatments used by patients with human immunodeficiency virus (HIV) infections. Studies are also being conducted on the effects of herbs on endocrine functioning in menopausal women, and naturopathic treatment protocols for *Giardia* infection and weight loss and chronic diarrhea in patients with acquired immunodeficiency syndrome (AIDS).

DIAGNOSIS AND TREATMENT

A naturopathic physician obtains information about all aspects of a person's life and the medical and family history. Naturopathic physicians use conventional medical texts and modern scientific medical diagnostic procedures and standards of care in combination with many forms of complementary health practices.

A treatment program, as with all the complementary health care systems, is based on evaluation of all the information obtained and the results of the physical examination and tests. Specific recommendations for lifestyle changes are discussed, and the patient is taught about and supported in making these changes. Teaching the person how to live healthfully is the primary goal of the naturopathic physician. However, herbs and other complementary treatments are used, depending on the diagnosis.

HOMEOPATHY

Hippocrates said that through the like, disease is produced, and through the application of the like, it is cured. Homeopathy is derived from two Greek words: *homoios* (similar) and *pathos* (suffering).

HISTORICAL PERSPECTIVE

Homeopathy is a system of complementary health care based on the theory of the Law of Similars, or the belief that a substance that causes certain symptoms in a healthy individual can be used to treat someone who is experiencing those same symptoms.[51]

In the early 19th century, the practice of medicine included bloodletting, induced vomiting, purging of the intestines, and use of massive doses of poorly understood substances such as mercury and arsenic. In response to these drastic treatments, Dr. Samuel Hahnemann advocated exercise, nutrition, and fresh air to aid in healing. At that time, his health recommendations were considered a radical approach to health.

Dr. Hahnemann was a German physician, chemist, and author of a text widely used by pharmacists. He spoke seven languages, and was a translator of medical texts. It was during his translation of a book on medicinal agents that his attention was drawn to the Peruvian quinine-containing *Cinchona* bark. Dr. Hahnemann questioned why the bark worked as a treatment for malaria, and he began to experiment on himself by initially ingesting large doses of the bark until he experienced the symptoms of malaria. These symptoms resolved after the bark was discontinued. Because of this experiment, he theorized that, if the symptoms of malaria could be created by ingesting large doses of the treatment for it, a smaller dose might stimulate the body of a person suffering with malaria to fight the disease.

Expanding on this hypothesis, he continued to experiment with hundreds of natural substances from plants, minerals, and animals. He identified substances that, when taken in significant amounts, caused symptoms of specific health problems but that, when ingested in minuscule amounts, appeared to successfully treat the corresponding problems.

For example *sepia,* derived from squid ink, was used for writing with quill pens about 100 years ago. In those days, it was observed that persons who licked the quills of their pens developed symptoms such as hot flushes, irritability, and decreased libido. As a result, extremely small concentrations of sepia are often used as one of the treatments for these symptoms.

The development of the treatments discovered by Dr. Hahnemann involved taking the identified substance and exposing it to a serial dilution process. His experimentation led to formulation[51] of the following principles of homeopathy:

- Like causes like.
- The greater the dilution of a remedy, the greater is its potency (ie, Law of Infinitesimal Dose).
- An illness is specific to the individual (ie, holistic medical model).

Because homeopathic treatments proved so successful in the middle to late 1800s for the treatment of infectious diseases such as cholera, typhoid, yellow fever, and scarlet fever, they gained widespread acceptance in the United States. During the cholera epidemic in Cincinnati, the death rate was only 3% among patients treated with homeopathy compared with 40% to 70% among those treated with conventional medicine.[51] During the yellow fever epidemic in New Orleans, the death rate was 5.6% with homeopathy and 16% with conventional treatments.[52] Although we may question such statistics and recognize the limitations of conventional medical treatments at that time, the low mortality rates associated with homeopathic treatments nevertheless are impressive.

The first homeopathic college opened in the United States in 1836, followed in 1844 by the establishment of the first national homeopathic medical organization, The American Institute of Homeopathy. By the end of the century, 22 homeopathic medical schools, including Boston University, University of Michigan, and New York Medical College, and 15,000 practitioners existed in the United States.[11]

Homeopathy's place in American medicine was short lived. In the 1860s, the AMA took a stand against homeopathy and attempted to expel any physician who practiced it or consulted with a homeopath in the treatment of a patient.[52] Homeopathy had practically died out by the 20th century. Only two homeopathic medical schools remained in the United States by 1920. However, acceptance of homeopathy is again growing. Many pharmacies carry homeopathic remedies, and increasing numbers of health care professionals are accepting them as treatments for some health care problems. Annual sales of homeopathic remedies have exceeded $150 million in the United States and continue to grow rapidly.[53] In 1996, the first homeopathic hospital opened in Los Angeles. A few health maintenance organizations are providing access to homeopathy, and increasing numbers of health care providers are attending homeopathic postgraduate courses.

Homeopathic remedies have been recognized by the Food and Drug Administration (FDA) as official drugs since 1939. The FDA regulates manufacturing, labeling, and dispensing of these drugs. Any licensed health care professional can practice homeopathy. Increasing numbers of physicians, dentists, veterinarians, homeopaths, osteopathic and naturopathic physicians, chiropractors, and other complementary health care providers are practicing homeopathy. Many registered nurses, nurse practitioners, and physician's assistants practice homeopathy, but they can do so only under the supervision of a physician in some states. It is estimated that more than 3000 physicians and other health care practitioners in the United States use homeopathy, and approximately 2.5 million persons (1% of the population) sought assistance from a homeopathic physician in 1990.[5]

In Germany, Hahnemann's birthplace, there are at least 6000 homeopathic practitioners, and there are at least 5000 in France. The homeopathic treatment *Oscillococcinum* is the largest-selling flu remedy in France. Homeopathic hospitals and outpatient clinics are a part of England's national health system. Homeopathy is also widely practiced in India by more than 25,000 physicians and by many others in Mexico, Argentina, and Brazil.[9]

PRINCIPLES OF HOMEOPATHY

The Law of Similars was first recognized by Hippocrates during his study of the effects of herbs on disease. This law can also be considered the theoretical basis for immunizations, in which minute amounts of a disease component, often a virus, are used to strengthen the body's immune response to a disease. Various theories describe the ways in which homeopathic treatments work. Homeopaths, just as practitioners of TCM and Ayurvedic medicine, believe that a life force or vital force is the "inherent, underlying, interconnective, self-healing process of the organism."[51] Homeopaths theorize that this bioenergetic process is sensitive to the submolecular homeopathic medicines. The resonance (vibration) of the microdose is thought to affect the resonance of the person's life force.[51]

Homeopaths point to the overuse of pharmaceutical drugs as a major factor in what they consider to be an overall decline of health. For example, according to Dr. Michael Carlston, who is also a homeopath and assistant clinical professor of family and community medicine at the University of California, San Francisco,

> It's very clear in my mind that recurrent ear infections in kids are a result of the antibiotics that are used. Out of two to three hundred new kids per year with recurrent ear infections, I see maybe two who aren't helped by homeopathy. And that's better than surgery is. Part of it is putting the brakes on the cycle of giving them antibiotics all the time. They can be used selectively, but if you can get better in other ways, it makes a lot more sense.[54]

Dr. Sharma, professor of biophysics in India, theorizes that the microdoses of homeopathic medicines are probably able to cross the blood-brain barrier and cellular and nuclear membranes to deliver their therapeutic effects more profoundly and more deeply than other drugs with larger molecular structures.[51] Homeopathic substances give off measurable electromagnetic signals. This may convey an electromagnetic "message" that matches the specific electromagnetic frequency or pattern of an illness, which then stimulates the body's natural healing processes. Using magnetic resonance techniques, homeopathic medicines showed distinctive readings of subatomic activity, but the placebos did not.[55]

Eighty-one of the 107 controlled clinical studies of homeopathic remedies revealed that the remedies were beneficial in treating headaches, respiratory infections, diseases of the digestive system, ankle sprains, postoperative infections and symptoms, and other health related disorders.[56] Homeopathic treatments have also been found to be effective in treating hay fever[57] and other health problems, including Parkinson's disease, bronchitis, migraines,[58] and symptoms associated with the climacteric. Sepia is an example of a homeopathic remedy used for treating some climacteric symptoms, including hot flushes, headaches before or during menses, and emotional changes.[59] Another example is belladonna, which is used for symptoms such as migraine headaches, menorrhagia, and severe hot flushes.[60]

DIAGNOSIS AND TREATMENT

I have found homeopathy to be effective at least 80% of the time in relieving menopausal symptoms. With homeopathy, an incorrect remedy produces no response, but after the correct remedy is given, a woman should experience an improvement in her symptoms within a maximum of five to six weeks.[61]

As with all complementary health care practices, a practitioner of homeopathy takes a detailed medical and lifestyle history, including subtle information that reveals the patient's unique response to an illness. The patient's perception of her life and stressors and her reaction to them are also considered important information to obtain.

A practitioner of homeopathy does not diagnosis a problem. Instead, the treatment is based solely on information about the person and the unique physical, emotional, and mental symptoms of that person. A treatment that most closely addresses all of the symptoms of the individual is then prescribed. The treatments are individualized, so that one may be suitable for one individual with particular symptoms associated with an illness but not for another person with the same illness who has somewhat different symptoms. Vitamins, minerals, and herbal preparations also are used by some homeopathic practitioners.

"What homeopathic treatment does is stimulate the immune system and trigger the body's natural defense mechanisms so that the body understands what it needs to do to cure itself."[16] It is understandable why a practitioner of homeopathy, as with practitioners of all forms of complementary therapies, is reluctant to generalize treatments for symptoms of the climacteric or any other problem. If a woman is unable to work personally with a homeopathic practitioner, there are several homeopathic remedies available in health food stores and pharmacies, and sometimes, personnel trained in homeopathy are employed by these stores to help a woman select the treatment that is best suited for her. Names of various homeopathic treatments sold specifically for symptoms associated with the climacteric are found in the Guidelines section.

HERBALISM, PHYTOMEDICINE, BOTANICAL MEDICINE, AND PLANT MEDICINE

European phytomedicines are among the world's best studied medicines, researched in leading European universities and hospitals. Some have been in clinical use under medical supervision for more than 10 years, with tens of millions of documented cases.[17]

HISTORICAL PERSPECTIVE AND MODERN USE

From the burial site of a Neanderthal man some 60,000 years ago to the first known ancient compilation of the use of herbal medicines in 2000 BC in the Middle East to medical texts of China written before the end of the 3rd century BC, herbal medicine has played a major role in healing. European settlers in America grew their own herbs, brought over from their countries, and traded their knowledge with that of Native Americans. Until the 1940s, many physicians in the United States used plant and herbal preparations in their practice of medicine.

Herbal medicine (ie, phytomedicines) is standard fare in Europe, and the compounds are classified as prescription drugs used for life-threatening diseases and those prepared in injectable forms; over-the-counter phytomedicines; and traditional herbal remedies.[17] In Europe, Japan, and China, phytomedicines are used to treat serious, life-threatening conditions such as heart disease and cancer and for symptomatic relief of colds and flus and other conditions that are treated by over-the-counter drugs in the United States. According to the World Health Organization, herbal medicine is the primary medical therapy for more than three fourths of the world's population.[17] It is used as an integral and accepted aspect of health care in every part of the world except in the United States.

At least 40% of conventional medicines have been derived from plant and earth sources.[62] The cancer drugs vinblastine and vincristine are derived from the rosy periwinkle. Digitalis comes from the foxglove plant, and taxol comes from the bark of the rare Pacific yew tree. Reserpine originally was derived from Indian snakeroot, morphine from the opium poppy, and atropine from belladonna. Aspirin is derived from the salicin in willow bark.

Varro Tyler, the recently retired Lilly Distinguished Professor of Pharmacognosy at Purdue University and one of the country's leading experts on herbal medicine, believes that "the proper use of herbs can add another dimension to health care."[63] Botanicals are less expensive than drugs. For example, saw palmetto is used in Europe for the treatment of enlarged prostate glands and costs only 40 cents each day, whereas the cost of the drug finasteride is about $1.75.[64] The World Health Organization found that 74% of the 119 plant-derived pharmaceutical medicines are used in ways that correlate directly with their traditional uses as discovered by native cultures.[65]

Regardless of the herbalists' origin of practice, they view illness as occurring when the body is experiencing the effects of stressors, including nutritional deficiencies or excesses and toxins from tobacco, alcohol, other drugs, and the environment. Herbs are used in an attempt to regenerate health by eliminating toxins and tonifying (building up, nourishing, stimulating) the body. They are used for a variety of purposes, from supporting adrenal gland functioning so that resistance to stress is increased to directly reducing the inflammatory response without inhibiting the natural inflammatory reaction. Some herbs help the body destroy or resist pathogenic microorganisms, reduce cramping in smooth and skeletal muscles, soothe and protect irritated and inflamed tissue, stimulate the digestive system, and have a diuretic action. Some herbs stimulate menstrual flow and improve the general functioning of the reproductive system, decrease uterine contractions, lower elevated blood pressure, promote bowel movements, reduce anxiety and tension, and enhance metabolic functions.

RESEARCH AND REGULATION

One obstacle in the research of herbal remedies is that they contain a multitude of active ingredients whose interactions are extremely complex. This adds to the difficulty in conducting research, which typically focuses on a single ingredient. Another obstacle is cost. To bring a new pharmaceutical drug to market costs $140 to $500 million.[66] What pharmaceutical company wants to spend that kind of money on an unpatentable product, and what herbal medicine manufacturer, without the major budgets of the pharmaceutical companies, can afford it?

Europe has dealt with these issues in ways that could be a model for the United States. The "Quality of Herbal Remedies," developed by the European Economic Community, outlines standards for quality, quantity, and production of herbal remedies.[17] It provides labeling requirements that member countries must meet. The standards are based on the World Health Organization's Guidelines for the Assessment of Herbal Medicines (1991).

Three categories of herbal remedies have been developed: rigorously controlled prescription drugs, including injectable herbal medicines and those for treatment of life-threatening diseases; over-the-counter phytomedicines, equivalent to our over-the-counter pharmaceuticals; and traditional herbal remedies consisting of those remedies that are judged safe on the basis of generations of use without serious incident, even though they have not undergone extensive clinical studies.

In France, the labels on these remedies include "traditionally used for," which for the consumer means that indications have not been confirmed by modern scientific experimentation and instead are based on historical evidence.[67] The "rule of prior use," followed in England, states that a herbal product is safe in lieu of scientific data if there is associated with it hundreds of years of use without evidence of detrimental side effects.[17]

Herbal products are considered as a single active ingredient in Germany, which makes it simpler to define and approve these products.[17] The regulation of herbal products is conducted through the German Federal Health Office by using a monograph system. Because the monographs are compiled from scientific literature, this system results in products whose potency and manufacturing processes are standardized. When research does not exist, as in France and other countries, traditional remedies are made available based on the history of use of the herbs for herbal remedies.

REACTIONS AND MEDICINAL USE

There are 10,000 to 20,000 deaths each year from gastric hemorrhages from nonsteroidal antiinflammatory drugs used for arthritis.[68] Conventionally trained health care professionals are concerned about possible toxic effects of herbs, and justifiably so, because they are used to dealing with pharmaceutical drugs that have the potential of exhibiting such effects. However, the good news is that adverse reactions to herbal medicines are likely to be idiosyncratic in nature because the concentration of the active ingredients is very low.[69] They are also composed of several ingredients that act synergistically, minimizing the possibility of toxicity. Dr. Andrew Weil, a physician and botanist and Director of the Programs for Integrative Medicine at the University of Arizona College of Medicine, has stated that there is no comparison between the relative dangers of pharmaceutical drugs and herbal medicine.[69] He also believes that the cases of deaths from herbal medicine can be counted on one or two hands and are rare, isolated cases.[69]

The concept of low concentration and multiple ingredients is a foreign one to conventionally trained health care professionals. They are used to dealing with concentrated, single-ingredient pharmaceuticals that have associated with them more powerful and intense effects. The level of concentration of drugs is directly associated with the potential for side effects and toxicity.

Perhaps the greatest concerns regarding herbs are quality control and use. Because herbs may be contaminated, it is important to use only those that are manufactured by reputable companies. This issue is addressed in more detail in the Guidelines section.

Another problem that results from the lack of quality control is the quality of herbs and methods of preparation of herbs, which affects their potency and the amount of herb contained in a product. Some products may contain such a small amount of the herbs or the herbs are of such poor quality that they are ineffective.

Some persons may use herbs as poorly as they often do pharmaceuticals and may not complete a full course of treatment. More importantly, they may assume that, because an herb is a "natural" form of treatment, it cannot harm them, and they may increase the recommended dosage in an attempt to "get better as soon as possible." Toxic effects are more likely to result from misuse through increasing the dosage beyond what is recommended on the packaging. Toxic effects may also result if a particular herbal program is used beyond the recommended period of time.

James Duke, a Department of Agriculture botanist, said, "Herbal medicine is like any other medicine. It should be used with discretion."[70] Duke explains that each herb has its own safe dose, and some herbs used for extended periods can harm the liver. Women who use herbal therapies must follow instructions carefully.

Hundreds of textbooks for health care professionals and pharmacists about herbal medicine are available in the United States. Many can be obtained by mail order through Herbalgram (see Appendix C). Studies of and publications about herbal research are growing, and attention is being given to well-conducted studies performed in other countries. A few examples of such research follows.

Patients treated with feverfew for migraines experienced a decrease in the frequency of migraines, had less severe symptoms, and had less vomiting.[71] Serum cholesterol was lowered by 9% through daily ingestion of the equivalent of one-half to one clove of garlic.[72] Another study found garlic to decrease total cholesterol by 20%, decrease low-density lipoprotein and triglyceride levels, and increase high-density lipoprotein levels.[73]

Daily intake of gingko biloba resulted in improved scores for memory, attention, and social functioning among patients with Alzheimer's disease.[74] Seven placebo-controlled trials showed ginkgo to be effective for a variety of complaints, including loss of memory, difficulty with concentration, headaches, depression, and dizziness.[75] Fifty percent of men who previously had not been helped by conventional treatment for impotency caused by arterial flow problems regained potency after 6 months of treatment with ginkgo.[76]

A meta-analysis of 23 randomized trials with a total of 1767 patients concluded that St. John's wort was superior to placebos and comparatively effective to standard antidepressants while producing fewer side effects.[77]

Cranberries have long been recommended as a medicinal herb for problems ranging from gastrointestinal disturbances to cancer, and it is commonplace to recommend cranberry juice to patients with urinary tract infections. The reason usually given for this is the herb's effect on altering the pH of the urine and thereby suppressing bacterial growth. However, the benefit of cranberry therapy results from a substance it contains that prevents adherence of bacteria to the lining of the bladder and urinary tract.[78–81]

HERBS AND THE CLIMACTERIC

Many herbs in addition to dong quai and ginseng can be used for the treatment of climacteric-related symptoms. One of these is St. John's wort, traditionally used as an antiinflammatory and for healing of wounds and valued for its ability to reduce pain and act as a mild sedative. It is used for symptoms of anxiety and irritability and has been recommended for the treatment of depression.[82,83]

Vitex is used for treatment of various symptoms, including emotional changes, hot flushes, vaginal dryness, hormonally related constipation, and digestive distress.[84] It can also be effective for the treatment of dysmenorrhea and fluid retention.

Black cohosh is used for the treatment of hot flushes, vaginal dryness, sleep disturbances, irritability, strengthening of pelvic musculature, and prevention and treatment of uterine prolapse. A study conducted in Germany gave 110 women (mean age of 52 and who had not received HRT for at least 6 months) a pharmaceutical preparation of this herb, Remifemin (which is found in many health food stores and pharmacies in the United States).[85] After 2 months of treatment, luteinizing hormone (LH) and follicle-stimulating hormone (FSH) levels were measured. FSH levels remained similar in the Remifemin and placebo groups, but LH levels were significantly reduced in the treated group. Women treated with black cohosh (Remifemin) experienced relief of climacteric-related symptoms similar to that experienced by women using estrogen.

Several other herbs are used to treat symptoms associated with the climacteric:

- Motherwort for nervousness and irritability
- Damiana for hot flushes, anxiety, nervousness, and decreased libido
- Devils club for constipation, aching joints, hot flushes
- Sage for mental clarity, improvement of memory, dysmenorrhea and menorrhagia, and prevention and reduction of inflammation of the joints

These are only a few examples of the many herbs that can be used by women during the climacteric. Ideally, a woman should seek the assistance of an herbalist to be evaluated to determine the most appropriate herbs for her and to learn how to take them and the duration of use. As Amanda McQuade Crawford states in The Herbal Menopause Book, "sometimes herbs help problems, sometimes they worsen them, and it is therefore the reason herbalists repeat ad nauseam that we have to see each woman rather than prescribe an herb for a condition."[86]

If a woman has any contraindications for using an estrogen-containing treatment, it is unknown whether phytoestrogenic herbs are safe for her. However, in this situation, a herbalist would be able to prescribe other herbal treatments that are not estrogenic.

A herbalist would also be able to discuss the interaction of herbs and vitamins and minerals. For example, vitamin C may inhibit the action of ginseng if ingested at the same time, but its action may be enhanced if taken with vitamin E. The action of vitamin E may be inhibited when taken with dong quai. However, if the woman is unable to afford the services of an herbalist, she can refer to various books about herbal therapies (see Appendix C) and can purchase various herbal products that contain a combination of several herbs. Any woman interested in herbal therapies should be encouraged to make every attempt to learn about herbal medicines and their effects on the climacteric.

Appendix C includes the names of some products that the manufacturers have been determined to be reputable through scrutiny by various pharmacists and herbalists. This is by no means a comprehensive list of all available products and all reputable companies that manufacture herbs. However, it is a good starting point from which you can provide recommendations, if you choose to do so, to your patients who wish to use herbal therapies.

OSTEOPATHIC MEDICINE

Osteopathic medicine is not considered a true complementary medical system, because the curriculum for osteopathic physicians is identical to that of conventional medical schools, with the exception of additional training in preventive medicine and treatment of the musculoskeletal system and in manipulative therapies. However, to the lay public, because osteopathy integrates specific complementary practices, it represents an alternative to conventional medicine.

HISTORICAL PERSPECTIVE

In 1892, the first school of osteopathy was founded by Dr. Andrew Taylor Still. As a conventionally trained physician, his goal was to search for better medical treatments than those that then existed.[87] Still believed that the musculoskeletal system played more of a major role in health than conventional physicians of that time believed. He believed that the vascular and nervous systems were influenced by the actions of muscles, ligaments, joint surfaces, and joint motion. He also believed that, through manipulation of the musculoskeletal system and the effect on the vascular and nervous systems, the body could be assisted in restoring health. The key to the development of disease was the relation between structure and function of the spinal column and organs.

Osteopaths believe that misalignment can directly affect an organ or system, and they believe it can indirectly produce serious effects. For example, a person with lower back problems may bend forward, resulting in a compromise in the movement of the rib cage. This restricts the functioning of the lungs, and continuous forward bending may cause muscles in the neck to spasm, which can result in headaches.

As one of the earliest health care systems in the United States to use manual healing methods, osteopathy emphasized the cause of disease at a time when conventional medicine was focused on control of symptoms through drugs and surgery. Osteopathic physicians at this time practiced the same full range of medicine and surgery as conventional physicians, but they were not allowed to practice in conventional medical hospitals. Separatism of osteopathic and conventional hospital and medical schools continued until the 1940s, and osteopaths were considered cultists by members of the AMA. Today, osteopathic physicians are allowed to join the AMA. There are approximately 50,000 osteopathic physicians and more than 15 osteopathic medical colleges in the United States, some of which are university affiliated.[12]

Four major principles constitute the philosophy of osteopathic medicine[17]:

@ Structure and function are interdependent. Behavior is an intermingled complex in which psychosocial influences can affect anatomy and physiology. All of these relationships are fundamentally designed to work in harmony.
@ The body has the ability to heal itself, and the role of the osteopathic physician is to enhance the healing process as much as possible.
@ Diseases, impairments, and disabilities arise from disruptions of the normal interactions of anatomy, physiology, and behavior.
@ Appropriate treatment is based on the ability to understand, diagnose, and treat—by whatever methods are available, including manually applied procedures. Hands-on procedures are used to identify somatic dysfunction; the osteopathic physician

then determines whether the pattern of somatic dysfunction can be related to the internal body organs, neuromusculoskeletal system, or (occasionally) behavioral dysfunction.

Many osteopathic therapy studies, although primarily conducted on a small scale, have demonstrated positive effects on neurophysiology, neurochemistry, and the clinical course of many medical conditions. Osteopathic manipulation has decreased blood pressure in hypertensive patients,[88] decreased the length of hospitalization and antibiotic therapy for patients with pneumonia,[89] and decreased asthma attacks and the need for medication.[90,91] For patients with chronic obstructive lung disease, osteopathic manipulation provided a significant improvement in pulmonary carbon dioxide levels, oxygen saturation, total lung capacity, and residual volume.[92] It has also relieved low back pain and muscle spasm[93] and headaches.[94] Carlisle Holland, an osteopathic physician, offers the following perspective:

> We have the advantage of knowing medicine, so we can be critical while looking at situations clinically and looking at alternatives. We know ways to get around medication or avoid surgery and do it in a way that is responsible. We know the consequences, and we know medicines and their power. If we choose to avoid prescribing medicine or to do homeopathy, we do it from a solid grounding in medicine and in understanding the musculoskeletal system. We have the best of all worlds.[95]

DIAGNOSIS AND TREATMENT

In addition to a comprehensive medical and lifestyle history, posture and gait are observed, and an orthopedic examination of the spine and hips is performed. Muscles and joints are evaluated, and a neurologic examination is conducted. Radiographs, magnetic resonance imaging, and bloods tests are ordered, if indicated, to exclude pathology.

When a woman in her climacteric is treated by an osteopathic physician, she is provided a comprehensive health care program, including spinal manipulation and perhaps manipulation of other areas of the body, and a nutritional and exercise program; relaxation techniques may also be prescribed.

CHIROPRACTIC

A patient finally went to a chiropractor for her back pain after finding no relief with the orthopedist. After three adjustments and a week of no symptoms, she had a follow-up visit with her M.D. On learning about the success of the chiropractic treatment, the orthopedist stated, "That was just the placebo effect." The patient responded, "If it works so well, why didn't you use it?"[96]

Chiropractic (ie, "done by hands") holds the same views about the spinal column as osteopathic medicine. The spine is considered "the seat of intelligence" of the body, and all physiologic functions depend on the "communication" between the nervous system and all other systems. By adjusting the spinal column, a disease can be cured and normal function restored to the organs, muscles, joints, and other tissues.

HISTORICAL PERSPECTIVE

Daniel David Palmer of Davenport, Iowa, was a healer who primarily used laying on of hands and faith healing. One day, he was approached by a janitor to heal deafness that had developed several years before this meeting. The janitor recalled that his deafness began shortly after he felt something "give way" in his back while stooped over to perform heavy labor. Palmer felt a lump on the janitor's back that he attributed to a misplaced vertebra. By applying firm pressure, he slipped it back into place; shortly thereafter, the janitor's hearing was restored.[12]

As a result of these experiences and the direct influence osteopathic medicine had on him, Palmer developed the first type of chiropractic care in the late 1800s. He believed that the root of most disease resulted from misalignment of the spine. He agreed with osteopathic physicians that displaced vertebrae resulted in a physical blockage that interfered with normal nerve transmission and normal functioning of the organs. He also believed in "man the spiritual" and "man the physical."[12] By manipulating the spine, interference to the flow of "Innate Intelligence" would result, thereby connecting the spiritual and physical aspects of the person. Palmer believed that this Innate Intelligence flowed through the nervous system, and by keeping the nervous system "healthy," the Innate Intelligence would be able to express itself, and the organs and entire body would then be in a state of health.

Palmer founded the first school of chiropractic in 1897. Chiropractic practices continued to be used throughout the United States, but in the 1960s chiropractic was classified as a cult by the AMA. A federal suit was filed against the AMA, the American Hospital Association, and six other medical associations by five chiropractors. The charges were antitrust violations by conspiring to eliminate chiropractic and by refusal to associate professionally with its practitioners. The chiropractors won this suit in 1987, which greatly contributed to the acceptance of the practice of chiropractic.

Chiropractors represent the second largest group of health care providers (the first is conventional physicians) and are licensed to practice in every state and Canada. More than 45,000 chiropractors are practicing in the United States, receiving two thirds of all health care visits for back pain.[12] Chiropractic training includes 4 years of study and uses many of the same texts as conventional medical schools. Unlike osteopathic physicians, chiropractors do not perform major surgery or prescribe medications, nor do they treat fractures, rapidly deteriorating medical conditions, or acute infections. They also do not treat life-threatening diseases or conditions that require invasive procedures.

Research in the area of chiropractic is in its early stages. Studies are underway to determine the effects of chiropractic treatment on dysmenorrhea; backache associated with pregnancy; head, neck, and shoulder pain; migraine headaches; carpal tunnel syndrome; and infant colic.

STRESS REDUCTION TECHNIQUES, GUIDED IMAGERY, AND MASSAGE

It is surprising how little Americans know about the art of relaxation. Relaxation is more than getting away from the daily grind, and it is more than the absence of stress. It is something positive and satisfying; it is peace of mind. True relaxation requires becoming sensitive to the basic needs for peace, self-awareness, thoughtful reflection and the willingness to meet these needs rather than ignoring or dismissing them.[97]

Almost all forms of complementary therapies integrate methods of reducing stress and many include various massage techniques. Guided imagery is a technique that can be helpful in the prevention and treatment of climacteric symptoms, cardiovascular disease, and other health problems.

Stress reduction techniques can include taking a few minutes to breathe deeply with the eyes closed or practicing any one of the several meditative techniques for 20 or more minutes each day (see Chapter 6). The choices are as endless as the applications.

MEDITATION

Dr. Bhagwan Awatramani, an Indian physician who travels internationally presenting workshops in meditation, believes health comes from a state of mental peace. He finds that most persons, however, have continuous mental distractions (ie, stress). His prescription for this problem is meditation. "It boosts the immune system and energizes the body. Regardless of one's physical health, with a quite mind there is well being. And quieting the mind can be learned."[98]

Meditation is an ancient form of healing used as a means to find inner peace. It is not daydreaming, nor is it a way of thinking logically about a problem and solving it. Instead, it is a way, as psychologist Robert Ornstein described it, to "turn down" conscious thought to allow more subtle sources of information to be perceived.[99]

Essential to meditation are a quiet environment, a comfortable position that allows the person to be relaxed yet alert, an object to focus on (eg, sound, phrase, word, breathing), and a passive, receptive attitude. If the mind wanders, the person gently reminds herself to go back to meditating. It serves as a means to keep the attention pleasantly anchored in the present moment.

There are several forms of meditative practices, ranging from repetitive and deep breathing exercises, praying, and Zen and transcendental meditation to ones that integrate movement, including yoga, tai-chi, and ch'i kong. It is not unusual for persons to try various forms of meditation before they find the one best suited to their beliefs and lifestyle. It is also not unusual for persons to use more than one form, depending on their needs at any given time. During the course of each day, a person may want to meditate and stretch in combination to gain a somewhat cardiovascular effect and may therefore practice one of the various forms of yoga. At another time of that day or another day, a person may choose to quietly sit and focus on deep breathing.

The key to meditation, regardless of the type practiced, is regularity, in which at least 20 to 30 minutes are spent quieting the mind. Meditation can be one of the healthiest complementary techniques used by women. It can help to relieve pain and symptoms associated with the climacteric, and it can strengthen the immune and endocrine system. It can be an aid in making lifestyle changes, enhance creative and intellectual abilities, reduce anxiety, and generate feelings of self-control, self-understanding, and peacefulness.

GUIDED IMAGERY AND VISUALIZATION

Guided imagery can be used for stress reduction and healing. Dr. M. Rossman, cofounder of the Academy of Guided Imagery, believes that it is probably a person's least used health resource. "It can be used to remember and recreate the past, develop insight into the present, influence physical health, enhance creativity and inspiration, and anticipate possible futures."[100]

The imagination is quite powerful. Most persons, often without realizing it, are experienced "practitioners" of imagery—sometimes in ways that cause them to experience stress reactions without even realizing it. For example, it is not uncommon for persons to worry about things that have already taken place, are currently taking place, or have not yet taken place. It is through this "worrying" that the physiologic reactions associated with stress occur.

Anyone who has experienced "goose bumps" when being told a scary story, experienced chills just thinking about or visualizing fingernails scraping across a blackboard, or felt sexually aroused by visualizing or thinking about something sexual knows the power of the imagination. Some athletes use imagery, seeing themselves successfully practicing a maneuver or performing in an event. Visualizing a color or scene that is relaxing is another example of imagery. It is through imagery that the nervous system naturally stores, accesses, and processes information, making it an especially effective vehicle for dialogue between the mind and body and ultimately contributing to the healing process.

A person can learn how to imagine (visualize) a healing process in the affected area of the body, such as creating a picture of a narrowed coronary artery expanding and plaque being removed from the body. A woman can develop imagery techniques to effectively deal with stressors, thereby preventing the harmful emotional and physiologic effects they can create. Even when imagery does not cure a disease, patients still reap great benefits, including relief of anxiety and an increase in self-esteem and sense of control over their bodies—ideal benefits for women as they approach or have passed menopause.

MASSAGE

Massage is the third most frequently used form of complementary care in the United States. There are at least 50,000 massage therapists representing various forms of massage in the United States.[12] With the growing acceptance of massage, combined with its ability to aid in relaxation and the healing processes, hospitals in the United States may one day have massage wards, as do hospitals in China. Health insurance companies in the United States may follow Germany's lead and reimburse for massage, as does the national health insurance system in that country.

Various methods of massage are used to help to reduce stress and to aid in the healing process. They have been used since ancient times in TCM and Ayurvedic medical practices and in other complementary healing systems. In the United States, massage was usually a unique privilege of the affluent during their day at a health spa or after a game of golf, but times have changed. Books and video tapes on the art of massage abound. Massage is encouraged as a form of intimate communication among lovers or a way that a friend can help another relieve shoulder tension or neck pain. Hands are massaged during a manicure, as are the feet during a pedicure. Massage is frequently integrated into physical and rehabilitative therapies.

The benefits of massage appear to be reaching the masses, and the effects of human touch are being evaluated by the scientific community. Research conducted at the University of Miami's School of Medicine Touch Research Institute has demonstrated that premature babies given regular massages had a 6-day shorter hospital stay and a 50% greater weight gain than babies who did not receive the massages.[101]

An increase of natural killer cells, lowered serotonin levels, and less anxiety were experienced by men infected with HIV who received daily massages for 1 month. A decrease in depression and lower levels of stress hormones in urine and saliva have been reported in hospitalized depressed and adjustment-disordered children and adolescents who received massage therapy.[102]

A buildup of lactic acid and other waste products in chronically overworked or tense muscles can cause stiffness, soreness, and spasm. Massage improves circulation to the area and aids in the elimination of toxins. Massage can enhance the healing process after injury by increasing the blood supply and oxygen to an area while helping the patient relax. Relaxation results in part from the release of endorphins and enkephalins, imparting a natural tranquilizing effect.[103] Research has also shown that massage can reduce acute and chronic pain and increase muscle flexibility and tone in patients with traumatically induced spinal pain[104] and reduce the frequency of episodes of pain and disability in patients with inflammatory bowel disease.[105]

The Touch Research Institute is conducting studies on the effects of massage in areas such as infants with cancer, pregnancy, and persons with asthma, diabetes, hypertension, and eating disorders.[12] The National Institutes of Health's Division of Alternative Medicine has awarded grants to study the benefits of massage in areas such as immune system functioning in AIDS patients taking antiviral drugs, reduction of anxiety and depression in bone marrow transplant patients, and reduction of anxiety and need for follow-up care in women undergoing surgery for uterine cancer.[12]

Even if a woman is unable to afford the cost of a professional massage therapist or does not have a partner, she can be encouraged to "share" massages with a friend. Even a hand or neck massage can be extremely relaxing, and because it involves being touched by another person, it can be a nurturing and "healing" experience as well.

CONCLUSIONS

Past Surgeon General C. Koop wrote, "One must have an open mind about complementary therapies and understand belief systems that emphasize the mind-body connection. At a time when many Americans complain of stress, make poor nutritional choices, and are increasingly concerned about environmentally induced illnesses, these messages could hardly be more timely." He continued, "For years, we have attempted to export Western medicine to the developing world. The sad truth is that the persons we are attempting to help simply cannot afford it. I have doubts about how much longer we can afford some of it ourselves. It is possible that a decade from now, we may be more ready to ask the peoples of the developing world to share their wisdom with us. During the nineteenth century American medicine was an eclectic pursuit where a number of competing ideas and approaches thrived. Doctors were able to draw on elements from different traditions in attempting to make persons well. Perhaps there is more to this older model of American medicine than we in the twentieth century have been willing to examine."[106]

The discussion of some of the complementary health care practices has only briefly introduced you to the world of complementary medicine. These systems and practices and many others have "pearls" to offer women. They offer women choices for the relief of symptoms associated with the climacteric. They also offer choices about the ways in which women can improve their health in general that will ultimately affect the prevention and treatment of chronic diseases such as osteoporosis and coronary artery disease.

One of the most positive aspects of any complementary health care system is that the practitioner spends a considerable amount of time educating the patient about the specific nutrition, exercise, and stress reduction programs appropriate to the diagnosis. It is a level of education and counseling that is usually unavailable through conventional medical practices and clinics because of the financial or policy constraints of our health care delivery system. For many women, this level of education and support is essential in helping them make healthy changes in their lifestyle.

One woman may decide to use HRT with acupressure or use homeopathic remedies and practice yoga. Another may decide to deal with stress through Zen meditation and relieve hot flushes through use of dong quai and other herbs. Still another may decide to have a comprehensive evaluation and treatment program by a naturopathic or osteopathic physician. The choices are many, but they may be limited by available resources in the community and financial constraints, unless a woman has health insurance that pays for complementary health care practices. Fortunately, even these limitations need not prevent a woman from learning about these practices, nor do they have to be barrier to integrating some of the practices, such as meditation, into her life.

REFERENCES

1. Duhl L. Introduction. In: Collenge W, ed. The American Holistic Health Association complete guide to alternative medicine. New York: Warner Books; 1996:xxi.
2. Bezold C, et al. The future of work and health. Westport, CT: Auburn House; 1986.
3. Villaire M. Alternative medicine: integrating in a conventional world. LACMA Phys 1995;Feb 20:21.
4. Hufford DJ. Folk medicine in contemporary America. In: Kirland H et al, eds. Herbal and magical medicine traditional healing today. Durham, NC: Duke University Press; 1992.
5. Eisenberg DM, et al. Unconventional medicine in the United States: Prevalence, costs and patterns of use. N Engl J Med 1993;328:246–252.
6. Blumber D, et al. The physician and unconventional medicine. Altern Ther 1995;1:142.
7. Alternative medicine, expanding medical horizons: a report to the Institutes of Health on alternative medical systems and practices in the United States. Washington, DC: U.S. Government Printing Office; 1992.
8. Miller KL. Alternatives to estrogen for menopausal symptoms. Clin Obstet Gynecol 1992;35:884–893.
9. Alternative medicine: the definitive guide. Fife, WA: The Burton Goldberg Group; 1994.
10. Huxley A. Foreword. In: Mann F, ed. Acupuncture, the ancient Chinese art of healing. London, UK: William Heineman Medical Books; 1962.
11. Reader's Digest Association. Family guide to natural medicine. New York: Reader's Digest Association; 1993.
12. Collinge W. The American Holistic Health Association's complete guide to alternative therapies. New York: Warner Books; 1996.
13. American Association of Acupuncture and Oriental Medicine. General handout. Raleigh, NC: 1994.
14. Helms J. Physicians and acupuncture in the 1990s: a report for the Subcommittee on Labor, Health and Human Services and Education of the Appropriations Committee. Washington, DC: U.S. Government Printing Office; June 24, 1993.
15. Bienfield H. Personal communication. In: Collinge W, ed. The American Holistic Health Association complete guide to alternative therapies. New York: Warner Books; 1996.
16. Ito D. Without estrogen. New York: Crown Trade Paperbacks; 1994:59.
17. Alternative medicine, expanding medical horizons: a report to the Institutes of Health on alternative medical systems and practices in the United States. Washington, DC: U.S. Government Printing Office; 1992.
18. Gerber R. Vibrational medicine. Santa Fe, NM: Bear; 1988.
19. De Vernejoul P, et al. Study of acupuncture meridians using radioactive tracers [in French]. Bull Acad Natl Med 1985;Oct 22:1071–1075.
20. Zhu Z-X. Research advances in the electrical specificity of meridians and acupuncture points. Am J Acupunct 1981;9:203–215.

21. Jayasuraiya A. Open International University's textbook on acupuncture. Colombo, Sri Lanka: Open University; 1987.

22. Chatfield KB. The scientific basis of acupuncture. In: Pizzorno JE, Murray MT, eds. Textbook of natural medicine. Seattle: John Bastry College Publications; 1988.

23. Bullock ML, et al. Controlled trial of acupuncture for severe recidivist alcoholism. Lancet 1989;8652:1435–1439.

24. Xang X, et al. Clinical observation on needling extrachannel points in treatment of mental depression. J Tradit Chin Med 1994;14:14–18.

25. Coan RM, et al. The acupuncture treatment of low back pain: a randomized, controlled study. Am J Chin Med 1980;8:181–189.

26. Christensen PA, et al. Electroacupuncture and postoperative pain. Br J Anaeth 1990;62:258–262.

27. Qi-song, et al. Relieving effects of Chinese herbs, ear acupuncture, and epidural morphine on post-operative pain in liver cancer. Chin Med J 1994;107:289–294.

28. Naser M, et al. Acupuncture in the treatment of paralysis in chronic and acute stroke patients, improvement correlated with specific ct scan lesion sites. Acupunct Electrother Res Int J 1994;19:227–249.

29. Chan K. Progress in traditional Chinese medicine. Trends Pharmacol Sci 1995;16:182–187.

30. Li W, Lien EJ. Fu-zhen herbs in the treatment of cancer. Oriental Healing Arts Int Bull 1986;11:108.

31. Guo ZH, et al. Chinese herb "destagnation" series 1: combination of radiation with destagnation in the treatment of nasopharyngeal carcinoma (NPC): a prospective randomized trail on 188 cases. Int J Radiat Oncol Biol Phys 1989;16:297–300.

32. Sun Y. The role of traditional Chinese medicine in supportive care of cancer patients. Recent Results Cancer Res 1988;108:327–334.

33. Li L, et al. Observations on the long-term effects of "yi qi yang yin decoction" combined with radiotherapy in treatment of nasopharyngeal carcinoma. J Tradit Chin Med 1992;12:263–266.

34. Weng W, et al. Therapeutic effects of the Cratageus pinnatifida on 46 cases of angina pectoris: a double-blind study. J Tradit Chin Med 1984;4:293–294.

35. Shan P, et al. The beneficial effects of cyclovirobuxine D (CVBD) in coronary heart disease: a double blind analysis of 110 cases. J Tradit Chin Med 1984;4:15–19.

36. Chen YU, et al. Clinical observations on the effects of Radix rosae multiflora in reducing blood lipids. J Tradit Chin Med 1984;4:295–296.

37. Weed S. Menopausal years: the wise woman way. New York: Ash Tree Publishing; 1992.

38. Micozzi M. Fundamentals of complementary and alternative medicine. New York: Churchill Livingston; 1996:231.

39. Lonsdorf N. Personal communication. In: Alternative medicine, expanding medical horizons: a report to the Institutes of Health on alternative medical systems and practices in the United States. Washington, DC: U.S. Government Printing Office; 1993.

40. Lad V. Ayurveda: the science of self-healing. Santa Fe NM: Lotus Press; 1984.

41. Prasad KJ, et al. Ayurvedic (science of life) agents induce differentiation in murine neoblastoma cells in culture. Neuropharmacology 1992;31:599–607.

42. Engineer FH, et al. Protective effects of M-4 and M-5 on Adriamycin-induced microsomal lipid peroxidation and mortality. Biochem Arch 1992;8:267–272.
43. Dileepan N, et al. Priming of splenic lymphocytes after ingestion of an Ayurvedic herbal food supplement: evidence for an immunomodulatory effect. Biochem Arch 1990;6:267–272.
44. Arnold JB, et al. Chemopreventive activity of Maharishi Amrit Kalash and related agents in rat tracheal epithelial and human tumor cells [abstract]. Proc Am Assoc Cancer Res 1991;32:128.
45. Sharma HM, et al. Inhibition of human LDL oxidation in vitro by Maharishi Ayur-Veda herbal mixtures. Pharmacol Biochem Behav 1992;43:1175–1182.
46. Sharma HM, et al. Antineoplastic properties of Maharishi 4 against DMBA-induced mammary tumors in rats. Pharmacol Biochem Behav 1990;35:767–73.
47. Sharma HM, et al. Marahrishi Amrit Kalash (MAK) prevents human platelet aggregation. Clin Ther Cardiovasc 1989;8:227–230.
48. Janssen G. The application of Maharishi Ayur-Veda in the treatment of ten chronic diseases: a pilot study. Ned Tijdschr Geneeskd 1989;5:586–594.
49. Hudson T. Escharotic treatment for cervical dysplasia and carcinoma. Nat Med 1993;4:23.
50. Hudson T, Standish L. Clinical and endocrinologic effects of a menopausal formula. Presented at the American Association of Naturopathic Physicians Convention; Portland, OR, 1993.
51. Ullman D. Discovering homeopathy: medicine for the 21st century. Berkeley, CA: North Atlantic Books; 1988.
52. Coulter HL. Divided legacy: a history of the schism in medical thought, vol 2. Washington, DC: Wehawken; 1977.
53. Mcauliffe S. Homeopathy goes mainstream: new treatments for old ills. Longevity 1992;4:62.
54. Carlston M. In: Collinge W, The American Holistic Health Association complete guide to alternative therapies. New York: Warner Books; 1996:139–140.
55. Smith RB Jr, Boericke GW. Changes caused by succussion on NMR patterns and bioassay of bradykinin triacetate (BKTA) successions and dilution. J Am Inst Homeopathy 1968;61:1197–1212.
56. Kleignen J, et al. Clinical trials of homeopathy. BMJ 1991;302:316–323.
57. Reily DT, et al. Is homeopathy a placebo response: controlled trial of homeopathic potency with pollen in hay fever as model. Lancet 1986;2:881–886.
58. Zenner S, Metelmann H. Therapeutic use of lymphomyosot-results of a multicenter use: observation study on 3,512 patients. Biotherapy 1990;8:49, 79.
59. Beeley B. Herbal wisdom. Meno Times 1995;Winter:7.
60. Ullman R, Reichenberg-Ullman J. The patient's guide to homeopathic medicine. Edmounds, WA: Picnic Point Press; 1995.
61. Reichenberg-Ullman J. Menopause. Natural Health 1992;March/April:75.
62. Clayton C, McCullough VA. Consumers health guide to alternative health care. Holbrook, MA: Adams:1995.
63. Health 1995;May/June:80.
64. Champault G, et al. A double-blind trial of an extract of the plant *Serenoa repens* in benign prostatic hyperplasia. Br J Clin Pharmacol 1984;18:461–462.
65. Farnsworkth NR, et al. Medicinal plants in therapy. Bull World Health Organ 1985;63:964–981.
66. Wall Street J 1993.

67. Artiges A. What are the legal requirements for the use of phytopharmaceutical drugs in France? J Ethnopharmacol 1991;32:231–234.
68. Is it safe because it is natural? Presented at Herbal Medicine and Your Health, a program offered by the Rosenthal Center for Alternative/Complementary Medicine, Department of Rehabilitation Medicine, Columbia University College of Physicians and Surgeons. Chemical Marketing Reporter; Jan 2, 1989.
69. Weil A. Is it safe because it is natural? Presented at Herbal Medicine and Your Health, a program offered by the Rosenthal Center for Alternative/Complementary Medicine Department of Rehabilitation Medicine, Columbia University College of Physicians and Surgeons; 1996.
70. Long P. The naturals. Health 1995;May/June:89.
71. Murphy JJ, et al. Randomized double-blind placebo-controlled trial of feverfew in migraine prevention. Lancet 1988;2:189–192.
72. Warshafsky S, et al. Effect of garlic on total serum cholesterol: a meta-analysis. Ann Intern Med 1993;119:599–605.
73. Bordia A. Effect of garlic on human platelet aggregation in vitro. Atherosclerosis 1978;30:355–360.
74. Hofferberth B. The efficacy of EGb 761 in patients with senile dementia of the Alzheimer type: a double-blind, placebo-controlled study on different levels of investigation. Hum Psychoparmacol 1994;9:215–222.
75. Kleijen J, et al. Gingko biloba for cerebral insufficiency. Br J Clin Pharmacol 1992;34:352–358.
76. Sikora R, et al. Gingko biloba extract in the therapy of erectile dysfunction J Urol 1989;131:1013–1016.
77. Linde K, et al. St. John's wort for depression—an overview and meta-analysis of randomized clinical trials. BMJ 1996;313:253–258.
78. Avorn J, et al. Reduction of bacteriuria and pyuria after ingestion of cranberry juice JAMA 1994;271:751.
79. Sobata AE. Inhibition of bacteria adherence by cranberry juice: potential use for the treatment of urinary tract infections. J Urol 1984;131:1013.
80. Schmidt DR, Sobota AE. An examination of the anti-adherence activity of cranberry juice on urinary and non-urinary bacterial isolates. Microbios 1989;55:173.
81. Zafriri D, et al. Inhibitory activity of cranberry juice on adherence of type 1 and type P fimbriated *E. coli* to eucaryotic cells. Antimicrob Agents Chemother 1989;33:92.
82. Suzuke O, et al. Inhibition of monoamine oxidase by hypericin. Planta Med 1984;50:272–274.
83. Muldner H, Zoller M. Antidepressive effect of a *Hypericum* extract standardized to an active hypericin complex biochemical and clinical studies. Arzneimittelforschung 1984;34:918–920.
84. Hobbs C. Vitex: the women's herb. Capitola, CA: Botanica Press; 1990.
85. Düker EM, et al. Remifemin. Planta Med 1991;57:420–424.
86. Crawford A. The herbal menopause book, herbs, nutrition & other natural therapies. Freedom, CA: The Crossing Press; 1997:92.
87. Gevitz N. The DOS: a social history of osteopathic medicine. University of Chicago: Unpublished PhD dissertation; 1980.
88. Northrup TL. Manipulative management of hypertension. J Am Osteopath Assoc 1961;60:973–978.

89. Noll D, et al. The efficacy of OMT in the elderly hospitalized with acute pneumonia [abstract]. J Am Osteopath Assoc 1992;92:1179.
90. Wilson PT. Experimental work in asthma at the Peter Bent Brigham Hospital. J Am Osteopath Assoc 1925;25:212–214.
91. Koch RS. Structural patterns and principles of treatment in the asthmatic patient. Acad Appl Osteopath 1957;71–72.
92. Howell RK, et al. The influence of osteopathic manipulative therapy in the management of patients with chronic obstructive lung disease. J Am Osteopath Assoc 1975;74:757–760.
93. Krpan MF, et al. Low back pain (LBP) treatment by high velocity low amplitude (HVLA) osteopathic manipulative therapy and effectiveness measured by electromyography (EMG) plasma catecholamines and beta endorphin [abstract]. J Am Osteopath Assoc 1992;92:1283.
94. Hoyt WHF, et al. Osteopathic manipulation in the treatment of muscle contraction headache. J Am Osteopath Assoc 1979;78:322–325.
95. Holland C. Osteopathic medicine: structure and function. In: Collinge W, ed. The American Holistic Health Association complete guide to alternative therapies. New York: Warner Books, 1996:227.
96. Mootze RD. Chiropractic models: current understanding of vertebral subluxation and manipulable spinal lesions. In: Sweer JJ, ed. Chiropractic family practice: a clinical manual. Gaithersburg, MD: Aspen, 1992:2–8.
97. Cottrell R. Stress management. Guilford, CT: Dushken, 1992:186.
98. Awatramani B. Integrating medicine and meditation. Newslett Santa Fe Inst Med Prayer 1996:2.
99. Benson HJ, et al. The relaxation response. Psychiatry 1974;37:37–46.
100. Rossman M. Personal communication. In: Alternative medicine, expanding medical horizons: a report to the Institutes of Health on alternative medical systems and practices in the United States. Washington, DC: U.S. Government Printing Office; 1994:244.
101. Field TC, et al. Tactile/kinesthetic stimulation effects on preterm neonates. Pediatrics 1986;77:654–658.
102. Field TC, et al. Massage reduces anxiety in child and adolescent psychiatric patients. J Am Acad Child Adolesc Psychol 1992;31:125–131.
103. Kaard B, Tostinbo O. Increase of plasma beta endorphins in a connective tissue massage. Gen Pharmacol 1989;20:487–489.
104. Weintraub M. Shiatsu, Swedish muscle massage, and trigger point suppression in spinal pain syndrome. Massage Ther J 1992;31:99–109.
105. Yoachin G. The effects of two stress management techniques on feelings of well-being in patients with inflammatory bowel disease. Nurs Papers 1983;15:5–18.
106. Koop C. The art and science of medicine. In: Micozzi M, ed. Fundamentals of complementary therapy. New York: Churchill Livingston; 1996.

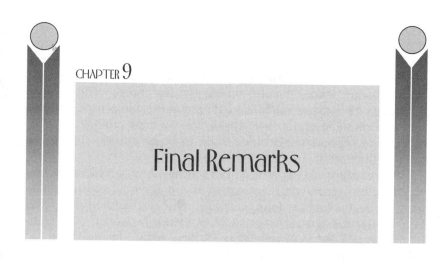

CHAPTER 9

Final Remarks

Even with an elaborate and expensive a system for the delivery of personal health care services, several studies conducted in Western industrialized nations have documented that it is self-care, not professional health care, that responds to most health care needs.[1] The amount of information about nutrition, exercise, stress reduction, and other preventive health care practices is vast, and I hope that the information selected from many sources has shown that viewing menopause as an "estrogen deficiency disease" that can only be treated by hormone replacement therapy is not acceptable.

Every woman, at some point during the climacteric, will experience a decline in estrogen, progesterone, and dehydroepiandrosterone. Some will also experience a decline in testosterone. The onset and rate of the decline in these hormone levels is variable.

Some women experience symptoms associated with the climacteric. The range of the symptoms and their effects on a woman's physical and emotional well-being depend on a multitude of factors. Other women remain free of symptoms.

Cardiovascular disease, cancer, and other chronic degenerative diseases account for 75% of American deaths. The stage for these diseases and for osteoporosis is often established early in life. However, this can be greatly ameliorated by a complement of lifestyle changes. Most women are probably deficient in several nutrients and have yet to integrate into their lives the basic lifestyle changes essential for the prevention and treatment of disease and climacteric-related symptoms.

More is unknown than is known about the climacteric. This is also true for many of the treatment choices available for related symptoms.

Serious consideration of these and other points leads to one major conclusion: If we are to have an impact on the way in which a woman experiences the climacteric and the course of her health, the "magic bullet" approach to treatment of the climacteric must be replaced with one of self-care. To do this, we must provide the education and support that women need to be able to practice these ideas to the fullest.

This concept is a departure from the way in which conventional medicine is practiced and the attitude of the public as a result of this practice. As the late Dr. John Knowles, who headed the Rockefeller Foundation and Massachusetts General Hospital, stated, "The people have been led to believe that national health insurance, more doctors, and greater use of high-cost, hospital-based technologies will improve health. Unfortunately, none of them will."[2]

When it comes to playing a major role in assisting your patients in their own self-care practices, you are faced with professional limitations, especially the lack of time that stems from financial realities. It is the rare health care provider who can say that he or she has enough time to take a history, perform an examination, and deal with immediate health issues, much less take a comprehensive lifestyle history and then provide adequate education and guidance based on what the history reveals. However, you are encouraged to do as your patients must do when they are considering the most beneficial ways to approach meeting their own health care needs and take some time to consider the best ways in which you can be instrumental in helping your patients obtain the information and support they must have:

- Do you provide you patients a comprehensive lifestyle history or self-assessment tool that they can complete in their leisure time to help them and you to identify areas of need?
- Do you have patient education materials that focus on preventive health measures and a list of community and health resources that you can give to your patients?
- Is it possible to offer monthly health promotion programs through your practice or clinic covering topics ranging from the climacteric in general to exercise, nutrition, hormone replacement therapies, and complementary therapies?
- Can experts in these areas from your community be persuaded to give a couple of hours of their time every few months to offer such programs for your patients?

These are examples of questions that you may want to consider when determining the best strategies to meet the needs of your patients.

Another problem that may confront you is your own lack of knowledge about preventive health care practices such as nutrition. This is true for most conventionally trained health care professionals, because such practices were not a primary focus in medical and nursing schools and clinician training programs and because so much has changed since the Basic Four Food Group was taught.

If you have not done so already, consider taking advantage of the increasing number of continuing education programs, books, and journals devoted to these areas. Two excellent resources are the National Institutes of Health's *Alternative Medicine: Expanding Medical Horizons* and *The Kellogg Report: The Impact of Nutrition, Environment, and Lifestyle on the Health of Americans.* You may also want to consider subscribing to journals such as *Nutrition Today, Alternative Therapies in Health and Medicine, Clinical Pearl News,* and *Herbalgram.* Journals such as these can help you to learn about and direct you to other resources that discuss the promising and exciting research in the areas of preventive medicine and complementary health care practices.

Consider meeting with complementary health care practitioners in your community. The wealth of information and clinical experiences that you and they can share should not be underestimated. Relationships can evolve with these practitioners and with nutritionists, physical therapists, or even a local yoga instructor, which can ultimately lead to developing a system that can meet the needs of your patients.

REFERENCES

1. DeFreise, et al. Medical self-care instructions for laypersons: a new agenda for health science. Continuing education. Mobius 1982;2:45–51.
2. Knowles J. Doing better and feeling worse: health in the United States. New York: WW Norton; 1977.

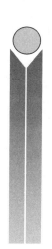
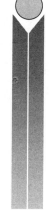

Guidelines for the Care of Women Over Thirty

These guidelines, developed in an outline format, provide recommendations for history taking and evaluation of perimenopausal and postmenopausal women. They highlight the major components of a total wellness program, as discussed in Chapters 3 through 8, and include suggested treatment regimens for hormonal and drug therapies and for herbal and homeopathic treatments.

I. HISTORY TAKING AND SCREENING PROCEDURES

Because the perimenopause can begin in the middle thirties to early forties, consider having all of your patients in this age group as well as your postmenopausal patients complete a comprehensive climacteric questionnaire before meeting with you. It can be sent to them before their appointments or completed at your office or clinic. This approach can facilitate discussion of sensitive areas, because some women are reluctant to disclose verbally certain types of information, particularly about sexuality, substance abuse, and eating disorders. They may feel more comfortable writing about their problems and concerns. The questionnaire can serve as an opening for a dialogue, and it may allow you to cover a greater range of issues within your time constraints. Appendix A provides samples of questions that can be used for patient assessments of osteoporosis, cardiovascular disease (CVD), nutritional intake, physical activity, stress, sexual activities, and climacteric-related symptoms.

A. Routine Information for All Women Older Than 30

1. Familial and personal medical, obstetric, and gynecologic history and information about substance abuse, domestic violence, sexual abuse, and sexuality

2. Risk factors for osteoporosis (see Chapter 4)

3. Risk factors for CVD (see Chapter 3)

4. Age at menopause of close relatives on maternal side and symptoms experienced by these relatives

5. Assessments of the following

    a. Nutritional intake

    b. Level of physical activity

    c. Level of stress

    d. Assessment of sexual life

    e. Presence and degree of climacteric-related symptoms

    f. Ways in which the woman may be treating her symptoms

B. Physical Examination

Women should receive a complete physical examination every 1 to 2 years, depending on health status and personal and family history.

1. Blood pressure

2. Height

3. Weight and determination of waist-hip ratio (fat distribution around waist is a risk factor for CVD). The ratio is determined by dividing the waist measurement by the hip measurement. The target ratio is 0.8.

4. Calculation of body mass index (BMI) should be considered. Multiply the weight by 700, divide the total by the height in inches, and divide again by the weight. According to the National Women's Health Resource Center, a BMI of around 25 or less is considered to be within a healthy weight range.

5. Pelvic examination

6. Rectal examination (all women age 40 and older)

7. Breast examination

8. Skin examination

9. Thyroid examination

10. Heart and lung examination

11. Examination of the extremities

12. Skin cancer screening (every 3 years)

C. Laboratory Tests

1. Papanicolaou smear

2. Rubella titer (if not previously performed)

3. PPD test for tuberculosis (if high risk)

4. Sexually transmitted infection screening, as appropriate

    a. Gonorrhea

    b. Syphilis

    c. Chlamydial infection

    d. Human immunodeficiency virus infection

5. Urinalysis

6. Fecal occult blood (all women age 40 and older)

7. Complete blood cell count

8. Thyroid stimulating hormone (TSH). All women at age 45 or younger should have TSH levels tested if they are experiencing climacteric-related symptoms. Thyroid dysfunction can present symptoms similar to some of those associated with the climacteric, such as fatigue, poor memory, and decreased libido. Hypothyroidism can elevate cholesterol and cause hypertension. This test should be repeated every 2 years after age 50.

9. Fasting plasma glucose (after at least an 8-hour fast). The American Diabetes Association's new protocol advises this test at age 45, and if results are normal, it should be repeated every 3 years. Persons younger than 45 should be tested if they are more than 20% above ideal weight; have a parent or sibling with diabetes; are African American, Hispanic, native American, or Asian (high-risk ethnicities); have a baby born weighing 9 pounds or have had gestational diabetes;

have blood pressure at or above 140/90 mm Hg; have a high-density lipoprotein (HDL) cholesterol level of 35 mg/dL or less or triglyceride level of 250 mg/dL or more; and have impaired fasting glucose or impaired glucose tolerance determined in previous testing. The Association estimates that these guidelines could identify 2 million of the approximately 8 million adults with undiagnosed diabetes.

10. Levels of total cholesterol, HDL, low-density lipoprotein (LDL), and triglycerides (preferably after a 12- to 14-hour fast). These tests should be performed every 5 years as long as results remain normal.

11. A hematocrit test should be performed every 5 years as long as results remain normal.

12. An FSH test should be performed at the onset of significant climacteric-related symptoms.

13. Dehydroepiandrosterone sulfate (DHEAS) level testing is recommended at the onset of significant climacteric-related symptoms if considering DHEA therapy. Repeat the test after 6 months of therapy to assess dosage response.

D. Other Procedures

1. Mammogram

   a. Baseline at age 35 to 40. If high risk, begin screening 5 years before the age at diagnosis of breast cancer of a family member.

   b. Every 2 years until age 50 if low risk and every year if high risk

   c. Once each year after age 50

2. Bone density screening

   a. If a woman is in a high-risk category according to family and personal health history (eg, osteoporosis on maternal side, eating disorders, substance abuse, corticosteroid therapy, past and current poor diet, sedentary lifestyle, stress), the baseline should be determined at age 25 to evaluate evidence of osteopenia or osteoporosis. If the baseline is normal, screening does not have to be repeated until menopause, unless a woman experiences a situation that could negatively affect bone density, such as a course of corticosteroid therapy or a prolonged period of restricted physical activity, or if a woman continues to live an osteoporosis-causing lifestyle.

b. Baseline for women in their forties or at onset of perimenopausal symptoms for women in low-risk category. Repeat screening should be performed after menopause (a time of rapid bone loss) and at 5-year intervals after menopause.

3. Electrocardiogram (at age 30 and every 2 years thereafter)

4. Chest radiograph (at age 50)

5. Exercise stress test, possibly with echocardiographic imaging or a radionuclide tracer. Testing is often recommended for women age 50 and older who are asymptomatic, have a few risk factors, and have some family history of coronary heart disease.

6. Flexible sigmoidoscopy (initially at age 50 and repeated every 3 to 5 years if results remain normal). Contrast barium enema and colonoscopy are recommended for women considered to be at high risk for colorectal cancer.

7. Hearing and visual acuity tests (all women age 50 and older every 1 to 3 years)

F. Additional Evaluations

1. Perimenopausal women may be interested in observing fertility signs such as cervical mucus or basal body temperature changes (see Appendix B)

2. Postmenopausal women may be interested in mental status and lifestyle assessment. Although anxiety, depression, and other changes in mental or emotional status can strike any person at any age, they are particularly worrisome during midlife and later years. You can use any one of several excellent questionnaires developed by specialists in the field of geriatric medicine to evaluate the mental status of your post-

menopausal patients, or you can refer them to someone with expertise in this area. The woman's lifestyle, her support systems, diet, and financial issues should be evaluated, and items for this evaluation are included in many of the questionnaires developed by geriatric specialists. The same questionnaires, with modifications, can be used with perimenopausal patients.

II. DIETARY RECOMMENDATIONS

The recommendations listed here are based on the U.S. Department of Agriculture (USDA) guidelines. Intake of all foods that are fresh and free of preservatives, pesticides, antibiotics, and hormones should be emphasized. The use of cooking methods that minimize nutrient loss, such as light steaming and baking, should be emphasized. The consumption of a diet that consists of a variety of foods, particularly vegetables and whole grains, should also be emphasized to maximize the possibility of an adequate intake of all nutrients. Serving sizes are calculated to meet the daily needs of complex carbohydrates, protein, fiber, total fats, and basic nutrients.

A. Calorie Consumption

   1. Complex carbohydrates (eg, grains, beans, vegetables, fruits) should represent approximately 50% of a woman's daily calorie consumption.

   2. Protein should represent 20% to 30% of a woman's daily calorie consumption. If she works out at least three times per week, her protein requirement probably should be increased by approximately 20%.

   3. Total fats (less than 10% from saturated fats and cholesterol [less than 300 mg]) should represent 30% of a woman's daily calorie consumption or 15% to 20% if she is overweight or at high risk for CVD.

B. Serving Sizes

   1. Bread, cereal, pasta: 6 to 11 servings (serving size = 0.5 cup; 1 slice of bread = 1 serving)

   2. Vegetables: 2 to 3 servings = 1 to 1.5 cups

3. Fruit: 3 to 5 servings (1 serving = 1 medium piece of fruit, 0.5 cup cut fruit, or 0.75 cup of unsweetened fruit juice)

4. Low-fat or nonfat dairy products: 2 to 4 servings (1 serving = 1 cup of milk, 8 ounce of yogurt, or 1 to 2 ounce of cheese)

5. Lean meat, skinless poultry, fish, soy products (40 g/day), legumes, eggs, nuts: 2 to 3 servings (1 serving = 1 egg or 10 nuts)

6. Oils are to be used sparingly (eg, 2 teaspoons/day on salads or vegetables), with emphasis on unrefined, cold-pressed oils, particularly olive and canola oils for consumption of essential fatty acids.

7. Sugars are to be used sparingly, with emphasis on maple syrup and honey because of the nutrients they contain.

8. Eight 8-ounce glasses of water each day

C. Substances to Be Minimized or Avoided

1. Foods and substances to be minimized or avoided because of CVD, osteoporosis, and other chronic health problems

   a. Caffeinated beverages

   b. Beverages with high phosphorus levels

   c. Excessive sodium-containing foods (intake should be limited to approximately 2500 mg/day)

   d. *Trans*-fatty acids in margarines, convenience foods, and oils made from partially hydrogenated vegetable oils

   e. Alcoholic beverages

2. Foods and substances to be avoided for prevention or reduction of hot flushes

   a. Spicy foods

   b. Sugar

   c. Highly acidic foods such as oranges, grapefruits, tomatoes, and berries

   d. Alcoholic beverages and caffeine-containing beverages

D. Spacing of Meals

Small, easily digestible, protein-containing meals and
snacks (ie, three meals and two snacks) should be consumed every 2 to 3 hours to maintain stable glucose levels
and maximize digestion, absorption, and assimilation of
nutrients.

E. Ratio of Carbohydrates, Fats, and Proteins

Proteins, fats, and carbohydrates should be consumed at
the same time to maintain stable glucose levels and maximize digestion, absorption, and assimilation of nutrients.
For example, eating some fruit or a carrot as a snack is not
advised; eating a piece of fruit with a piece of low-fat soy
cheese or low-fat cottage cheese is a more reasonable and
healthful choice.

III. NUTRITIONAL SUPPLEMENTATION RECOMMENDATIONS

The following recommended dosages include a suggested
range for most of the vitamins and minerals listed. The
dosages ultimately depend on the amount of nutrients a
woman is consuming through her diet and the quality of her
diet; her general health status; presence or absence of climacteric symptoms; and degree of physical activity and stress
in her life. They also depend on her ability to make changes in
her lifestyle. For example, if a woman is consuming a high-
sugar diet but does not decrease her sugar intake, she will
probably be more nutrient deficient than a woman whose
sugar intake is minimal, and she should supplement with
doses in the higher range. This is also the case for a woman
who is experiencing considerable stress in her life but is
unable or unwilling to practice stress reduction methods. She,
too, could benefit from supplementing with the maximum recommended dosages. Vitamins and minerals should be taken
with meals or shortly thereafter. When more than the minimum recommended amount is taken, supplementation should
be taken in divided doses.

A. Vitamins

1. B_1, B_2, B_3 (niacin), B_6, B_{12}: 50 to 150 mg

2. B_5: 250 to 1000 mg (Increase by 250 mg every 2 weeks until the maximum of 1000 mg for hot flushes. If this maximum dosage provides no relief, reduce the dosage at the same rate it was increased. If relief is experienced, gradually decrease after 1 month from the maximum dosage to an amount that maintains relief.)

3. Folic acid: 400 to 800 μg

4. Vitamin E: 50 to 800 IU (More than 100 IU may not be advisable for women with diabetes, hypertension, or rheumatic heart disease or those who are using anticoagulant therapy; use 200 to 1200 IU for hot flushes; use 400 IU for cardiovascular protection for women 22 to 50 years old and 800 IU for women older than 50.)

5. Vitamin D: 100 to 400 IU

6. Vitamin A: 5000 to 10,000 IU, or 6 to 16 mg of beta-carotene

7. Vitamin K: 100 to 500 μg (not to be taken by women on anticoagulant therapy with Coumadin or warfarin but can be taken with heparin therapy)

8. Vitamin C: 200 to 3000 mg (average dose, 1000 mg)

9. Bioflavonoids: 500 to 1000 mg; 250 mg five to six times each day for hot flushes

B. Minerals

1. Calcium citrate: 250 to 1000 mg for perimenopausal women, 500 to 1500 mg for perimenopausal women, and 500 to 1500 mg for postmenopausal women (should be taken in divided doses, with the last dose taken at bedtime)

2. Magnesium aspartate or citrate: 600 to 1000 mg (calcium-magnesium ratio of 2:1, or with a magnesium-deficient diet, a ratio of 1:1)

3. Zinc: 10 to 50 mg

4. Copper: 1 to 3 mg

     5. Manganese: 2 to 15 mg

     6. Boron: 1 to 3 mg

     7. Silicon: 1 to 2 mg

     8. Selenium: 50 to 200 μg

     9. Chromium: 200 μg

   10. Iron: 10 to 23 mg

C. Essential Fatty Acids

Flax seed is considered one of the best essential fatty acids (EFAs) because it also rich in the phytochemical lignan, an estrogen modulator with estrogenic and antiestrogenic properties. EFA supplements can be expensive, and a good option is to buy the much less expensive flax seeds. One teaspoon of flax seeds can be crushed and placed in a small glass with enough water added to cover them. The covered glass should be refrigerated overnight and the mixture drunk the next day. Flax seeds can also be crushed and sprinkled on cooked vegetables and salads. There is little research on the long-term use of omega-3 and omega-6 essential fatty acids or the most appropriate ratio to consume. Some suggest 1 teaspoon every 3 days for 2 weeks per month is an adequate and safe dosage for health maintenance. For perimenopausal and postmenopausal women, the following recommended doses are taken until symptoms are relieved, and then the amount is reduced to 1 teaspoon every 3 days for 2 weeks per month.

     1. Organic flax seed, black currant, and borage oils: 1 tablespoons each day

     2. Evening primrose oil: 500 mg twice each day

     3. Essential oil formula by Internal Building Systems: taken as directed (contains flax seed, black currant seed, pumpkin seed oils and safflower oil, and vitamin E)

D. Digestive Enzymes

     1. Highly recommended to improve vitamin and mineral absorption, protein, carbohydrate, and fat use and for women with digestive disorders

    2. Contraindicated for women with gastritis or gastric or duodenal ulcers

    3. Several good brands of digestive enzymes are available from any pharmacy or health food store.

       a. Similase by Tyler Encapsulations

       b. Digestion by Scientific Bio-Logics

       c. Premier Enzyme Formula by Primary Resource

       d. Vitase Digestion Formula by Prevail Corporation

IV. EXERCISE RECOMMENDATIONS

The following recommendations represent the ideal goal for a woman. However, anyone with physical limitations or who has been sedentary should initiate a considerably modified program, such as walking for 15 minutes three times each week. As strength and stamina improve, the intensity and duration of exercises should be increased gradually.

A. Stretching and Warm-up Exercises

    1. To help prevent injuries

    2. For upper and lower body

    3. To be performed for 10 minutes

B. Strength-Training and Bone-Loading Exercises

    1. For osteoporosis prevention and treatment

    2. To help decrease or prevent climacteric-related symptoms

    3. To help reduce effects of stressors

    4. To be performed for 20 minutes 3 times each week

C. Aerobic Exercises

    1. For cardiovascular system

    2. To decrease or prevent climacteric-related symptoms

    3. To help reduce effects of stressors

    4. Low to moderate intensity to be performed 30 minutes each day (ideal) *or* 60 minutes every other day

    5. To be performed between 45% and 80% of maximum heart rate (calculation of range: subtract age from 220; multiply result by 0.45 and by 0.80)

D. Cool Down

   1. To help prevent injury and muscle cramping

   2. For upper and lower body

   3. To be performed for 10 minutes

V. STRESS REDUCTION RECOMMENDATIONS

Meditation and strengthening and cardiovascular exercises can be derived from yoga. Meditation and strengthening exercises can be obtained through chi kong and tai' chi.

A. Physical exercises, as in previous section

B. Deep breathing exercises, performed for at least 1 minute periodically throughout the day

C. Meditation

   1. To be performed every day (ideal) *or* every other day

   2. To be performed for 60 minutes (ideal) *or* for 10 to 30 minutes

D. Therapy, Counseling, and Group Support

E. Additional Activities

Any activity such as reading, listening to music, or a hobby that reduces stress and provides relaxation is beneficial and should be experienced on a regular basis.

VI. HORMONAL THERAPY RECOMMENDATIONS

Chapter 7 describes the types of and rationales for hormonal replacement therapies. Patience, good communication, and some experimentation with dosage and formulations usually result in an acceptable, side-effect-free regimen. For women sensitive to the standard dosage of estrogen, a lower one may still offer some cardiovascular and osteoporosis protection and usually reduces or eliminates climacteric-related symptoms. Begin with the lowest dose possible and slowly increase it to determine the woman's response and comfort level with the therapy. Plant-based estrogens, progesterone, and testosterone are available in different routes of administration and dosages. Pharmacists can provide more information about these hormone therapies (see Appendix C).

A. Estrogen

Regardless of the brand, dose, and route of administration of estrogen, it is essential that a progestin or natural progesterone be used in combination with estrogen to prevent endometrial hyperplasia and cancer. Some clinicians use the combined approach with natural progesterone for women who have had a hysterectomy because of its potential bone building effects. The combined approach also may be used for women with a history of endometriosis to minimize the possibility of a recurrence. If a woman has not had a hysterectomy and cannot or does not want to use a progestin or progesterone, unopposed estrogen therapy can be used in combination with an endometrial biopsy performed before initiation of therapy and annually thereafter.

1. Treatment regimens

The minimum dosage that appears to offer protection against CVD and osteoporosis is 0.625 mg of conjugated equine estrogen or an equivalent dosage of other available estrogen preparations. For treatment of climacteric-related symptoms of women who do not want to use estrogen, cannot tolerate a higher dose, or are not comfortable taking estrogen indefinitely, short-term estrogen therapy equivalent to approximately one half of the recommended dosage for prevention of cardiovascular and osteoporosis prevention can be taken for 1 to 2 months. Therapy is repeated if symptoms recur. Compliance is increased if the lowest dose of estrogen is initially prescribed. If well tolerated after 1 month of use, the dose can be increased.

a. For CVD and osteoporosis prevention:

(1) 0.625-mg oral dose of conjugated equine estrogen

(2) 1 mg of micronized estradiol (Estrace)

(3) 0.625 mg of piperazine estrone sulfate (Ogen, Ortho-Est)

    (4) 1 mg estradiol valerate

    (6) 0.05 mg transdermal estradiol patch (Estradiol)

    (7) 0.625 mg esterified estrogen (Estratab)

  b. Schedule of treatment with the oral forms

    (1) Daily (sequential regimen) from the 1st to the 25th day of each month: progestin or progesterone therapy as outlined in part B

    (2) Continuously (uninterrupted regimen), every day of each month: progestin or progesterone therapy as outlined in part B (The uninterrupted regimen eliminates the symptoms experienced when hormonal therapy is discontinued for a week and therefore increases compliance.)

2. Transdermal estrogen patches

  a. Applied every 3.5 days or once each week, depending on the product used

  b. Minimum dosage to prevent osteoporosis and CVD is 0.5 mg, but 0.1 mg may be necessary if symptoms are not relieved.

3. Vaginal estrogen preparations

Vaginal estrogen preparations (eg, Premarin, Estrace, natural estrogen creams) can relieve symptoms such as decreased vaginal lubrication, dyspareunia, irritation, pruritus, vulvovaginitis. Although minimal systemic absorption occurs, some women report improvement in hot flushes and other climacteric-related symptoms when using vaginal estrogen therapy in the following standard treatment regimen.

  a. One third of applicator two times/week for first week

  b. One third of applicator once daily for second week

  c. One third of applicator every other day for third week

  d. One third of applicator every 3 to 7 days

  e. One third of applicator weekly as a maintenance dose

4. Plant-based oral estrogen therapy
   a. Tri-Est or Bi-Est can be taken sequentially or continuously.
   b. Tri-Est contains 80% estriol, 10% estradiol, and 10% estrone. Bi-Est contains 80% estriol and 20% estradiol.
   c. Usual starting dose of 2.5 mg appears equivalent in relieving climacteric-related symptoms to 0.625 mg of conjugated estrogen.
   d. Progesterone can be added to these products at the dose prescribed by the clinician or taken separately.

5. Gels and creams
   a. Creams and gels are available that contain estriol-only and estriol, estrone, and estradiol (Tri-Est) or estriol and estradiol (Bi-Est).
   b. Pharmacies can compound various formulas and dosages per request and offer instructions for use.
   c. Dosages and instructions for use depend on the stage of the climacteric and symptoms.

B. Progestins and Natural Progesterone

1. Treatment Regimens
   a. Standard, older regimen: with the sequential estrogen therapy program (days 1–25 with 1-week interruption), a progestin or natural progesterone is taken during the last 14 days of estrogen therapy.
   b. Newer regimen: cyclic progestin or progesterone is taken for the first 12 days of each month in combination with an estrogen. Vaginal bleeding usually begins after the 9th day following this regimen.
   c. Starting dosages for the sequential program
      (1) 5 mg of medroxyprogesterone acetate (MPA)
      (2) 0.7 mg of norethindrone
      (3) 200 to 400 mg of micronized oral progesterone (The hormone is taken as equally divided morning and evening doses. If 300 mg is prescribed, 100 mg is taken in the morning and 200 mg in the evening.)

    d. For continuous or uninterrupted hormone therapy, a progestin or progesterone is taken with estrogen every day of the month. This regimen tends to decrease side effects and bleeding.

      (1) 2.5 mg of MPA

      (2) 0.35 mg of norethindrone

      (3) 100 to 200 mg of natural progesterone. (Dosage must be divided in half and taken in the morning and evening.)

    e. Another regimen is the use of a progestin from days 12 through 25 in combination with 85 days of continuous estrogen therapy. With this program, a woman experiences bleeding four times per year.

    f. Progesterone therapy can be used without any form of estrogen for relief of some symptoms associated with the climacteric and osteoporosis prevention (see Chapter 7).

2. Creams and gels

    a. Progest cream can be purchased without a prescription. One 2-ounce jar contains 960 mg of progesterone.

    b. Progesterone-based creams and gels are also available in higher doses (eg, 25 mg, 50 mg) and are available by prescription through pharmacies.

    c. Pharmacists can provide instructions for use.

3. Pro-Gest liquid

    a. Pro-Gest liquid contains three times the concentration found in the cream. It is used as sublingual drops, resulting in a more rapid absorption of the progesterone.

    b. It can be used alone or with an estrogen cream. The dose necessary to prevent hyperplasia or endometrial cancer when used in combination with an estrogen cream has not been established.

4. Oral progesterone

Micronized oral progesterone can be used alone at doses ranging from 25 to 100 mg daily.

C. Testosterone

Because the long-term effects of testosterone therapy, particularly in altering lipid profiles, are unknown (see Chapter 7), the best approach is to use the least amount possible and slowly increase the dose as needed. When testosterone is used alone, it is usually continued until the woman's libido returns to an acceptable level. Pharmacists can discuss instructions for use and modifications of therapies, and most will send a clinician's packet of information, including several research articles.

1. 1.2 to 10 mg tablets of synthetic testosterone capsules taken on a daily basis (most common form)

2. Forms derived usually from soybeans or wild Mexican yam:

a. Tablet or sublingual forms at 2.5 mg, 5 mg, or higher (if specifically ordered from pharmacies that compound natural testosterone); starting dose is usually taken once daily and increased to twice daily if the libido and energy level have not improved.

b. A 1% cream applied to the clitoris and labia may be adequate to increase libido in some women.

D. Combination Products

1. Estrogen with methyltestosterone (MeT): 0.625 mg conjugated equine estrogen (CEE) with 5 mg of MeT, or 1.25 mg of CEE with 10 mg of MeT (a progestin or progesterone must be added)

2. Esterified estrogen (EE) and MeT: 1.25 EE with 2.5 mg of MeT, or 0.625 mg of EE with 1.25 mg of MeT 1.25 (a progestin or progesterone must be added)

3. Estradiol (2.5 mg) and micronized progesterone (400 mg) capsules

E. Dehydroepiandrosterone

The issue of whether DHEAS levels should be obtained before initiation of DHEA therapy is controversial (see Chapter 7). For some women after age 30, when DHEA levels begin to steadily decline, low-dose DHEA therapy (eg, 2.5 mg/day) is prescribed initially. Symptoms of excessive DHEA and relief of climacteric symptoms are monitored, and if appropriate, the dose may be increased to 5 mg after 3 months of therapy. Doses may continue to be increased every 3 months to a maximum of 25 to 50 mg/day. is carefully monitored and increased as appropriate. If affordable, another approach is to obtain a DHEAS baseline level, prescribe an increasing DHEA schedule, and assess levels every 3 months for a year, until a dose compatible with normal levels and relief of symptoms is established.

1. The usual starting dose is 2.5 mg of DHEA, which can be obtained from a pharmacy that compounds DHEA. Dosages are manipulated based on the woman's response and blood levels (if taken).

2. Higher doses (eg, 50 to 100 mg) that are available for purchase in health food stores and elsewhere may not be of the same quality or have the same degree of bioavailability. Moreover, these doses may be higher than needed for physiologic replacement of DHEA, and side effects may be experienced.

3. Women with health problems such as lupus erythematosus, chronic fatigue syndrome, or cancer should use low-dose therapy initially, slowly increasing the dosage every 2 to 3 months based on symptoms and the potential side effects of DHEA. They may eventually require doses in the 50- to 100-mg range and should have DHEAS levels monitored every 3 months for 1 year and annually thereafter.

4. A DHEAS level that is midway or slightly above the normal level for adult women, as established by the laboratory, should be the goal of therapy for perimenopausal women.

5. The therapeutic goal for postmenopausal women at the time are DHEAS levels that are midway or slightly above the normal level for postmenopausal women, as established by the laboratory. It is recommended that you discuss with a pharmacist who compounds DHEA.

VII. OTHER DRUG THERAPIES

Check the *Physician's Desk Reference* for information about side effects and contraindications for these drugs.

A. For Hot Flushes

1. Bellergal-S: Dosage is usually one tablet taken twice a day. Each tablet contains 40 mg of phenobarbital.

2. Clonidine (Catapres-TSS): Initial recommended dose is the lowest available. The Catapres-TTS-1 patch is used once each week. Clonidine tablets can also be taken at a dose of 0.1 mg twice daily. Dose can be increased to 0.2 mg if hot flushes are not relieved and side effects are not experienced.

3. Bromocriptine: Initial dosage is 0.5 mg daily.

B. For Postmenopausal Osteoporosis

1. Alendronate (Fosamax): 10 mg in the morning

2. Calcitonin: available as salmon-calcitonin (injectable) for postmenopausal osteoporosis. Dosage is 100 IU/day, administered intramuscularly or subcutaneously.

VIII. HERBAL AND HOMEOPATHIC THERAPIES

Ideally, a woman should receive a complete evaluation, such as by a practitioner of TCM, a naturopathic physician, homeopathic practitioner, or herbalist, who can develop a comprehensive program. When this is not feasible, herbal, naturopathic, and homeopathic treatments developed specifically for the climacteric can be used and are available through mail order, health food stores, and homeopathic or herbal and conventional pharmacies (see Chapter 8 and Appendix C). The following treatments for climacteric-related symptoms are primarily those recommended by the Santa Monica Homeopathic Pharmacy and other excellent herbal, homeopathic, and nutritional supplementation programs that are available through Transitions for Health. Herbal, naturopathic, and homeopathic treatments are often used in combination with a plant-based progesterone cream or gel, an essential fatty acid, and vitamin and mineral therapy. All herbal and homeopathic treatments are taken at the lowest dosage possible for relief of symptoms and should be discontinued when symptoms are relieved. They are repeated if symptoms recur. If significant relief of symptoms does not result within 2 to 3 months, the woman should consider changing products or consulting a

practitioner with expertise in herbal or homeopathic therapies.

A. Herbal Treatments

The following treatments are not to be taken during menses.

1. Changes for Women by The Zand Formulas is used by
    women older than 30 who are beginning to experience
    hot flushes and other symptoms.

2. Female Formula by The Zand Formulas is used by
    premenopausal and perimenopausal women to help
    relieve symptoms of premenstrual syndrome (PMS)
    and dysmenorrhea.

3. Female Harmony by Crystal Star is used by peri-
    menopausal women who are beginning to experience
    PMS symptoms for the first time or an exacerbation of
    these symptoms.

4. EST-AID by Crystal Star is used by perimenopausal or
    postmenopausal women with minimal to severe
    symptoms. Pro-Gest or other progesterone creams or
    gels should be taken with this product when moderate
    to severe symptoms are experienced.

5. Vitex and an essential fatty acid supplement such as
    flax seed or evening primrose oil should be taken with
    EST-AID and other herbal therapies if relief of symp-
    toms is marginal or when moderate to severe symp-
    toms are experienced.

6. Fem-Esterro by Metagenics contains a combination of
    herbs, vitamins, and raw adrenal for symptoms asso-
    ciated with the climacteric and for women in need of
    adrenal support (eg, women with chronic or acute
    stress).

7. Lunar Formula Types 1 and 2 by Transitions for
    Health are used by perimenopausal women with var-
    ious premenstrual and other symptoms. The formula
    is based on cycle length. (The company offers infor-
    mation on assessing which formula to use.)

8. Solar Formulas 1 and 2 by Transitions for Health are
    used by women experiencing symptoms associated
    with the climacteric and for prevention of symptoms.

B. Homeopathics

Most of the following homeopathic remedies contain several substances that can provide relief for at least 50% of women who use them. If they do not provide significant relief, the woman probably should seek the assistance of a homeopathic practitioner who can recommend the treatments best suited for her.

1. Bioron homeopathics are excellent products, often sold as single remedies.

2. Natural Phases for perimenopausal women experiencing an exacerbation of PMS symptoms or who are experiencing them for the first time and Cyclease for dysmenorrhea (both by Bioron)

3. Menopause by Natra-Bio

4. Estrex by NF Formulations

5. Menopause by BHI

6. Menopause by Hylands

IX. TREATMENTS FOR VAGINAL DRYNESS AND DYSPAREUNIA

In addition to the herbs and homeopathics that can be taken orally for vaginal dryness and dyspareunia, other nonhormonal treatments can be used to relieve these symptoms.

A. Treatments Unassociated With the Time of Intercourse

1. Kegel exercises: An instructional cassette tape is available from HIP-PME, Box 8310, Spartanburg, SC 29305 (800 BLADDER).

2. Intravaginal therapies

a. Oils: vitamin E (100 IU starting dose) or cold-pressed castor, sesame, or coconut oil can be massaged around the introitus and into the vaginal tissues.

b. Aloe vera gel can be massaged around the introitus and in the vaginal tissues.

c. Calendula cream (without a petroleum base)

d. Replens or other vaginal moisturizers

B. Treatments Used With Intercourse

    1. Any of the lubricants specifically prepared for intravaginal use

    2. Egg white

X. SUMMARY OF RECOMMENDATIONS TO HELP RELIEVE OR PREVENT HOT FLUSHES AND OTHER CLIMACTERIC-RELATED SYMPTOMS

A. Exercise

B. Healthy diet

C. Deep breathing and meditative techniques

D. Avoidance of certain foods, substances, or medications that can cause or aggravate hot flushes, such as tobacco, marijuana (and other recreational drugs), caffeine, alcoholic beverages, sugar, spicy foods, hot foods and beverages, and antihistamines

E. Vitamin supplementation, particularly vitamins E and B_5 and bioflavonoids

F. Essential fatty acids, particularly flax seed

G. Avoidance of an environment in which temperature is too warm, including hot tubs and saunas

XI. INITIATION OF A TOTAL WELLNESS PROGRAM

A. Recommend to your patients that they keep a record of the following data during a typical week.

    1. All types and amounts of foods they eat and when they are consumed

    2. Types, duration, and frequency of activities

    3. Situations in which they found themselves feeling "stressed out"

    4. Ways in which they relaxed; frequency and duration

    5. Climacteric-related symptoms and degree to which they were experienced (eg, mild, moderate, severe)

B. Working With Professionals

If possible, your patients should work with one of your staff or be referred to a health care professional who can evaluate the week's worth of information to assist them in establishing realistic, obtainable goals.

C. Working Without Professionals

If your patients are unable to work with a health care professional, ask them to review the information they have recorded about their lifestyle for the week. If they find there are areas in which changes should be made for their health or climacteric-related symptoms, they should be encouraged to develop a plan for initiating the changes. For some women, "seeing their lives recorded" is the best impetus for change. It is important to encourage them to do the following:

1. Read materials that can help them to evaluate their lifestyle
2. Plan realistic goals that minimize stress
3. Not feel impatient or to try to change everything overnight
4. Recognize that the slower and more consistent the changes in lifestyle, the greater is the probability of success
5. Understand and accept that it is "okay" to take several months or years to reach their goals or change the unhealthy habits of a lifetime
6. Seek the support of friends, family, and programs available in their community

D. Staff Functions

If possible, assign one of your staff to the following tasks.

1. Identify local programs for women, such as exercise, stress management, nutrition, and vegetarian and low-fat food cooking classes, and support groups.
2. Contact your local library to determine whether they carry books about menopause, exercise, stress reduction, nutrition, cooking, and complementary therapies. If not, request that they do so.

3. Request that a local health food store or pharmacy carry the products (if they do not already) that are recommended in this guide.

4. Identify complementary health care practitioners in your area. Meet with them to discuss their practice, costs, and how referrals may best be facilitated. Because many women are not able to afford the usual cost of such a practitioner, discuss the possibility of their willingness to offer a sliding fee scale based on the women's income. (One women's clinic in Santa Monica serves women at or below poverty level, and a doctor in TCM has agreed to volunteer his time once each week to work with their patients.)

E. Collaborative Programs

If possible, have available in your office or clinic staff who have the expertise to evaluate your patients' lifestyles issues and who can work with them to develop a comprehensive health program. If this is not feasible, consider getting together with various professionals in your community to offer a series of wellness programs.

F. Pointers for Health Promotion[1]

1. Provide balanced information about the menopause to women and their families.

2. Discuss attitudes toward menopause, with reassurance about overly pessimistic beliefs.

3. Offer health promotion sessions focusing on diet, exercise, and smoking.

4. Offer stress management sessions.

5. Conduct group discussions of personal, health, and social issues encountered by women during midlife.

XII. CONCLUSION

All of these recommendations may be as stressful for you to consider as making lifestyle changes can be for your patients. Please take the time to consider what is realistic in the setting in which you are working. Offering a comprehensive wellness program may be out of the question, as may having staff available to help your patients develop their nutritional programs.

Whatever you are able to do, even if it must be limited to providing a list of educational materials and lifestyle recommendations, when combined with your support, will be extremely beneficial for and most appreciated by your patients.

REFERENCE

1. Hunter MS. Predictions of menopausal symptoms: psychological aspects. Baillieres Clin Endocrinol Metab 1993;7:33–45.

Sample Assessments of Nutritional Intake, Levels of Physical Activity and Stress, Sexual History, and Climacteric-Related Symptoms and Treatments

SAMPLE ASSESSMENT OF NUTRITIONAL INTAKE

1. In general, how would you describe your diet?
   Very healthy
   Sometimes healthy
   Rarely healthy

2. How many servings of the following do you have each day?
   Fresh fruit
   Fresh vegetables
   Meat
   Poultry
   Fish
   Dairy products
   Soy products
   Whole grains foods
   White flour products (eg, pasta, bread)
   Calcium-rich foods

3. Do you drink beverages with caffeine in them? If   (Yes/No)
   yes, what is the amount that you drink each day?

4. Do you feel that you have too much of
   the following items in your diet?   (Yes/No/Sometimes)
   Sugar
   Salt
   Fat
   Caffeine

5. How often do you drink alcoholic beverages?

6. If you drink alcoholic beverages, what quantity
    of them do you usually consume?

7. How many glasses of water do you drink each day?

8. Do you take vitamins?   (Yes/No)
    If yes, which ones do you take and
    in what amounts?

9. Do you take minerals?   (Yes/No)
    If yes, which ones do you take and
    in what amounts?

10. Do you take any other type of nutritional
    supplements? If yes, what are they?

11. Have you ever been on a diet to lose or
    gain weight?   (Yes/No)

12. Would you like some assistance in planning
    a healthy diet for yourself?   (Yes/No)

13. Is there any information about nutrition
    you would like to learn?   (Yes/No)

SAMPLE ASSESSMENT OF LEVEL OF ACTIVITY

1. Do you exercise to increase your heart rate?   (Yes/No)
    If yes, how many times each week do you do this?
        1 or 2
        3 or 4
        5 or more

2. If you exercise to increase your heart rate,

    Do you know how high your rate becomes
    during exercising?   (No/How high)
        What exercises do you perform?
        How long do you perform them?

3. Do you increase your level of activity when
    you can, such as by walking rather than driving
    or taking a bus or by climbing stairs rather
    than taking an elevator or escalator?   (Yes/No)

4. Do you perform stretching exercises?   (Yes/No)
    If yes, how often do you perform them?

5. Do you lift weights or use weight machines or
    other equipment to increase the strength
    of your muscles?   (Yes/No)
    If yes,
        How often do you perform these exercises?
        How long do you perform them?

6. When you exercise, do you feel
    pain in any part of your body?   (Yes/No/Do not exercise)

7. If you exercise, do you want to change
    your exercise program in any way?   (Yes/No)
    If yes, how would you like to change it?

8. Certain types of exercises performed in specific
    ways increase muscle strength, improve your heart
    and lungs, and help you to build strong bones.
    Do you feel that you know what these exercises
    are and how often and for how long they should
    be performed?   (Yes/No)
    Would you like to have this information?   (Yes/No)

9. If you do not exercise, what is the reason for this?

10. Would you like to receive assistance in
    beginning an exercise program?   (Yes/No)

SAMPLE ASSESSMENT OF LEVEL OF STRESS

1. Do you like your neighborhood?   (Yes/No)
    If no, please explain your answer.

2. Do you like the place (eg, home, apartment) in
    which you are living?   (Yes/No)
    If no, please explain.

3. Do you like the work you are doing?   (Yes/No/Sometimes)
    If no or only sometimes, please explain.

4. If you have a personal relationship with
    someone, is it a satisfying relationship?   (Yes/No)
    If no, please explain.

5. During the past 5 years, have you done or experienced any of the following?
   Moved
   Experienced the death of a family member or friend
   Has a family member of friend experienced a serious illness or accident
   Ended a close personal relationship
   Changed jobs
   Gone to school or a training program
   Been seriously ill or physically limited
   Had financial difficulties
   Been a victim of a crime or accident
   Any other major life changes

6. I feel that   (Yes/No/Sometimes)
   My life is good.
   I have enough time to relax and to do
      the things that I like to do.
   I have enough time to spend with family
      and friends.
   I have special, fulfilling friendships.
   I have support and love from friends and
      family.
   I get enough sleep.
   I am experiencing too much stress in my life.
   I am able to handle stress well.

7. How do you deal with stress or tensions in your life?
   Perform deep breathing exercises
   Meditate
   Listen to music
   Pray
   Laugh
   Talk with someone about how I feel
   Exercise
   Sleep
   Have an alcoholic beverage
   Use tranquilizers or other prescription or nonprescription drugs
   Use herbal or homeopathic treatments for stress
   Eat more than I should
   Other ways (please list)

8. When you are feeling stress, do you
      Eat too quickly
      Feel muscle tension in neck, shoulders, or elsewhere
      Get headaches
      Feel sick to your stomach
      Get diarrhea or become constipated
      Find it difficult to eat
      Have difficulty sleeping
      Become impatient with others
      Rush around, trying to do too many things at the same
         time
      Experience other effects (explain)

9. Would you like to learn about healthy ways
   that can help you effectively deal with stress?   (Yes/No)

HISTORY OF LIFESTYLE DURING ADOLESCENCE

1. During your teenage years through your twenties, did you
   consume a diet that contained
      Excessive sugar
      Excessive fatty foods
      Excessive protein (especially red meats)
      Soft drinks on a regular basis
      Caffeine on a regular basis
      Alcoholic beverages on a regular basis
      Adequate amount of calcium-rich foods
      Regular intake of fresh fruits and vegetables

2. In general, do you think your diet was, very
   healthy, somewhat healthy, or not healthy?

3. Were you a smoker during those years?   (Yes/No)

4. Did you exercise vigorously for at least
   three times each week for a minimum
   of 30 minutes?   (Yes/No/Sometimes)

5. In general, would you say you had a
   physically active lifestyle during
   those years?   (Yes/No/Sometimes)

6. In general, would you say your life during
   those years was very stressful, somewhat
   stressful, or not stressful?

SAMPLE SEXUAL HISTORY

1. Do you have any questions, problems, or concerns about your sexual life that you would like to talk about?

2. If you are currently having a sexual relationship, are you satisfied with this relationship? If you are not satisfied, what do you feel is the cause of this?

3. If you are not having a sexual relationship currently, is it because you prefer to not have one, there is no one in your life right now with whom to have this type of relationship, or some other reason (please explain)?

4. Are you comfortable sexually pleasuring
    yourself (masturbating)?   (Yes/No)
    Is there anything about this form of sexual
    activity you would like to talk about?   (Yes/No)

5. Have you ever experienced pain or
    discomfort with sexual intercourse   (Yes/No/
    or any other form of sexual activity?   Never had intercourse)
    If yes,
        Where was the pain (eg, vaginal opening,
            inside the vagina, in the pelvis [lower
            belly], other)?
        Why do you think you experienced this pain?
        Have you ever talked with a health care
            professional about this?

6. Have you ever been asked to do something
    sexual against your will?   (Yes/No)

7. Have you ever done or had anything done
    sexually against your will?   (Yes/No)

8. Are you using anything to prevent pregnancy?   (Yes/No)
    If yes,
        What method of contraception are you using?
        Are you satisfied with this method?
        Do you have any questions about this method
            or any other method?

9. Do you know when you no longer have to use
    a method of contraception?

10. How many times have you needed to
    use an over-the-counter medication   (Number of times/
    for a vaginal infection in the past year?   Have never used)

11. Do you have any questions or concerns
    about sexually transmitted diseases? (Yes/No)

12. It is important that you consider whether
    you need to be tested for sexually transmitted
    diseases. Answering the following questions
    can help you to determine this need. (Yes/No)
    I have had more than one sexual partner
        in the past year.
    I have had more than one sexual partner
        in the past 10 years.
    I have had a sexual relationship with a man
        who is bisexual or homosexual.
    I have had a sexual relationship with a woman
        who is bisexual.
    I have always used condoms during intercourse
        (vaginal and anal).
    I have been treated for a sexually transmitted
        disease.
    I feel that I have put myself at risk for getting
        a sexually transmitted disease.
    I have shared a needle or injection equipment
        with another person.
    I have a tattoo.
    I had a blood transfusion before 1985.
    I have had sexual contact with someone who
        has had or has a sexually transmitted disease
        (eg, herpesvirus infection, *Chlamydia* infection,
        human immunodeficiency virus infection,
        gonorrhea, syphilis, venereal warts)

13. As you become older, you may experience or may
    already be experiencing changes in the way in
    which your body responds during sexual activity.
    Lack of knowledge about these changes may cause
    a woman to experience problems in her sexual life.
    As a man ages, his body also changes in the way it
    responds during sexual activity. Would you like to
    learn about the changes that you may experience
    and/or the man experiences? (Yes/No)

14. Is there anything about sexually related issues
    or your sexuality that you would like to discuss? (Yes/No)

SAMPLE LIST OF CLIMACTERIC-RELATED SYMPTOMS AND WAYS IN WHICH SYMPTOMS ARE OR HAVE BEEN TREATED

The following list of symptoms may or may not be related to menopause. Please note how often you have any them and how much they bother you by placing a check mark in the appropriate column. *Mild* means the symptom does not really bother you, but you are aware of it. *Moderate* means that the symptom bothers you to some degree. *Severe* means that the symptom is very bothersome and can even disrupt your life.

1. Daily, weekly, or monthly experiences
    Heavier than usual menstrual bleeding
    Lighter than usual menstrual bleeding
    Spotting of blood
    Worsening of premenstrual syndrome symptoms
    Hot flushes
    Night sweats
    Fatigue
    Emotional changes
    Restlessness
    Poor concentration
    Forgetfulness
    Headaches
    Hair loss
    Joint and muscle pain
    Swelling in joints
    Backaches
    Cold hands and feet
    Feelings of suffocation
    Heart pounding fast or hard
    Pressure or tightness in head or body
    Dizziness
    Insomnia
    Loss of appetite
    Food cravings
    Tender or painful breasts
    Change in sexual feelings
    Changes in how you physically feel during a sexual time
    Vaginal dryness
    Vaginal itching
    Frequent or painful urination

Problems holding urine or leaking urine
Pain with intercourse
Dry skin
Frequent bruising
"Prickly" sensations (like ants crawling over the skin)
Change in body scent
Pain in the mouth, with or without bleeding gums
Dry mouth
Metallic, sour, salty, or peppery taste or burning sensations
    in mouth
Tingling in the hands or feet
Constipation or diarrhea
Difficulty digesting foods

2. Are you experiencing any other symptoms? (Yes/No)
   If yes, what are they?

3. Treatments and lifestyle changes you have used in
   the past or are currently using to relieve your symptoms:
   Hormone therapy
   Diet
   Exercise
   Vitamins
   Minerals
   Herbs
   Homeopathics
   Stress reduction techniques
   Acupuncture
   Other (please explain)

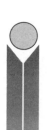

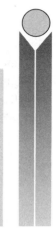

Instructions for Observing Cervical Mucus and Basal Body Temperature

WHAT IS CERVICAL MUCUS?

1. Cervical mucus is a substance made in the cervix, which is the bottom part of the uterus. Mucus can be seen and felt by a woman and can be used to know on which days she can and cannot become pregnant.

2. Sometimes the mucus is the infertile kind, and sperm cannot travel through or live in it.

3. As ovulation approaches, the mucus becomes the fertile kind. Sperm can travel and live easily in fertile mucus for 3 to 5 days.

HOW DOES CERVICAL MUCUS CHANGE?

1. If a woman wipes the vaginal opening with toilet tissue, she usually does not see any mucus on the tissue for 1 to a few days after her menstrual bleeding ends. Her vaginal area feels dry during these days. However, some women see mucus right after bleeding ends, and this probably is normal for them.

2. Mucus, described as pasty, sticky, and crumbly looking, is usually seen next. This mucus does not feel wet, and the vaginal area (by thinking about it) "feels" sticky or dry. The mucus may be white to yellow and lasts for 1 to a few days.

3. As ovulation nears, the mucus becomes wet. It is described as creamy to slippery and stretchy. It may be cloudy to clear and

usually lasts for 2 to a few days. When wet mucus is being made, the vaginal area feels wet.

4. Shortly after ovulation, the mucus loses its wet feeling, and the vaginal area again feels sticky or dry. Some women do not see any mucus for the rest of the menstrual cycle.

HOW DO I CHECK MUCUS?

1. Begin checking for mucus after menstrual bleeding ends.

2. Before checking for mucus, ask yourself whether the area around and in the vaginal opening feels wet. This is not done by touching the area. Instead, it is done by thinking about it: "Does my vaginal area feel wet or dry?"

3. Wipe the vaginal opening with toilet tissue before or after urinating.

4. Look at the toilet paper for mucus. If mucus is seen, place it between two fingers and feel the mucus. Open the fingers slowly to see whether the mucus stretches. Ask yourself whether the mucus feels wet, whether it is stretchy or slippery, and whether it is sticky or pasty.

5. Check for mucus each time you go to the bathroom throughout the day. Use these symbols to record mucus changes:
    *   *   Bleeding
    *   S   Spotting
    *   D   Dry days; no mucus is seen; vaginal area feels dry all day
    *   M   Sticky, pasty mucus that does not feel wet; vaginal area feels sticky or dry
    *   Ⓜ   Creamy or stretchy, slippery, wet mucus; vaginal area feels wet

6. Remember to do the following:
    Fill in every part of the fertility awareness chart you can.
    Mark every day you have intercourse with a check mark
    Use the notes column to write down anything you think may affect your basal body temperature, mucus, or menstrual cycle, such as a fever, taking medications, or traveling.
    If you have any questions about how to check or chart your fertility signs, please talk to your clinician.

FERTILITY AWARENESS CHART

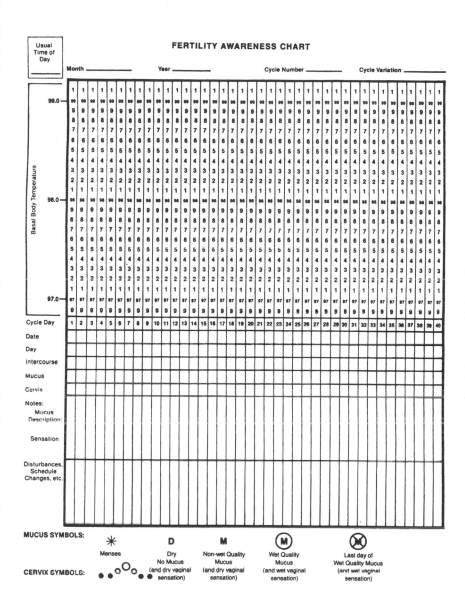

MUCUS SYMBOLS:

✳	D	M	Ⓜ	⊗
Menses	Dry No Mucus (and dry vaginal sensation)	Non-wet Quality Mucus (and dry vaginal sensation)	Wet Quality Mucus (and wet vaginal sensation)	Last day of Wet Quality Mucus (and wet vaginal sensation)

CERVIX SYMBOLS: ● ● ○ O O ● ●

You may also want to attend a fertility awareness or natural family planning class. If so, contact a local church, Department of Public Health, family planning program, or Planned Parenthood office about classes in your area.

WHAT IS BASAL BODY TEMPERATURE AND HOW DOES IT CHANGE?

Basal body temperature (BBT) is the temperature of the body at rest. It changes under certain conditions:

1. The BBT is usually low during menstrual bleeding.
2. It stays low for a few to several days.
3. It rises 0.3 to 1 degree around the day of ovulation.
4. After the temperature rises, it stays high for about 12 to 16 days or until menstrual bleeding starts again.
5. The temperature usually rises on the day of ovulation or 1 to 2 days after ovulation.

The BBT can be evaluated by following these steps:

1. Begin taking your temperature on the first day of menstrual bleeding or at least by the time menstrual bleeding ends.
2. Take your temperature as soon as you wake up and before any activity, such as eating, drinking, or smoking.
3. Place the silver end of the thermometer under your tongue and leave it in place for 5 minutes. You can also take your temperature rectally or vaginally. Because these temperatures may be about 1 degree higher than the oral temperatures, try to take the temperature the same way throughout the menstrual cycle.
4. After 5 minutes, read the thermometer, and record the temperature on your chart.
5. If you cannot read and record the temperature after 5 minutes, place the thermometer in a safe place, away from any type of heat, and read it later. If the temperature is between two lines on the thermometer, record the *lowest* of the two temperatures.

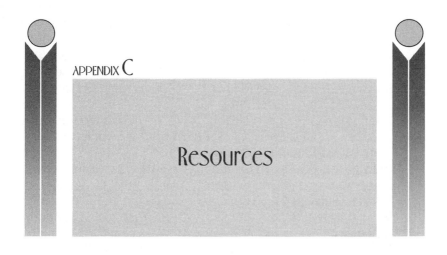

Resources

The following list includes an ample representation of the information available about climacteric-related issues and complementary health care practices. Some of the books, journals, newsletters, and organizations emphasize conventional medical approaches, and others focus on a holistic approach.

BOOKS

This section contains the names of the books used as references for this text, and others have been included because they can help in expanding your knowledge of conventional and complementary approaches to the care of women during the climacteric. To avoid showing favoritism, this section does not include the names of the many wonderful books written for the lay public about the climacteric. We suggest that you scan the bookstores to become familiar with these and select a few that would be appropriate for your patients.

Alternative Medicine, Expanding Medical Horizons: A Report to the Institutes of Health on Alternative Medical Systems and Practices in the United States. Washington, DC: U.S. Government Printing Office; 1995.

Assessment of Fracture Risk and its Application to Screening for Postmenopausal Osteoporosis: Report of a WHO Study Group. Geneva: World Health Organization; 1994. (1211 Geneva 27, Switzerland)

Beasley J, Swift J. *The Kellogg Report: The Impact of Nutrition, Environment, and Lifestyle on the Health of Americans.*

Annandale-on-Hudson, NY: The Institute of Health Policy and Practice of the Bard College Center; 1989. (800/787-0230)

Borysenko J, Borysenko M. *The Power of the Mind to Heal.* Carson, CA: Hay House; 1994.

Bronner F. *Nutrition and Health, Topics and Controversies.* Boca Raton, FL: CRC Press; 1995. (200 Corporate Boulevard, NW, Boca Raton, FL 33431)

Budwig J. *Flax Oil as a True Aid Against Arthritis, Heart Infarction, Cancer, and Other Diseases.* Vancouver, BC: Apple: 1994. (800/668-2775)

Butler R, Lewis M. *Love and Sex After 60.* New York: Ballantine Books; 1993.

Byyny R, Speroff LA. *Clinical Guide for the Care of Older Women: Primary and Preventative Care,* 2d ed. Baltimore: Williams & Wilkins; 1996.

Carr P, Freund K, Somani S. *The Medical Care of Women.* Philadelphia: WB Saunders; 1995.

Castleman M. *The Healing Herbs.* Emmaus, PA: Rodale Press; 1991.

Chopra D. *Ageless Body, Timeless Mind.* New York: Harmony Books; 1993.

Colgan M. *The New Nutrition: Medicine for the Millennium.* Vancouver, BC: Apple; 1995.

Collinge W. *The American Holistic Health Association Complete Guide to Alternative Therapies.* New York: Warner Books; 1996.

Cottrell R. *Stress Management* (Wellness Series). Guilford, CT: Dushken; 1992.

Davis M. *The Relaxation and Stress Reduction Workbook.* Oakland, CA: Metal New Harbinger Publications; 1988.

Dossey T. *Healing Words.* New York: HarperCollins; 1993.

Edelman D. *Sex in the Golden Years.* New York: Donald I. Fine; 1992.

Evans W, Rosenberg I. *Biomarkers: The Ten Determinants of Aging.* New York: Simon & Schuster, 1992.

Frawley D, Lad V. *An Ayurvedic Guide to Herbal Medicine.* Santa Fe: Lotus Press; 1986.

Frawley D, Lad V. *The Yoga of Herbs.* Santa Fe: Lotus Press; 1988.

Gaby A. *Preventing and Reversing Osteoporosis.* Rocklin, CA: Prima Publishing; 1994.

Golan R. *Optimal Wellness*. New York: Ballantine Books; 1995.

Goleman D, Gurin J. *Mind-Body Medicine*. New York: Consumer Reports Books, 1993.

Gordon J. *Manifesto for a New Medicine*. New York: Addison-Wesley; 1996.

Hudson T. *Gynecology and Naturopathic Medicine: A Treatment Manual*. Aloha, OR: TK Publications; 1994.

Ito D. *Without Estrogen*. New York: Crown Trade Paperbacks; 1994.

Mills S. *The Essential Book of Herbal Medicine*. New York: Penguin; 1991.

Mishell D. *Menopause, Physiology and Pharmacology*. Chicago: Year Book Medical Publishers; 1987.

Murray M. *Stress, Anxiety and Insomnia*. Rocklin, CA: Prima Publishing; 1995.

Murray M, Pizzorno J. *Encyclopedia of Natural Medicine*. Rocklin, CA: Prima Publishing; 1991.

Ornish D. *Dr. Dean Ornish's Program for Reversing Heart Disease*. New York: Random House; 1990.

Pelletier K. *Mind as Healer, Mind as Slayer*. New York: Dell; 1992.

Quillin P. *Healing Nutrients*. New York: Vintage Books, 1989.

Rector-Page L. *Healthy Healing: An Alternative Healing Reference*. Sonora, CA: Healthy Healing Publications; 1992.

Reed D. *The Complete Book of Chinese Health and Healing*. Boston: Shambhala; 1994.

Rosenthal S. *Sex Over 40, 50, 60, 70*. New York: St. Martin's Press, 1987.

Siegel R. *Six Seconds to True Calm*. Santa Monica, CA: Little Sun Books; 1995.

Simkin A, Ayalon J. *Bone Loading*. London: Prion; 1990.

The Burton Goldberg Group. *Alternative Medicine: The Definitive Guide*. Fife, WA: Future Medicine; 1994.

Weil A. *Health & Healing*. Boston: Houghton-Mifflin; 1988.

Williams R. *Anger Kills*. New York: Harper Perennial; 1993.

Wolensky F. *Nutritional Concerns of Women*. Boca Raton, FL: CRC Press; 1996. (2000 Corporate Boulevard, NW, Boca Raton, FL 33431)

Wolfe HL. Menopause, a Second Spring: Making a Smooth Transition With Traditional Chinese Medicine. Boulder, CO: Blue Poppy Press; 1992.

JOURNALS

Alternative Health Practitioner: The Journal of Complementary and Natural Care. Springer Publishing Co., 536 Broadway, New York, NY 10012-9904.

Alternative Therapies in Health and Medicine: A Peer-Reviewed Journal. Box 627, Holmes PA 19043-9650 (800/345-8112). (Articles examine a variety of disciplined inquiry methods, including high-quality scientific research in complementary therapies, and encourage integration of complementary therapies with conventional medical practices in a way that provides for a rational, individualized, comprehensive approach to health care.)

Clinical Pearls. IT Services, 3301 Alta Arden #2, Sacramento, CA 95825.

Complementary Therapies in Medicine: The Journal for all Health Care Professionals. Churchill Livingstone, 650 Avenue of the Americas, New York, NY 10011.

Herbalgram: The Journal of the American Botanical Council and The Herb Research Foundation. Box 201660, Austin, TX 72720-1660 (The journal provides excellent resources about herbal research and numerous herbal medicinal books for health care professionals.)

Nutrition Today. Williams and Wilkins, Box 23291, Baltimore, MD 21298-9325.

SEICUS Report. Sexuality Information and Education Council of the United States, 130 West 42nd Street, #2500, New York, NY 10036.

SYLLABUS

Herbal Medicine and Your Health. Rosenthal Center for Alternative/Complementary Medicine, Department of Rehabilitative Medicine, Columbia University, College of Physicians and Surgeons. (This is a syllabus from a program held in 1996 for physicians and other health care professionals at Columbia-Presbyterian Medical Center, New York.)

NEWSLETTERS

Alternative Medicine Integration and Coverage, St. Anthony's Publishing, Inc., P.O. Box 96561, Washington, DC 20090.

A Friend Indeed, Box 1710, Champlain, NY 12919-1710.

Dr. Andrew Weil's Self-Healing, P.O. Box 792, Mount Morris, IL 61054-0792.

Health Wisdom for Women. Christine Northrup, M.D., Phillips Publishing, 7811 Montrose Road, Box 60110, Potomac, MD 20897-5924.

Hot Flash, A Newsletter for Midlife and Older Women, Box 816, Stony Brook, NY 11790-0609.

Meno Times, The Menopause Center, P.O. Box 6558, San Rafael, CA 94903 (415/459-5430). (The center also offers video and cassette tapes of symposiums held to discuss complementary approaches to health care for women.)

Menopause News (800/241-MENO).

Mind-Body Health (800/222-4745).

National Menopause Foundation, Center for Climacteric Studies, Gainesville, FL 32601 (800/886-4354).

National Women's Health Report, National Women's Health Resource Center, 2440 M Street NW, #325, Washington, DC 20037 (202/293-6045).

Natural Solutions, Transitions for Health, 621 SW Alder Street, #900, Portland, OR 97205 (800/888-6814).

Newsletter of the American Institute of Stress, 124 Park Avenue, Yonkers, NY 10703.

Sex Over Forty, Box 1600, Chapel Hill, NC 27515.

Women's Health Connection, Women's International Pharmacy, Box 6338, Madison, WI 53716.

World Research News, 15300 Ventura Boulevard, #405, Sherman Oaks, CA 91403.

Women's Health Watch, Information for Enlightened Choices, Harvard Medical School, Box 420234, Palm Coast, FL 32142-0234 (904/445-4662).

ORGANIZATIONS

American Botanical Council, Box 201660, Austin, TX 78720-1660. (The group provides educational materials and their quarterly journal HerbalGram that includes articles about herbs and medicinal plant research.)

American Association of Naturopathic Physicians, 2366 Eastlake Avenue East, #322, Seattle, WA 98102 (206/323-7610). (They provide a list of licensed naturopaths throughout the United States.)

American Holistic Medical Association, 4101 Lake Boone Trail, #201, Raleigh, NC 27607 (919/787-5146). (Consider becoming a member! There is also an association for nurses. It provides a nationwide referral directory of physicians who use complementary therapies.)

American Menopause Foundation, 350 Fifth Avenue, New York, NY 10010 (212/714-2398). (This nationwide network of support groups deal with conventional and complementary treatments and other issues related to the menopause.)

National Center for Homeopathy, 801 N. Fairfax Street, #306, Alexandria, VA 22314 (703/548-7790). (The group provides a directory of practitioners and homeopathic study groups throughout the United States.)

National Women's Health Network, 1325 G Street NW, Washington, DC 20006 (202/223-2226).

The American Institute of Stress, 124 Park Avenue, Yonkers, NY 10703. (The staff conduct literature searches on request.)

The Herb Research Foundation, 1007 Pearl Street #200, Boulder, CO 80301 (303/449-2265). (The group offers packets of information about specific herbs on request.)

World Research Foundation, 15300 Ventura Boulevard, #405, Sherman Oaks, CA 91403 (818/907/5483). (The group offers packets of information about complementary therapies on request.)

PHARMACIES THAT COMPOUND PLANT-BASED HORMONE COMPOUNDS

The pharmacies that compound hormonal treatments provide literature describing their products and instructions for use for your patients. Some offer patient educational materials. They also have pharmacists available to discuss patient and prescribing issues. Contact at least a couple of these pharmacies in your area, chat with the pharmacists, and review the literature about their products and their company before deciding which to use.

College Pharmacy, 833 North Tejon Street, Colorado Springs, CO 80903 (800/888-9358). (In addition to several other hormonal therapies, this pharmacy compounds a progesterone gel and an estrogen and progesterone gel that its pharmacists feel has a better absorption rate than progesterone cream.)

Women's International Pharmacy, 5708 Monona Drive, Madison, WI 53716 (800/279-5708).

MANUFACTURERS OF NUTRITIONAL SUPPLEMENTS AND HERBAL AND HOMEOPATHIC TREATMENTS

The companies that manufacture vitamins and minerals, herbs, and homeopathics included in this section have been selected by various complementary practitioners and pharmacies in the Los Angeles area, based on their expertise in evaluating the quality of such products, cost, and customer and patient response. The following manufacturers' addresses and phone numbers have not been included, because their products can be ordered through health food stores and pharmacies for your patients.

Manufacturers of Nutritional Supplements
Ecological Formulas
Future Biotics
Metagenics
Natures Plus
Optimox
Progressive Labs
Rainbow Light
Solgar
Twin Labs

Manufacturers of Herbs
The Zand Company
Crystal Star
Born Again
Herb Farm
Gaia

Manufacturers of Homeopathics
Bioran
Compli Med
Manufacturers of Digestive Enzymes
Tyler
Primary Resource
Ness

OTHER RESOURCES

Aeron Lifecycles (800/631-7900). (They will send a list of the amount of progesterone contained in various progesterone based products.)

Brown and Benchmark Publishers Catalog, 25 Kessel Court, Madison, WI 53711. (They offer several books and manuals for use by health care professionals and patients in numerous areas ranging from fitness and nutrition to aging and gerontology. Their Wellness Series is particularly recommended for use by patients. It includes a wealth of information, several self-assessments, and beneficial tips about making health-promoting changes in lifestyle.)

Colgan Institute, 523 Encinitas Boulevard, #204, Encinitas, CA 92024 (619/632-7722). (The group offers several books about nutrition and nutritional supplementation programs.)

Health Choice Productions, 2554 Lincoln Boulevard, Suite 484, Marina Del Ray, CA 90291. (They offer patient education materials about the climacteric and health-promoting strategies.)

The Holistic Arts and Sciences Network, Inc., 3491 131st Avenue NE, Minneapolis, MN 55447. (The group offers video tapes in many areas, including several types of yoga and massage therapies, tai chi, Ayurvedic medicine, homeopathy, and herbal therapies.)

Transitions for Health (800/888-6814). (Their catalog offers a selection of essential fatty acid and vitamin and mineral supplements and naturopathic treatments.)

Women to Women, 1 Pleasant Street, Yarmouth, ME 04096. They offers educational materials about various aspects of women's health, including the climacteric.)

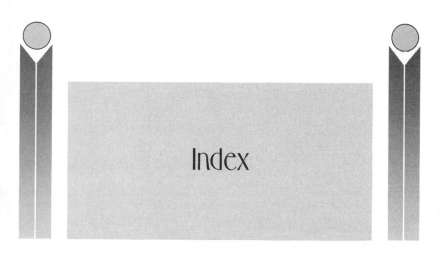

Index

The letter *t* before a page number indicates a table; the letter *f* indicates a figure.